精神障害の予防をめぐる最近の進歩

Recent Advances in Early Intervention and Prevention
in Psychiatric Disorders

小椋　力　編

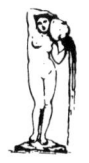

星 和 書 店

Seiwa Shoten Publishers

2-5 Kamitakaido 1-Chome
Suginamiku Tokyo 168-0074, Japan

はじめに

　本書は，第1回日本国際精神障害予防会議（First Japan International Conference on Early Intervention and Prevention in Psychiatric Disorders）で講演された内容を一冊にまとめたものである。会議の名称は，日本語としてなじみにくいと思ったが，英国人を中心とした国際会議「First UK International Conference on Early Intervention in Psychosis」に参加し，このような会議を目指していたので上記のごとく決めた。

　本会議は，2001年6月22～23日沖縄コンベンションセンターで開催された。参加者は475人で外国からは台湾，韓国，中国，フィリピン，インドネシア，オーストラリア，アメリカ合衆国，ノールウェーの計8か国であった。「International Conference on Early Psychosis」の代表者であるPatric McGorry教授等，この領域で活躍中の第一人者をお招きし講演をお願いした。日本からは日本精神障害予防研究会の世話人が中心となってプログラム委員会を組織した。参加者は，精神医学・医療・保健・福祉とその関連分野で活躍している医師，心理士，看護婦（士），精神保健福祉士，当事者等であった。

　内容についてみると，精神障害の予防に関する総論，この領域における先進諸国の現状などが特別講演として述べられた。シンポジウムとして「精神分裂病の危険因子，早期発見，予防」「精神分裂病の初回エピソードに対する治療」「地域精神保健システムと精神障害の予防」「アジアにおける精神障害に対する早期介入と予防」，トピックスとして「学校の精神保健とその問題の予防」「家庭の精神保健とその問題の予防」「職場の精神保健とその問題の予防」「アルコール・薬物乱用の予防」「痴呆の早期発見・治療・予防」が講演された。

　Welcome Party, Farewell Partyのいずれも盛況であり，本会議の件が第一面トップ記事として掲載された地元紙が会場に持ち込まれ紹介されるなど盛りあがった。この盛りあがりが，わが国における「精神障害の予防」に関する研究，活動等につながることを望んでいる。会議，パーティー等で強く印象づけられたのは，医師のみならず当事者，家族を含む関係者の連携とネットワークの重要性であった。

　本書のタイトルは「精神障害の予防をめぐる最近の進歩」としたが，国の内外における本領域の最近の進歩が読みとっていただけると思う。本書がこの分野におけるさらなる進展に貢献できることを願ってやまない。

平成13年11月
第1回日本国際精神障害予防会議議長
日本精神障害予防研究会　代表世話人
琉球大学医学部精神神経科学講座教授
　　　　　小　椋　　力

目　次

はじめに　iii

■精神障害の早期介入と予防
　……………Patrick D. McGorry　1

■精神分裂病の予防
　……………Ming T. Tsuang, 他　16

■精神病の予防に関するノルウェーの現状
　……………Tor K. Larsen　20

■精神病の予防に関するオーストラリア・メルボルンの現状…………Jane Edwards, 他　26

■精神分裂病患者に対する初期の心理社会的ならびに精神力動的治療……西園　昌久　34

■胎生期・周産期のストレス指標と精神分裂病との関係　……………今村　明, 他　39

■通知票による病前行動特徴と成績に関する研究　……………佐々木　司, 他　42

■脳画像による早期診断　川崎　康弘, 他　46

■高危険児研究の結果と早期介入プログラム
　……………原田　誠一, 他　50

■学校精神保健システムにおける予防的介入
　……………福治　康秀, 他　54

■精神分裂病の脆弱性指標としての探索眼球運動　……………松島　英介, 他　57

■日本における初回エピソード精神病患者への治療戦略　……………嶋田　博之　60

■長期転帰から見た初回エピソードに対する治療戦略　……………小川　一夫　64

■精神障害者の権利と予防　…大島アヤノ　68

■精神障害者地域生活支援と予防
　……………石川英五郎　70

■医療機関と地域の連携　……蟻塚　亮二　74

■日本における精神障害に対する早期介入と予防　……………山本　和儀　77

■学生の精神保健：台湾における精神障害に対する早期介入と予防　……Eng-Kung Yeh　80

■インドネシアにおける精神障害に対する早期介入と予防　……………Sasanto Wibisono　84

■韓国における精神障害に対する早期介入と予防　……………Sung Kil Min　88

■Early psychosis の早期発見と対応
　……………Patrick D. McGorry　93

■精神分裂病に対する早期マネジメントにおける最近の進歩……………Barry D. Jones　103

■初回エピソード患者の治療における新しい非定型抗精神病薬の役割　…Tim Lambert　107

■予防的観点からみた ADHD 児の治療
　……………岩坂　英巳, 他　112

■学校の精神保健とその問題の予防：注意欠陥多動障害（ADHD）…………原田　謙　116

■不登校の下位分類と対応　…笠原　麻里　121

■不登校の早期介入　…………山崎　透　124

■家庭の精神保健とその問題の予防
　……………白石　弘巳　128

■職場の精神保健とその問題の予防
　……………倉林るみい　132

■アルコール・薬物乱用の予防：内科と精神科の連携によるアルコール依存症早期治療と早

■期回復を目指して……渡辺　省三,他 136

■アルコール・薬物乱用の予防：BDIM(Before-Discharge Intervention Method)によるアルコール依存症の否認への気付効果について……………猪野　亜朗,他 140

■痴呆の早期発見・治療・予防
　………………………宇野　正威 144

■精神分裂病の性・年齢別分布
　………………………菊池　美紀,他 148

■精神分裂病発症とライフイベント
　………………………木下　裕久,他 150

■初発分裂病の発症前特徴
　………………………石崎　裕香,他 152

■日本における初発分裂病の精神病未治療期間(DUP)について………水野　雅文,他 154

■沖縄県における精神分裂病の未治療期間(DUP)に関する予備的調査
　………………………村上　忠,他 156

■分裂病の早期発見・早期治療
　………………………原田　誠一,他 158

■児童青年期発症精神分裂病患者の発症様式の検討……………………中谷　英夫,他 160

■The family attitude scale の日本での妥当性の評価………………藤田　博一,他 162

■精神病性の初発状況と早期介入
　………………………仲本　晴男 164

■単回エピソード分裂病
　………………………小林　聡幸,他 166

■複雑系における精神医学…佐藤　武 168

■精神分裂病患者の子供に対する治療的関わりについて…………………皆川　恵子,他 170

■分裂病の母と難聴の父から生れ中学生になって異常行動が出現した一女性例
　………………………田中　晋,他 172

■子どもを持つ分裂病利用者に対する作業所を中心とした地域トータル・サポート
　………………………友田奈津美,他 174

■精神分裂病患者の再入院調査
　………………………岡　敬,他 176

■精神分裂病患者の再入院因子についての考察
　………………………福田　耕嗣,他 178

■三次予防のための精神分裂病の治療を展望する………………………梅田　征夫,他 180

■再発予防……………中村　靖,他 182

■精神科病院薬剤科の機能と役割
　………………………石田　保美,他 184

■地域住民の精神障害者観に関連する要因の分析………………………田中　悟郎,他 186

■精神障害者支援のための健康教育を実施して
　………………………木﨑　晴美,他 188

■三次予防のための療養病棟におけるコミュニティミーティングの試み
　………………………庄司　恵美,他 190

■精神医療におけるインフォームド・コンセントについて……………古井　博明 192

■精神分裂病患者の自殺企図因子の検討
　………………………松村みゆき,他 194

■仙台市精神保健福祉総合センターの電話相談における精神医学相談の実態について
　………………………林　みづ穂,他 196

- ■電話相談による自殺予防活動に関する統計的評価 …………………影山　隆之　198

- ■精神疾患の一次，二次予防を目的としたこころの検診 ……………野田　哲朗，他　200

- ■U市職員に対するメンタルヘルスケア …………………衛藤　進吉　202

- ■全国の自治体職場におけるメンタルヘルス状況と対策の実態 ………吉岡　伸一，他　204

- ■児童養護施設における心理学的援助について …………………植田　聡美，他　206

- ■総合精神保健福祉センターにおける児童虐待家庭への取り組み ……小川　一夫，他　208

- ■中高校生の自尊感情，不安傾向と学校適応状況，親子関係との関連 …………………與古田孝夫，他　210

- ■私立中高等学校における精神科校医としての相談業務と役割について …………………中村　道子，他　212

- ■日本における自閉症圏障害の診断告知に対する親の満足度の決定因子 …………………納富　恵子，他　214

- ■大学生に多発する60項目版GHQの異常高値 …………………泉　慈子，他　216

- ■大学生における被害観念の発生予測 …………………森本　幸子，他　218

- ■精神障害（者）に対する医学生の非好意的態度を改善するための医学教育の方法についての研究 …………………山本　和儀，他　220

- ■感情表出（EE）と大うつ病の再発および再燃との関連についての研究 …………………植木　啓文，他　222

- ■うつ病の早期発見・早期治療 …………………福田　吉顕，他　224

- ■気分障害の症状・経過に与える自殺企図の影響 …………………福永　貴子，他　226

- ■高齢者の抑うつ症状と自殺念慮との関連について …………………田中江里子，他　228

- ■老年期鬱病の看護 ……兼本　恵美，他　230

- ■うつ状態や自殺念慮時の高齢者の援助希求行動 …………………坂本　真士，他　232

- ■郷土文化を媒介とした回想法 …………………赤嶺　政信，他　234

- ■老人性痴呆疾患治療病棟でのヒヤリハット …………………阿河　礼子，他　236

- ■二次予防のうえで重要な精神科急性期治療棟と分裂病の様態 …………佐々木勇之進　238

- ■大学保健管理センターにおける「精神障害の早期発見・早期対応プロジェクト」についての7年間の経験 ………福治　康秀，他　240

- ■前駆期が5年間継続した後に発症した精神分裂病の一女性例 ………備瀬　哲弘，他　242

- ■分裂病の1次・2次予防への寄与を目指す疾患教育プログラムの実施経験 …………………原田　誠一，他　244

- ■学校交流会に対する長期入院患者の意識調査 …………………赤崎恵理子，他　246

- ■精神科の病院に対する地域の小学生の意識調査 …………………宮川　由香，他　248

- ■児童青年期発症精神分裂病患者の保護者の意識調査 …………柳下　杏子，他　250

- ■症状改善の観点から見たデイケアの有効性

- ……………………志喜屋　昇，他 252
- ■精神科デイケアを切り口とした再発予防の取り組み ……………市来　真彦，他 254
- ■SSTが慢性分裂病者に及ぼす影響 ……………………大野　宏明，他 256
- ■関連施設連絡協議会の試み ……………………大月　紀子，他 258
- ■強固な妄想体系で全生活史を置き換えていたケースが地域で自らの人生を再発見するまで ……………………金子　忍，他 260
- ■精神障害者の就労支援と地域ネットワークの試み ……………一杉　光男，他 262
- ■精神分裂病圏障害者の人生形成と地域リハビリテーション機能 ……加藤　欣子，他 264
- ■お互いの語り合いの場が再発予防に ……………………金城　和代 266
- ■人格目録における自己制御の減退と補足運動野の体積減少との関係 ……………………松井　三枝，他 268
- ■精神分裂病の発症年齢とN200異常 ……………………王　継軍，他 270
- ■沖縄県名護市における脳検診4年間の報告 ……………………城間　清剛，他 272
- ■長寿県沖縄における健常高齢者の頭部MRIによる形態学的検討 …宮平　良尚，他 274
- ■事象関連電位P300は痴呆の予測，早期発見に役立つか ……………Yu Jin，他 276
- ■うつ病の脆弱性指標としての事象関連電位N200異常 ……………川崎　俊彦，他 278
- ■インドネシアのジャカルタ，ボゴール地区における精神分裂病患者の援助希求行動 ……………………Heriani，他 280
- ■バリにおける精神医学の概念 ……………Luth Ketut Suryani 282
- ■在日ラテンアメリカ精神障害者の治療と予防 ……………………阿部　裕，他 284
- ■東海村臨界事故に関連した適応障害の一例 ……………………中野　英樹，他 286
- ■パニック障害患者のcopingとQOL ……………………竹内　龍雄，他 288
- ■知的障害者の不適応予防のための施設の心理的機能についての若干の考案 ……………………平野　潔 290
- ■日本における周産期精神医学(1) ……………………山下　洋，他 292
- ■日本における周産期精神医学(2) ……………………上田　基子，他 294
- ■日本における周産期精神医学(3) ……………………吉田　敬子，他 296
- ■婚姻後に精神障害を発症または再発した離婚調停事件の当事者について ……………………神川千賀子 298
- ■月経前不快気分障害の診断基準(DSM-IV)を用いた検討 …………尾鷲登志美，他 300
- ■摂食障害の予防活動 …生野　照子，他 302
- ■女子大学生における摂食障害傾向と環境要因との関連 ……………石田　彩子，他 304
- ■青年期女性における摂食障害の早期徴候とSelf-esteemの関係 ………塚本　美奈 306
- ■医学生の喫煙開始防止には入学後早期の介入

■が必要 ……………………武田　裕子, 他　308

■医学生は構内の禁煙環境と禁煙教育カリキュラムを求めている ……武田　裕子, 他　310

■多飲水と水中毒に関する予防医学的考察
　…………………………徳田　毅, 他　312

■一般人群と精神障害者群の生活習慣病有病率の比較より障害者群の予防, 治療について
　…………………………角谷　嘉紀, 他　314

■精神分裂病患者の緩和ケア病棟における日常生活動作の低下の予測について
　…………………………上間　一, 他　316

■精神障害者の身体合併症の外科的治療に際しての危険因子に関する検討
　…………………………宮里　洋, 他　318

■一般在宅高齢者における認知障害とMRI所見 …………………………古賀　寛, 他　320

精神障害の早期介入と予防

The recognition and optimal management of early psychosis

Patrick D. McGorry*

Introduction

"The best progressive ideas are those that include a strong enough dose of provocation to make its supporters feel proud of being original, but at the same time attract so many adherents that the risk of being an isolated exception is immediately averted by the noisy approval of a triumphant crowd." Milan Kundera[1].

Over the past decade, there has been a growing sense of optimism about the prospects for better outcomes for schizophrenia and related psychoses, which has achieved the status of a "progressive idea". However, while there is a sociopolitical dimension to all successful reform, this one has an extremely solid basis. Clinicians and policy makers are enthusiastic about reform based on this idea because of the sound logic behind it, the unacceptably poor access and quality of care previously available to young people with early psychosis and the increasing evidence that better outcomes can be achieved.

Some of this optimism has flowed from the development of a new generation of antipsychotic medications with greater efficacy and fewer toxic side-effects, but a second major factor has been the belated recognition that a special focus on the early phases of illness could result in a substantial reduction in morbidity and better quality of life for patients and their families. This is not a new idea, having been formulated in the 19th century by the alienists (Scull) and further developed during the preneuroleptic era by Sullivan[2] in particular and others subsequently.[3,4] However, in the face of a number of severe obstacles, it remained dormant for decades, gradually reemerging during the 1980's as a result of some key research studies,[5,6,7] and growing exponentially during the 1990's.

The first episode research focus immediately revealed the special clinical needs of young people at this phase of illness, the iatrogenic effects of standard care and a range of secondary preventive opportunities. This was especially clear when the clinical care of the first episode and recent onset patients was streamed separately from chronic patients, something which is still difficult to engineer. The key failures in care are prolonged delays in accessing effective treatment which usually occurs in the context of a severe behavioural crisis, crude and typically traumatic and alienating initial treatment strategies, and subsequent poor continuity of care and engagement of the patient with treatment. Young people have to demonstrate severe risk to themselves or others to gain access and a relapsing and chronically disabling pattern of illness to deserve ongoing care. These features are still highly prevalent in most systems of mental health care even in developed countries with reasonable levels of spending in mental health.

The innovative work of Falloon[5] and the increasing devolution of mental health care into community settings has provided further momentum, as has a genuine renaissance in biological and psychological treatments for psychosis. An exponential growth in interest in neuroscientific research in schizophrenia has injected further optimism into the field with a new generation of clinician-researchers coming to the fore. Several countries have developed national mental health strategies or frameworks which catalyse and guide major reform and mandate a preventive mindset and linked reform. Around the world an increasingly large number of groups have established clinical programs and research intiatives focussing on early psychosis and it now constitutes a growth point in clinical care as well as research. This blend of science and sociology has the potential to lead to a sea change in the way these illnesses are conceived and managed.

While primary prevention is still out of reach, secondary prevention or "early intervention" is an excellent interim option. This means early detection of new cases, shortening delays in effective treatment, optimal and sustained treatment in the early "critical period" of the first few years of illness. To reduce the impact and burden of psychotic disorders in society as a whole would constitute a major achievement. It may even be possible to reduce the prevalence as well by shortening the duration of illness by delaying onset, reducing the period of time spent living with the symptoms and disability or accelerating recovery. However, none of this has occurred despite the development of highly effective treatments,[6] because we have failed to translate these advances to the real world beyond the randomised controlled trial. Even with existing knowledge, substantial reductions in prevalence and improved quality of life are possible for patients provided societies are prepared to pay for it. Early intervention, with its promise of more efficient treatment through an enhanced focus on the early phases of illness, is an additional prevalence reduction strategy which is now available to be tested and, if cost-effective, to be widely implemented.

Evidence is critical if there is to be a real world shift in attitudes and clinical practice and if we are to avoid a further false dawn in the history of this field. However, for each element, we need to determine how much evidence is required before a change in practice is warranted. In deciding where the onus of proof should lie, we should also remember that the alternative to early and optimal intervention is delayed and substandard treatment with all its human consequences (Lieberman and Fenton 2000). Even in developed countries, as consumers and carers will readily attest, the timing and quality of standard care is relatively poor, very much a case of "too little, too late". In developing countries, a significant proportion of cases never receives treatment.[7] While we do need evidence, there are obvious additional clinical and commonsense drivers for more timely and widespread treatment of better quality.

Conceptual framework for early intervention

While it is possible to discuss the preventive clinical management of early psychosis within the traditional framework of primary, secondary and tertiary prevention, there is now a superior alternative. Mrazek and Haggerty[8] developed a more sophisticated framework for conceptualizing, implementing and evaluating preventive interventions within the full spectrum of interventions for mental disorders.

They classified preventive interventions as universal, selective and indicated. Universal preventive interventions are focused upon the whole population eg. immunisation and prevention of smoking, while selective preventive measures are aimed at asymptomatic subgroups of the population whose risk of becoming ill is above average, eg. annual mammograms for women with a positive family history of breast cancer. Indicated prevention is concerned with subthreshold symptoms which confer high risk for a more severe disorder.

The other two (secondary) preventive foci identified are early case detection and optimal management of the first episode of illness and the subsequent "critical period". In summary these three foci can be collectively termed *early interven-*

tion'.

Prepsychotic intervention

This is the earliest possible phase for preventive intervention in psychosis and has great potential. At the present point in time it remains a clinical research issue, though guidelines must be developed to guide a clinical response to young people presenting for treatment with potentially subthreshold or prodromal symptoms, since they are distressing and disabling.

Indicated prevention is defined as follows:

'Indicated preventive interventions for mental disorders are targeted to high-risk individuals who are identified as having minimal but detectable signs or symptoms foreshadowing mental disorder, or biological markers indicating predisposition for mental disorder, but who do not meet DSM-III-R diagnostic levels at the current time.'

- In fact, subthreshold symptoms become a risk factor in their own right for more severe disorder. Although in reality patients present with more dimensional patterns of symptomatology, this preventive framework assumes a categorical model of illness, which underpins an epidemiological approach to mental disorders and our current nosological systems. Since universal and selective prevention remain out of reach at present, indicated prevention marks the current frontier of prevention in psychotic disorders.

"The best hope now for the prevention of schizophrenia lies with indicated preventive interventions targeted at individuals manifesting precursor signs and symptoms who have not yet met full criteria for diagnosis. The identification of individuals at this early stage, coupled with the introduction of pharmacological and psychosocial interventions, may prevent the development of the full-blown disorder." Mrazek and Haggerty (p.154)[16]

- The idea of intervening at this stage of illness raises conflicting concerns. Some regard it as an early form of treatment and hence a key opportunity, however the situation is not so clearcut. With the passage of time, some of these cases will be seen to have been manifesting an early form of the disorder in question, and the subthreshold clinical features will then turn out to have been "prodromal". On the other hand, others will not and some will therefore constitute "false positives" for the disorder in question. This has caused concerns about the effects of labelling.
- Nevertheless, it is necessary to respond since they have at least have crossed a clinical threshold where they either require or request treatment. This will either be because they have reached diagnostic threshold for other comorbid syndromes, or because the subthreshold symptoms of the putatively core disorder have become disabling or distressing. In any event, as any clinician knows, help-seeking and treatment need in psychiatry are not perfectly correlated with diagnostic threshold; not surprisingly, patients do not always conform to the DSM or ICD categories and thresholds.[9,10,11]
- Clinicians working with such a range of comorbidity potentially have two objectives. Firstly, they may treat what is already present, and secondly they can try to reduce the risk of the existing syndromes worsening or evolving into a more serious syndrome, such as acute psychosis. The first is not controversial and is merely good clinical care, the second is essentially a research endeavour. Partly because of the real need to respond to cases identified through early detection of first episode psychosis, many centres focusing on first episode patients have developed clinical and research

programs for help-seeking subthreshold cases.

1. Early detection of first episode psychosis
- Beyond the subthreshold or prodromal phase, there is the issue of timing of treatment. Early case detection aimed at shortening delays in accessing treatment should reduce prevalence and morbidity provided there is an effective form of treatment available.
- We know from a range of studies that the duration of untreated psychosis (DUP) is extremely prolonged in developed countries (refs) and averages around one year. Most studies have shown a significant correlation between DUP and early indicators of response to treatment and recovery. Hence it has become an attractive target for intervention.
- Even if response to treatment remains good after significant delay, there is still a powerful human and medical argument for making effective treatment available to young people as early as possible (Lieberman and Fenton 2000, Ho and Andreasen 2000).

2. The optimal management of the first episode and the critical period
- The third and most robustly evidence-based preventive focus is enhancing the *quality* of treatment. The notion that optimal treatment of the early phase of disorder could shorten the duration of illness and thus reduce the prevalence of the disorder, and further have a positive medium to long term effect on the course and outcome is an attractive idea.
- The idea of a 'critical period' during which the disorder is more responsive to intervention has recently been developed for psychotic disorders and fits with the patterns of illness severity found in recent follow-up studies as well as the developmental stage of life in which these illnesses emerge.[11,12,13,14,15,16] (add latest Harrison ref BJPsych 2001).
- If early detection provides one safety net to limit the psychosocial damage of these illnesses, then optimal and sustained treatment during this critical period when the vulnerability is at its peak can act as a second one, providing a degree of "damage control". This strategy is supported by the fact that the level of disability attained within the first 2 years or so after entry to treatment strongly predicts the level of disability many years later (Harrison et al 2001).

Optimizing and intensifying early phase treatment, including sophisticated recovery and relapse prevention strategies, is therefore a third subtype of secondary prevention which could be implemented and evaluated within mental health services even with the present level of knowledge. Given the alternative for patients and families, we really should ask ourselves why not? Even if the burden of disease is reduced during the period of active treatment yet the ultimate level of disability attained is not this is a highly appropriate treatment goal which is uncontroversial in other areas of health care, eg diabetes.

The basis for early intervention in the real world

1. Pre-psychotic intervention
- Deficits in social functioning are primarily established during the pre-psychotic or prodromal phase, the active period of illness proximal to attaining diagnostic threshold. The level of psychosocial development achieved by the end of the prodromal phase, when the first psychotic symptom appears, strongly influences the further social course of the disorder by setting a 'ceiling' for recovery.[17,18]
- This means it is a "prodromal" change not a "premorbid" one, since during childhood, most people with subsequent schizophrenia

are only very subtly, if at all, different from their peers, and even less so from those who later develop an affective illness.[19,20]

- In childhood the disorder is rarely clinically active, and it is far too early to make any accurate predictions regarding subsequent psychosis in adolescence or adulthood. While an early vulnerability may exist in a proportion of cases, other environmental risk factors[21] and putative problems with adolescent brain development processes (a second stage process, termed neurodegenerative or neurotoxic by some)[22] clearly come into play during adolescence or later, though months or years prior to the emergence of the diagnostically defining features of psychotic disorder.[25]

- Recently it has become possible to identify those at incipient (ultra high) risk (UHR) of transition to psychosis, through an approach termed the 'close-in' strategy[23]. These young people are already distressed and functioning poorly, and are willing to accept professional help.[24,25,26,27,28] Even with good psychosocial care, 41% of operationally defined UHR patients make the transition to first episode psychosis within a 12-month follow-up period.

- Several clinical features, such as depression and various negative and positive symptoms, further enhance the capacity to predict transition to psychosis within this group even though a very diverse range of clinical features are present.[29,30,31] The risk of progression is also higher for those with a longer duration of symptoms, but there is clearly a less specific early prodromal phase where prediction will be much less feasible. Non-specific psychosocial interventions helpful in the reduction of risk for a range of disorders may find a place during this less differentiated phase.

- A recent randomised controlled trial in this clinical population has shown a significant reduction in transition rate to psychosis for patients receiving specific treatment (ST) - very low dose risperidone (1-2mg/day) and cognitive therapy - in comparison to non-specific treatment (NST) - supportive psychotherapy and symptomatic treatment Ref under review).[41]

- A range of ethical and conceptual issues need to be considered in relation to this emerging field (new issue of schiz research coming out in August 2001), However it is important to note that these patients have experienced a recent change in subjective experience, have emerging and significant disability and are seeking help. As defined in Table 2, they also have a very substantial risk of developing a frank psychotic illness, usually, but not always, schizophrenia. They must be distinguished from a subgroup of the general population who report isolated psychotic symptoms in the apparent absence of distress, disability or progressive change, and who do not desire assistance[32].

- Further research is urgently required to clarify the range of treatments which will alleviate their distress and disability and reduce their risk of subsequent psychosis.

- In the interim there is a need for a clinical response from psychiatrists, community mental health services and primary care, since these young people are highly symptomatic and at increased risk of suicide, substance abuse and vocational failure. What should the clinician do when approached by a young person or by the family of a young person who appears to be at high risk?

- Firstly, if the symptoms are very non-specific, especially if they are of recent-onset, and there is no family history of psychosis, then the approach should be a general and supportive one. This could include treating any specific features, such as depression, panic or OCD, with a psychosocial approach initially, com-

bined with the use of an SSRI, if symptoms are persistent or severe.
- For those meeting the criteria for ultra high risk (UHR) as defined above, the offer, at least, of initial psychosocial treatment, including the emerging range of cognitive therapies, with or without syndrome-based drug treatments, aimed at the relief of such distress and disability in young people seems eminently justifiable as a component of youth-oriented mental health care. What the patient and family should be told about the level of risk of future psychosis has been debated, however in our experience, an open approach of disclosure, guided by the curiosity of the patient and family has worked well.
- If this offer of intervention is initially refused, as it may well be in this age group, this can usually be accepted, although some kind of assertive follow-up is also justifiable, combined with family contact because, in addition to the risk of psychosis, there is, as mentioned, a higher than expected rate of substance abuse, deliberate self-harm and suicide in this potentially prepsychotic population.[33]
- Not uncommonly, the parents of the young person will be concerned about vocational failure and social withdrawal in their relative, but will be unable to persuade them to attend for assessment. This is partly because of problems relating to stigma and self-stigmatisation. In this situation, rather than retreat behind the usual barriers erected by more traditional clinical approaches, it is more appropriate to ensure that a way is found for the young person to be assessed and offered help in a non-stigmatising manner. This can be accomplished through home visits by the family doctor, by the school counsellor, or by mobile youth mental health teams linked to specialist youth health services or specialist mental health services. Early intervention teams can also be located in mainstream community facilities to facilitate such assessments and avoid stigma.
- Naturally a good understanding of the range of normal psychology of adolescents and young adults, and of appropriate interviewing and engagement strategies is invaluable. Engagement is more than half the battle in early intervention in psychosis and a youth mental health orientation is critical. It effectively deals with the false positive issue, which recedes when a broader focus on youth mental health with all of its comorbidity is embraced.
- Even if psychosis does emerge and the symptoms cross the threshold for antipsychotic therapy, a key advantage of this focus on vulnerable, prepsychotic or potentially prodromal people is that a therapeutic relationship has been established when it is much more possible to do so. The young person has been less severely ill and more accessible to relationships generally. This means that recommendations re drug therapy are more likely to be accepted when they are made by patient and family, and, in our experience, that hospitalisation can be avoided in most cases, hence reducing the costs and trauma associated with treatment of the first psychotic episode. Furthermore, the duration of untreated psychosis (DUP) is reduced to an absolute minimum. Even if only a minority of first episode cases can be engaged prior to psychosis and no transitions to psychosis can be prevented, the advantages are still potentially great. Treatment will be commenced "on the right foot" in atmosphere of trust rather than fear and disruption, and with fewer complications.
- The final clinical issue in this phase of illness is whether there is a role for antipsychotic medications prior to reaching the threshold for diagnosis of a frank psychotic disorder. Despite the lower risks of disabling side-effects

and better efficacy of the novel antipsychotic drugs, and the positive early research findings described above, caution is required here. If the indications for broadening the use of antipsychotic medications beyond frank and persistent psychosis as reflected in the DSM-IV psychotic disorders are not very carefully defined and supported by high quality research, then it is likely that much harm could be done. While we await such guidance from research, it seems reasonable for clinicians to proceed as follows.

- The conservative engagement and monitoring strategies outlined above could be offered, and each syndrome, eg depression, as it manifests could be specifically treated with pharmacological and psychosocial interventions within a youth mental health model
- Antipsychotic medications should be withheld except in the following situations when they could be considered. Patients who meet the ultra high risk (UHR) criteria as defined, and who are rapidly deteriorating (but have not become frankly psychotic in a persistent manner such that they meet criteria for schizophreniform disorder or another major DSM-IV psychotic disorder) with increasing suicidality or risk of violence, or with increasingly disorganised, stigmatising or embarrassing behaviours, could be offered a trial of low dose antipsychotic medication which could be reviewed after say 6 weeks.
- If substantial improvement occurred then it would seem reasonable (as if the patient had had a first psychotic episode) to continue the treatment for 6-12 months and then, provided remission was maintained, to withdraw the medication cautiously and slowly at that point. If the first drug used were to have little beneficial effect, then the situation is less clearcut, though other antipsychotic treatment trials could be considered especially if the patient's condition continued to worsen.
- In the future a range of other strategies may prove to worth trying such as cognitive remediation, cognitive behaviour therapy, and putative neuroprotective agents, such as lithium and essential fatty acids. This proposed approach is clearly based on emerging clincial experience with such patients and its validity needs to be thoroughly tested through further clinical research. The value of such research cannot be overestimated given the critical nature of this phase of illness in relation to outcomes for patients.

2. Early case detection in first episode psychosis
- Once the currently accepted threshold for treatment with antipsychotic medication - the first clear and sustained emergence of psychotic features - is reached, there is a firmer foundation for early intervention. Despite this and the severity of these disorders, for a substantial proportion of people, such treatment is surprisingly delayed, often for very prolonged periods.[34,35] Hence for the typical case, the above description of the pre-psychotic treatment strategy is a long way from present reality. Indeed for others, especially in the developing world,[14] treatment is never accessed.
- The duration of untreated psychosis (DUP), as a marker of delay in delivering effective specific treatment, is a potentially important variable in relation to efforts to improve outcome in first episode schizophrenia, and more widely in first episode psychosis.[36]
- DUP is important because, unlike other prognostic variables such as genetic vulnerability, gender and age of onset, it is a potentially malleable variable which can become the focus of intervention strategies.
- Psychosis may be an easier and less conflicted target to detect than schizophrenia.[37,38] Schizophrenia, which requires a period of frank psy-

chotic features for diagnosis, may take time to emerge as a stable diagnosis, and our primary treatment target is positive psychotic symptoms for which we prescribe antipsychotic medications (notwithstanding their effects on other symptom domains).

- A strong and extensive literature supports a correlational link between DUP and both short and long term outcome,[42,39] although two recent studies have cast doubt on the link.[40,41]
- Assuming the link is as robust as it seems, there is one further question. Is the association causal? That is, is delay (prolonged DUP) in treatment a risk factor for worse outcome? Or is the link due to a common underlying factor, namely a more severe form of illness, which has a more insidious onset with more negative symptoms, more paranoid ideation, less salience and awareness of change and less willingness to seek and accept treatment? Even if this is so, DUP may still be a key intervening variable through which these clinical features influence outcome, and hence reducing it may mitigate their effect.
- Although it is not yet clearly proven that reducing DUP improves outcome, there is a strong prima facie case, as McGlashan[42] has emphasized, that delayed treatment is already a major public health problem:
 "(prolonged) DUP, by itself, is reason enough for early intervention on a large and intensive scale" (p.901).
- What justifies such a statement is a clinical appreciation derived from patients and families directly of the destructive effects of delay and the range of negative psychosocial outcomes which accumulate during the period of untreated psychosis.[47,42] These include vocational failure, self-harm, offending behaviour, family distress and dysfunction, aggression, substance abuse, and victimization by others.
- Mental health services in partnership with local communities, primary care and individual clinicians could therefore embark upon a range of strategies to reduce delays in treatment onset. This is not a process which is seen as part of the mandate of clinicians or clinical services, indeed depending on the funding system, it is more common for the latter to regulate their workload by restricting access to new patients. There may be a reluctance to widen access because of a lack of resources, due to inadequate funding, to cope with a feared influx of referrals. This is a real issue since it is quite true that the effect of early detection strategies in community psychiatry settings (eg community education and mobile detection teams) will probably be twofold, as witnessed in recent Scandinavian studies.[42]
- Firstly, if intensive efforts are made to improve mental health literacy in the general community, recognition skills among general practitioners through training and consultation-liaison, and access to and engagement with specialist mental health services, then the duration of untreated psychosis for the average case should be substantially reduced, especially the relatively small subgroup with a very long DUP. This should make the work of the service easier and result in a reduced need for inpatient care and involuntary treatment.
- Secondly, there will be an increase in treated incidence of psychosis and hence workload. Nevertheless, there would be a corresponding reduction in the prevalence of hidden psychiatric morbidity in the community.
- Clearly these effects will be complex to measure and monitor. To achieve them, an initial change in the culture of clinical practice will be required with reciprocal effects upon the complexion of the service. More resources will be required for services to become proactive in this way, to undertake the detection

role and cope with the additional caseloads. Such a role should be built into part of the mandate of modern community-based mental health services and requires leadership from within psychiatry, but needs to be developed in partnership with communities and primary care. It also needs to be added to the existing budgets for health services on a regional basis rather than expecting direct service budgets to absorb such costs.

3. Optimal and intensive phase-specific intervention in first episode psychosis and the 'critical period'

- Since it does not require as much of a change in role as the previous two preventive foci, more intensive phase-specific treatment during the first episode of psychosis, and beyond into the critical period, is the most feasible proposition for most clinicians and researchers interested in secondary prevention. Several monographs have appeared on this subject recently.[24,43,44,45]
- In general, there is some evidence that such intensive treatment of young people at this phase of illness is effective;[24,47,53,46] and cost-effective[47] in real world settings at least in the short-term, though more research is certainly required to examine the longer term impact and to determine the most appropriate service models.
- Whether it is possible to reduce the intensity of treatment over a longer time frame or not,[21] is an important secondary research question. Recent studies would suggest that treatment intensity should not be reduced within the first 5 years for the majority of patients.

First episode psychosis

The key elements of management in first episode psychosis are described in detail elsewhere.[27,51,52,53,48] They can be summarised as follows.

1. *Access and engagement*

- Most people, though not all, who develop psychotic disorders are young people with little or no experience of mental health services. They lack knowledge and carry the same fears and prejudices as the rest of the community regarding mental illness and will generally be reluctant to seek or accept help. This is not specific to first episode psychosis but is a common problem in adolescent psychiatry, exaggerated by the sense of invulnerability which is part of normal adolescence.
- The presence of psychotic symptoms, particularly delusions, may further inhibit awareness and help-seeking.
- Access and engagement with services are processes that can be markedly enhanced by the way services are designed and operated. Mobile assessment available around the clock in a setting that suits the individual patient and family is a key advance in improving access to care. This should ideally be offered even prior to a crisis or high risk situation having developed so that a calm and careful process of assessment and initial management can be undertaken.
- Engagement with services is made more difficult if a traumatic crisis and involuntary treatment is the initial experience of the young patient and family. Many services still shield themselves behind concrete and self-serving interpretations of local mental health legislation requiring patients who are not actively seeking help on their own behalf or who reject it, especially first episode cases, to develop suicidal or violent behaviour before even direct assessment is offered. Although crises cannot always be avoided, the frequency can be reduced substantially if resources are devoted to a mobile early detection and assessment service.[49]

2. *Assessment*
- The assessment process is of major importance at the point of first entry to specialist mental health care for obvious reasons. Ultimately this should be comprehensive and include a developmental and family perspective. However, the goal of detailed assessment should not undermine the goals of engagement and initial management of the distressed young patient and their family, so it should be carried out in a stepwise fashion.
- The initial assessment should focus on the major diagnostic issues and levels of risk of harm to self or others. The rest can be pieced together over time. A key issue is to determine whether is patient is clearly psychotic, and if so whether there is also a major mood syndrome present. Substance abuse and dependence are frequently comorbid with positive psychotic symptoms, and it is important to identify the small proportion of cases where the psychosis represents a simple acute intoxication, rather than the more common scenario where each disorder acts as a risk factor for the other.
- As early detection strategies begin to bite, it is also likely that more subthreshold cases, including those with isolated psychotic symptoms,[40] will be assessed. Some of these patients have psychotic symptoms that are not typical of the textbook or diagnostic manual and may confuse clinicians. Many of these patients do request and require treatment, many with antipsychotics and often with other drug therapies as well, however further research may be required to carefully define the range of appropriate treatment for such patients. Our existing treatment strategies are most clearly indicated when they are offered to severe acute cases or patients with prolonged untreated illness and significant disability, though the onset of clearcut and sustained positive psychotic symptoms represents a watershed for any given patient.
- Although the novel antipsychotics have broader effects than positive symptoms alone, the clear emergence of frank and sustained (at least 1 week) positive symptoms is currently a necessary step to considering their use in clinical settings. Hence in detection and diagnosis *psychosis* is an appropriate target. Secondary targets then become mania, depression, and a range of other comorbid syndromes and syndromes, rather than DSM or ICD diagnoses per se, because they constitute a better guide to drug therapy.[45,50]

3. *Acute treatment*
- The initial decision is whether inpatient care is required. This will be influenced by patient factors, the degree of family and social support, and by the range of services available and local policies. Where this is possible, home-based acute care is preferred for a range of reasons and can be achieved in over 50% of cases with a highly structured and intensive approach.[51,52]
- An antipsychotic-free period of at least 48 hours is usually advisable, during which benzodiazepines only are prescribed to alleviate the distressing symptoms of agitation, anxiety and insomnia. If sustained psychosis is confirmed then antipsychotic medication may be commenced.
- The second generation or novel antipsychotics are indicated as first, second and even third line therapy because of their greater efficacy and better tolerability. The starting dose should be very low (eg 0.5mg risperidone or 2.5mg olanzapine) and be increased to an initial "step" and held there for the effect to be evaluated (eg 2mg risperidone or 7.5mg olanzapine). Further increases should only occur in the setting of poor response and only then

at intervals of approximately 3 weeks to allow the effect of the change in dose to become clear. The all-too-familiar weekly doubling of the dose at ward rounds should become a thing of the past.

- We now know that these dosages are sufficient to produce sufficient levels of D2 blockade in the CNS to bring about a clinical response and that the threshold for clinical response is lower, albeit narrowly so, than the threshold at which neurological and other side-effects begin to manifest. Classic research conducted at the Karolinska Institute in Sweden and at the Clarke Institute in Canada for the demonstration of this narrow therapeutic window.[53,54]

- These low doses of antipsychotics are not intended or expected to deal with the behavioural disturbances and associated symptoms frequently seen in this acute phase. The latter should be managed if at all possible with benzodiazepines and psychosocial strategies during this period, since the use of parenteral or sedating oral typical neuroleptics will inevitably produce aversive neurological side-effects and undermine, perhaps terminally, an already fragile process of engagement and adherence to treatment.

- Emergency situations requiring urgent sedation can be managed with intramuscular benzodiazepines such as midazolam or lorazepam in most cases. In occasional cases this will be ineffective and a short-acting sedating neuroleptic, droperidol 5mg intramuscularly is the next best option.

- Longer-acting depot preparations such as zuclopenthixol acetate ("Acuphase") seem superficially appealing because they purport to avoid the necessity for repeated injections during the acute phase, but their delayed onset of action and the almost inevitable production of distressing neurological side-effects mean that the risks outweigh the benefits for nearly all first episode patients. Repeated injections are in any case very rarely required with good nursing care, a supportive milieu and liberal use of benzodiazepines in the acute phase.

- Naturally intensive psychosocial support is essential for the patient and family during this highly stressful period, though services are often unable to provide this due to inadequate funding, low morale and poor skills, combined with an unfortunate lack of awareness or acknowledgement of its critical role. This is a deficiency in urgent need of reform.

- Home-based care is less stressful for the patient in particular and usually results in a reduced need for acute medication.

- The identification and treatment of the major affective syndromes, especially mania, is a key issue in the treatment of first episode psychosis. A manic syndrome is present in up to 20% of cases of first episode psychosis and should be rapidly treated with a mood stabiliser, ideally lithium carbonate or alternatively sodium valproate, to promote full recovery while minimising antipsychotic dosages.

- Depression, unless clearly dominating the clinical picture, commonly resolves in parallel with the positive psychotic symptoms, however if it persists or worsens during the post-psychotic period, it should be actively treated with a combination of SSRI and psychological intervention. More detailed descriptions of the principles and practice of acute care can be found in Kulkarni and Power,[60] Aitchison et al[53] and the Australian Clinical Guidelines for Early Psychosis[56].

4. *The recovery phase*
- Up to 85-90% of first episode patients will achieve a remission or partial remission of their positive psychotic symptoms within the 12 months following entry to treatment,

though some potentially responsive patients will fail to engage with treatment or rapidly cease adherence to medication.
- A range of psychosocial strategies can augment and broaden the scope and depth of the recovery process, and these include psychological interventions,[55,56,57,58] family interventions[59] and group based recovery programs[60]. Some of these will increase the remission rate for positive symptoms and they all aim to improve negative symptoms, functioning and quality of life.
- Rapid discharge of responding patients following an acute first episode of psychosis to unsupported general practitioners is a poor practice. It represents a missed opportunity for maximising and consolidating recovery and for secondary prevention. An integrated shared care model with the GP and other agencies is likely to prove more beneficial.

The critical period
- This term can be regarded as covering the period following recovery from a first episode of psychosis and extending for up to five years subsequently. This is based on the notion[23] that this is the phase of maximum vulnerability. A number of recent research studies have focused on the treated course of early psychosis. These have shown that the early course of illness for both schizophrenia and affective psychosis is turbulent and relapse prone with up to 80% of patients relapsing within a five year period. These findings suggest that drug therapy should be continued for most if not all patients for longer than 12 months after recovery from a first psychotic episode.
- However, it should be remembered that a subsample, at least 20%, never relapse, that some will not relapse for a prolonged period, and that relapse prevention is not the sole consideration in treatment but rather a means to an end. Adaptation to illness is a challenging often overwhelming task for these young people and they usually need to be given time and special help to come to an acceptance of the need for maintenance treatment.[61]
- A concerted effort should be made to maintain the engagement of most patients with clinical care during the early years after onset and to have in place a written relapse plan so that action can be taken if symptoms reemerge whether on or off medication. A good therapeutic and personal relationship with the patient and family is the key to success and should be nurtured, though continuity of care is at a premium in public psychiatry in developed countries. This deficiency is the Achilles' heel of the system, leaving patients, who often have significant problems with trust and in forming social relationships with no safety net.
- Even with standard care however, it has been shown that outcome at 13 years is much more positive than expected, supporting the notion of an early critical period, which may be turbulent but seems to abate after 2-5 years. With optimal care such outcomes could be substantially improved.

Conclusion

There is growing support for a more preventive stance in the treatment of schizophrenia and psychotic disorders. Primary prevention, specifically universal and selective preventive interventions, is beyond our capacities at the present stage of knowledge. However, indicated prevention for subthreshold symptoms has been endorsed as the frontier of prevention in schizophrenia,[16] and early detection and optimal early treatment are clearly within the mandate of clinicians and services, and can be justified despite predictable academic skepticism. This skepticism must be appropriately addressed through rigorous clinical research, but it may prove difficult to fully dissipate, and should not be allowed to snuff out precious therapeutic optimism which can improve morale within services as well as patient outcomes. Evidence will be a vital guide because a range of new clinical and ethical issues are being brought to light as the frontier advances, and it is important that changes in mental health care are based on solid foundations, not shifting sands, as so often in the past. Nevertheless, dispersing the mists of pessimism which have shrouded the clinical care of people with schizophrenia and encouraged stigma is an overdue and worthwhile endeavour. The treatment objectives and approaches described in this chapter characterise recent early steps in this direction, with the hope that further progress will rapidly occur.

References

1) Kundera, M. : The Book of Laughter and Forgetting. Faber and Faber, London, p.273, 1996.
2) Sullivan, H. S. : The onset of schizophrenia. Am. J. Psychiatry, 151 ; 135-139, 1992. (1994 : reprinted)
3) Cameron, D. E. : Early schizophrenia. Am. J. Psychiatry, 95 ; 567-78, 1938.
4) Meares, A. : The diagnosis of prepsychotic schizophrenia. Lancet, i ; 55-59, 1959.
5) Falloon, I. R. H. : Early intervention for first episode of schizophrenia : A preliminary exploration. Psychiatry, 55 ; 4-15, 1992.
6) Hegarty, J., Baldessarini, R., Tohen, M. et al. : One hundred years of schizophrenia : a meta-analysis of the outcome literature. Am. J. Psychiatry, 151 ; 1409-1416, 1994.
7) Padmavathi, R., Rajkumar, S., Srinivasan, T. : Schizophrenic patients who were never treated --a study in an Indian urban community. Psychol. Med, 28(5) ; 1113-1117, 1998.
8) Mrazek, P. J., Haggerty, R. J., eds. : Reducing risks for mental disorders : frontiers for preventive intervention research. National Academy Press, Washington D.C., 1994.
9) Regier, D. A., Kaelber, C. T., Rae, D. S. et al. : Limitations of diagnostic criteria and assessment instruments for mental disorders. Arch. Gen. Psychiatry, 55 ; 109-115, 1998.
10) Spitzer, R. L. : Diagnosis and need for treatment are not the same. Arch. Gen. Psychiatry, 55 : 120, 1998.
11) Frances, A. : Problems in defining clinical significance in epidemiological studies. Archives of General Psychiatry, 55 ; 119, 1998.
12) Birchwood, M., MacMillian, F. : Early intervention in schizophrenia. Aust. N.Z.J. Psychiatry, 27 ; 374-378, 1993.
13) Birchwood, M., Todd, P., Jackson, C. : Early intervention in psychosis : The critical period hypothesis. Br. J. Psychiatry, 172 (Supplement 33) ; 53-59, 1998.
14) Loebel, A., Lieberman, J. A., Alvir, J. M. et al. : Duration of psychosis and outcome in first-episode schizophrenia. Am. J. Psychiatry, 149 ; 1183-1188, 1992.
15) McGorry, P. D., Singh, B. S. : Schizophrenia : Risk and possibility. In : Raphael, B., Burrows, G. D., eds, Handbook of Studies on Preventive Psychiatry. Elsevier Science Publishers : Amsterdam, The Netherlands, 1995.
16) McGorry, P. D., Jackson, H. J., eds. : The Recognition and management of Early Psychosis : A Preventive Approach. Cambridge University Press, Cambridge, England, 1999.
17) Häfner, H., Nowotny, B., Löffler, W. et al. : When and how does schizophrenia produce social deficits? Eur. Arch. Psychiatry Clin. Neurosci, 246 ; 17-28, 1995.
18) Häfner, H., Löffler, W., Maurer, K. et al. : Depression, negative symptoms, social stagnation and social decline in the early course of schizophrenia. Acta Psychiatr Scand, 100 ; 105-118, 1999.
19) Jones, P., Rodgers, B., Murray, R. et al. : Child developmental risk factors for adult schizophrenia in the British 1946 birth cohort. The Lancet 1994 ; 344 ; 1398-1402.
20) Van, Os J., Jones, P., Lewis, G. et al. : Developmental precursors of affective illness in a general population birth cohort. Arch. Gen. Psychiatry, 54 ; 625-631, 1997.
21) Mahy, G., Mallett, R., Leff, J. et al. : First-contact incidence rate of schizophrenia on Barbados. Br. J. Psychiatry, 175 ; 28-33, 1999.
22) Rapoport, J., Giedd, J., Blumenthal, J. et al. : Progressive cortical change during adolescence in childhood-onset schizophrenia. Arch. Gen. Psychiatry, 56 ; 649-654, 1999.

23) Bell, R. Q. : Multiple-risk cohorts and segmenting risk as solutions to the problem of false positives in risk for the major psychoses. Psychiatry, 55 ; 370-81, 1992.
24) McGorry, P., Phillips, L., Yung, A. : Recognition and treatment of the pre-psychotic phase of psychotic disorders : Frontier or fantasy?. In : Mednick, S., McGlashan, T., Libiger, J. Johannessen, J., eds, Early intervention in psychiatric disorders. Kluwer : Netherlands, in press.
25) McGorry, P. D., Yung, A. R., Phillips, L. J. : "Closing in" : what features predict the onset of first episode psychosis within a high risk group? In : Zipursky, R. B., ed, The Early Stages of Schizophrenia. American Psychiatric Press, US, in press.
26) Yung, A., Phillips, L., McGorry, P. et al. : Prediction of psychosis. Br. J. Psychiatry, 172 (Supplement 33) ; 14-20, 1998.
27) Yung, A., McGorry, P., McFarlane, C. et al. : Monitoring and care of young people at incipient risk of psychosis. Schizophr Bull, 22(2) ; 283-303, 1996.
28) McGorry, P., Jackson, H., Edwards, J. et al. : Preventively-oriented psychological interventions in early psychosis. In : Psychological Treatments for Schizophrenia. Institute of Psychiatry, The University of Manchester, Oxford, England, 1999.
29) McGorry, P. D., Phillips, L. J., Yung, A. R. et al. : The identification of predictors of psychosis in a high risk group. Schizophr Res, 36(1-3) ; 49-50, 1999.
30) Schultze-Lütter, F., Klosterkötter, J. : What tool should be used for generating predictive models? Schizophr Res, 36(1-3) ; 10, 1999.
31) Phillips, L., Yung, A., Hearn, N. et al. : Preventive mental health care : Accessing the target population. Aust. N.Z.J. Psychiatry, 33 ; 912-917, 1999.
32) Van, Os. J., Bijl, R., Ravelli, A. : Can the boundaries of psychosis be defined? Schizophr Res, 41 (1) ; 8, 2000.
33) Phillips, L., McGorry, P., Yung, A. et al. : The development of preventive interventions for early psychosis : Early findings and directions for the future. Schizophr Res, 36(1-3) ; 331-332, 1999.
34) McGlashan, T. : Duration of untreated psychosis in first-episode schizophrenia : Marker or determinant of course? Biol Psychiatry, 46 ; 899-907, 1999.
35) Carbone, S., Harrigan, S., McGorry, P. et al. : Duration of untreated psychosis and 12-month outcome in first-episode psychosis : The impact of treatment approach. Acta Psychiatr Scand, 100 ; 96-104, 1999.
36) Harrigan, S. M., McGorry, P. D., Krstev, H. : Does treatment delay in first-episode psychosis really matter? Schizophr Res, 41 ; 175, 2000.
37) McGorry, P. : A treatment-relevant classification of psychotic disorders. Aust. N. Z. J. Psychiatry, 29(4) ; 555-558, 1995.
38) Driessen, G., Gunther, N., Bak, M. et al. : Characteristics of early- and late-diagnosed schizophrenia : Implications for first-episode studies. Schizophr Res, 33(1-2) ; 27-34, 1998.
39) McGorry, P., Edwards, J., Mihalopoulos, C. et al. : EPPIC : An evolving system of early detection and optimal management. Schizophr Bull, 22 ; 305-326, 1996.
40) Ho, B. C., Andreasen, N. C. : Duration of initial untreated psychosis - methods and meanings. Paper presented at the 2nd Interntional Confernece on Early Psychosis "Future Possible", 31 March and 1-2 April, New York, 2000.
41) Craig, T. J., Bromet, E. J., Fennig, S. et al. : Is there an association between duration of untreated psychosis and 24-month clinical outcome in a first-admission series? American Journal of Psychiatry, 157(1) ; 60-66, 2000.
42) Lincoln, C., Harrigan, S., McGorry, P. : Understanding the topogaphy of the early psychosis pathways. Br. J. Psychiatry, 172 (Supplement 33) ; 21-25, 1998.
43) McGorry, P., Edwards, J., eds. : Early Psychosis Training Pack. Gardiner-Caldwell Communications Ltd : Cheshire, UK, 1997.
44) McGorry, P. D., ed. : Preventive strategies in early psychosis : verging on reality. Br. J. Psychiatry, 172 (Supplement 33) ; 1-136, 1998.
45) Aitchinson, K., Meehan, K., Murrary, R. : First episode psychosis. Martin Dunitz Ltd, London, 1999.
46) Power, P., Elkins, K., Adlard, S. et al. : Analysis of the initial treatment phase in first-episode psychosis. Br. J. Psychiatry, 172 (Suppl 33) ; 71-76, 1998.

47) Mihalopoulos, C., McGorry, P., Carter, R. : Is phase-specific, community-oriented treatment of early psychosis an economically viable method of improving outcome. Acta Psychiatr Scand, 100 ; 47-55, 1999.
48) National Early Psychosis Project Clinical Guidelines Working Party, Australian Clinical Guidelines for Early Psychosis. National Early Psychosis Project, University of Melbourne, Melbourne, 1998.
49) Yung, A. R., Jackson, H. J. : The onset of psychotic disorder : clinical and research aspects. In : The recognition and management of early psychosis : A preventive approach. (Eds McGorry, P. D., Jackson, H. J.), Cambridge University Press, New York, 1999.
50) Bermanzohn, P. : Hierarchical diagnosis in chronic schizophrenia : A clinical study of co-occurring syndromes. Schizophr Res, 41(1) ; 43, 2000.
51) Fitzgerald, P., Kulkarni, J. : Home-oriented management program for people with early psychosis. Br. J. Psych., 172(Suppl 33) ; 39-44, 1998.
52) Kulkarni, J., Power, P. : Initial management of first-episode psychosis. In : McGorry, P. D., Jackson, H. J., eds, Recognition and management of early psychosis : A preventive approach. Cambridge University Press, New York, 184-205, 1999.
53) Kapur, S., Zipursky, R., Jones, C. et al. : Relationship between dopamine D_2 occupancy, clinical response, and side effects : a double-blind PET study of first-episode schizophrenia. Am. J. Psychiatry, 157(4) ; 514-520, 2000.
54) Nyberg, S., Farde, L., Halldin, C. Dahl M-L : D_2 dopamine receptor occupancy during low-dose treatmnt with haloperidol decanoate. Am. J. Psychiatry, 152 ; 173-178, 1995.
55) Edwards, J., Maude, D., McGorry, P.D. et al. : Prolonged recovery in first-episode psychosis. Br. J. Psychiatry, 172(Suppl.33) ; 107-116, 1998.
56) Lewis, S. W., Tarrier, N., Haddock, G. et al. : The SOCRATES trial : A multicentre, randomised, controlled trial of cognitive-behaviour therapy in early schizophrenia. Schizophr Res, 41(1) ; 9, 2000.
57) Power, P., Bell, R., Mills, R. et al. : A randomised controlled trial of a suicide preventative cognitive oriented psychotherapy for suicidal young people with first episode psychosis. Schizophr Res, 36(1-3) ; 332, 1999.
58) Edwards, J. : Cannabis and psychosis project : Intervention and client group. Inaugural Interntional Cannabis and Psychosis Conference. Melbourne, February 1999.
59) Gleeson, J., Jackson, H. J., Stavely, H. : Family intervention in early psychosis. In : McGorry, P. D., Jackson, H. J., eds, The recognition and management of early psychosis. Cambridge University Press, New York, 376-406, 1999.
60) Albiston, D. J., Francey, S. M., Harrigan, S. M. : A group program for recovery form early psychosis. B. J. Psychiatry, 172(Supp 33) ; 117-121, 1998.
61) Jackson, H., McGorry, P. D., Dwards, J. et al. : Cognitively-oriented psychotherapy for early psychosis(COPE). Preliminary results. British Journal of Psychiatry, 172(suppl.33) ; 93-100, 1998.

---

*Patrick D. McGorry : University of Melbourne Department of Psychiatry.

精神分裂病の予防

Preventing schizophrenia

Ming T. Tsuang[*1,*2,*3,*4]　　William S. Stone[*1,*2,*3]

One of the most important questions in schizophrenia research is whether prevention is possible. The concept of prevention is itself complex, but is meant here to refer to the prevention of psychotic and prodromal symptoms. Before we begin to address the question of prevention, however, we must first solve the more fundamental issue of determining how to identify the individuals who stand the greatest risk of developing schizophrenia. This is critical for at least two reasons. First, it will facilitate the development of homogeneous groups for treatment, and second, identification of the liability to schizophrenia will facilitate the development of more specific treatment targets. The accumulated evidence from research with first-degree biological relatives of patients with schizophrenia shows that the liability to schizophrenia, called "schizotaxia", is associated with deficits in a variety of domains, even in the absence of psychosis or prodromal symptoms. This paper will review the concept of schizotaxia briefly, and consider evidence for its validation as a syndrome.

Schizotaxia

Meehl (1962) introduced term schizotaxia in 1962 to describe the unexpressed genetic liability to schizophrenia. He described a condition that manifested itself as a subtle, neural integrative defect that always resulted in either a 'compensated' schizotypy, or in schizophrenia. Whether such individuals developed schizotypy (the more moderate outcome) or schizophrenia (the more severe outcome) depended on the protection or risk afforded by environmental circumstances. While Meehl proposed later that schizotaxia need not progress into either of these more overt conditions (Meehl 1989), he suggested that the majority of cases would do so. The concept of schizotypy entered the psychiatric nomenclature eventually in the form of schizotypal personality disorder, but the notion of schizotaxia did not. It did remain in use among researchers, however, to describe the concept of liability to schizophrenia. Now, however, almost four decades after Meehl introduced the term, a large body of research with the nonpsychotic relatives of patients with schizophrenia supports the idea that schizotaxia is also a meaningful clinical condition, and a risk factor or marker for subsequent psychosis (Erlenmeyer-Kimling 2000 ; Erlenmeyer-Kimling et al 2000 ; Faraone et al 2001).

We reformulated Meehl's view of schizotaxia recently to integrate newer findings (Faraone et al 2001 ; Tsuang et al 2000). While our reformulation retains Meehl's core notion of a liability to schizophrenia, it differs in several ways. First, we consider the etiology of schizotaxia to derive from both genetic factors and from the biological consequences of adverse environmental factors (e.g., pregnancy or delivery complications), consistent with a polygenic, multifactorial model (Gottesman 1991). By contrast, Meehl proposed that the etiology was solely genetic, and the result of a single, major gene. Second, unlike Meehl, we do not view schizotypy or schizophrenia as the only, or even the most likely, outcomes of schizotaxia. Instead, we view schizotaxia as a stable condition in a majority of cases. Third, unlike Meehl, we have begun to identify the components of schizotaxia based on psychiatric and neuropsychological attributes found in first-degree relatives of schizophrenic patients, which has led to an operational definition of the concept.

Our initial research criteria for schizotaxia focuses on negative symptoms and neuropsychological deficits (in attention, long-term verbal declarative memory, and executive functions) that occur in both patients with schizophrenia and in their non-psychotic relatives (Faraone et al 2001 ; Gottesman 1991 ; Tsuang 1991). This conceptualization is similar to 'negative' schizotypal personality disorder, (i.e., schizotypal personality disorder minus the positive symptoms), although it is broader in that more relatives of patients with schizophrenia show core symptoms of schizotaxia than meet the diagnostic criteria for schizotypal personality disorder (SPD). Our approach owes much to Venable's emphasis on cognitive approaches to schizophrenia (Venables 1964), which has helped the field to focus attention on both cognitive and neurobiological features of schizophrenia and related disorders.

Tsuang et al. (1999) defined specific definitions for negative symptoms and neuropsychological deficits in first-degree, non-psychotic relatives of patients with schizophrenia, along with other inclusion and exclusion criteria for a research diagnosis of schizotaxia. Consistent with steps proposed by Robins and Guze (1970), our current efforts focus on efforts to establish the validity of schizotaxia as a syndrome. Thus far, 3 lines of evidence are supportive of this proposed designation.

First, evidence of concurrent validation for schizotaxia was obtained recently by comparing relatives of patients with schizophrenia who met criteria for schizotaxia with relatives who did not meet criteria, on independent measures of clinical function (Stone et al 2001). Twenty-seven adults were compared on the Social Adjustment, Physical Anhedonia, Global Assessment of Functioning, and the Symptom Checklist-90 Scales. Eight subjects met criteria for schizotaxia, while 19 did not. The groups did not show significant differences on age, gender, level of education, level of paternal education, estimated IQ, or reading levels. Both groups functioned within normal levels of academic achievement and overall cognitive ability, and neither group showed evidence of a "downward drift" from their parents. Group differences in comorbid psychiatric diagnoses were not significant. Thus, schizotaxia was reflected more in subtle and selective problems than in global deficits. The results showed that the schizotaxic group was more impaired than the non-schizotaxic group in each measure of clinical function. These findings provided the first evidence of concurrent validation for the proposed syndrome of schizotaxia.

Second, we treated 6 non-psychotic, first-degree adult relatives of patients with schizophrenia who met our criteria for schizotaxia, with low doses of risperidone for 6 weeks. Our reasoning was that since : a) the pattern and of psychiatric and cognitive difficulties in relatives share etiological and psychopathological elements with schizophrenia ; b) newer antipsychotic medications such as risperidone reduce at least some negative symptoms and neuropsychological deficits in schizophrenia (e.g. Carpenter et al 1995 ; Green et al 1997 ; Rossi et al 1997 ; Stip 1996) ; and c) such medications produce fewer adverse side effects (at least at lower doses) than more typical neuroleptics (Tamminga 1997), then they might also reduce symptoms of schizotaxia safely. The results were encouraging. Five out of six cases showed improvements in attention and reductions in negative symptoms. Interestingly, the subject who did not respond to treatment had a lower IQ (75) than the other subjects (92-111), which may have limited potential treatment effects. Side effects of risperidone were temporary and mainly mild. Thus, clinical deficits in schizotaxia may be identifiable, and to a significant extent, reversible. From the viewpoint of validity, it will be important to determine whether similar symptoms in non-schizotaxic subjects respond to risperidone in similar ways. A larger, double-blind study is currently underway to determine whether our initial findings can be replicated.

The third line of evidence that is relevant to validation efforts involves analyses of data from the NIMH Genetics Initiative for Schizophrenia, which is a collaborative study of the genetics of schizophrenia at Columbia, Harvard and Washington Universities. In this project, families with at least two affected relatives (one with DSM-III-R schizophrenia and one with either schizophrenia or schizoaffective (depressed) disorder) were included. Subjects received SANS/SAPS and SIS ratings. Genotyping was performed by the NIMH-Millennium consortium using a genome-wide scan with 459 short-tandem repeat markers, with 10cM average spacing.

In one ongoing project, SANS/SAPS data were used (Stone et al in preparation). After a nonparametric data reduction was performed, a two-stage cluster analysis was implemented. In the first stage, all subjects diagnosed with psychotic disorders were excluded; in the second stage, all subjects with any schizophrenia-related diagnosis, including a schizophrenia-related personality disorder (i.e., schizotypal, schizoid and paranoid personality disorders), were removed. The main finding was that even when all subjects with schizophrenia-related diagnoses were excluded, a stable cluster comprised of first-degree, non-psychotic relatives remained. The cluster differed significantly from a larger, 'non-affected' cluster, and was characterized by a collection of SANS/SAPS symptoms that included (but was not limited to) negative symptoms. These findings thus showed the presence of clinical symptoms consistent with schizotaxia in a subgroup of relatives, in the absence of any schizophrenia-related, DSM-IV diagnostic disorder. Additional analyses are underway to determine whether membership in this cluster is predictive of other psychiatric diagnoses, or whether it will demonstrate genetic linkage.

Thus far, these findings are preliminary, and are based on either small numbers of subjects, or on subjects who were not diagnosed specifically with schizotaxia. Nevertheless, the results are both consistent and converging, and provide initial evidence for the notion that schizotaxia is a valid clinical syndrome. While additional validation studies are clearly needed, there is reason for cautious optimism that we are honing in on a working model of the liability to schizophrenia. In so doing, we continue to advance towards the larger goal of developing strategies to prevent this devastating disorder.

Preparation of this article was supported in part by the National Institute of Mental Health (NIMH) Grants 1 R01MH 4187901, 5 UO1 MH4631802 and 1R37MH4351801, by the Veterans Administration's Medical Research, Health Services Research and Development and Cooperative Studies Programs, and by a National Alliance of Research in Schizophrenia and Depression (NARSAD) Distinguished Investigator Award.

References

1) Carpenter, W. T., Conley, R. R., Buchanan, R. W. et al.: Patient response and resource management: another view of clozapine treatment with schizophrenia. American Journal of Psychiatry, 152; 827-832, 1995.
2) Erlenmeyer-Kimling, L.: Neurobehavioral deficits in offspring of schizophrenic parents: Liability indicators and predictors of illness. American Journal of Medical Genetics (Neuropsychiatric Genetics), 97; 65-71, 2000.
3) Erlenmeyer-Kimling, L., Rock, D., Roberts, S. A. et al.: Attention, memory, and motor skills as childhood predictors of schizophrenia-related psychoses: the New York High-Risk Project. American Journal of Psychiatry, 157; 1416-1422, 2000.
4) Faraone, S. V., Green, A. I., Seidman, L. J. et al.: "Schizotaxia": Clinical Implications and New Directions for Research. Schizophrenia Bulletin,

27 ; 1-18, 2001.
5) Gottesman II : Schizophrenia Genesis : The Origin of Madness. New York : Freeman, 1991.
6) Green, M. F., Marshall, Jr. B. D., Wirshing, W. C. et al. : Does risperidone improve verbal working memory in treatment resistant schizophrenia? American Journal of Psychiatry, 154 ; 799-804, 1997.
7) Meehl, P. E. : Schizotaxia, schizotypy, schizophrenia. American Psychologist, 17 ; 827-838, 1962.
8) Meehl, P. E. : Schizotaxia revisited. Archives of General Psychiatry, 46 ; 935-944, 1989.
9) Robins, E., Guze, S. B. : Establishment of diagnostic validity in psychiatric illness : Its application to schizophrenia. American Journal of Psychiatry, 126 ; 983-987, 1970.
10) Rossi, A., Mancini, F., P. S, al. e : Risperidone, negative symptoms and cognitive deficit in schizophrenia : an open study. Acta Scandinavica Psychiatrica, 95 ; 40-43, 1997.
11) Stip, E. : The effect of Risperidone on cognition in patients with schizophrenia. Canadian Journal of Psychiatry, 41 ; S35-S40, 1996.
12) Stone, W. S., Faraone, S. V., Seidman, L. J. : Concurrent validation of schizotaxia : A pilot study. Biological Psychiatry, 50 ; 434-440, 2001.
13) Stone, W. S., Wilcox, M. A., Faraone, S. V.(in preparation) : Genetic epidemiology of multiplex families.
14) Tamminga, C. A. : The promise of new drugs for schizophrenia treatment. Canadian Journal of Psychiatry, 42 ; 265-273, 1997.
15) Tsuang, M. T. : Morbidity risks of schizophrenia and affective disorders among first-degree relatives of patients with schizoaffective disorders. British Journal of Psychiatry, 158 ; 165-170, 1991.
16) Tsuang, M. T., Stone, W. S., Faraone, S. V. : Towards reformulating the diagnosis of schizophrenia. American Journal of Psychiatry, 147 ; 1041-1050, 2000.
17) Tsuang, M. T., Stone, W. S., Seidman, L. J. et al. : Treatment of nonpsychotic relatives of patients with schizophrenia : Four case studies. Biological Psychiatry, 41 ; 1412-1418, 1999.
18) Venables, P. H. : Input dysfunction in schizophrenia. In Maher B(ed), Progress in experimental personality research. New York : Academic Press, pp 1-41, 1964.

[*1]Ming T. Tsuang, M. D., Ph. D., William S. Stone, Ph. D. : Harvard Medical School Department of Psychiatry at Massachusetts Mental Health Center.
[*2]Harvard Institute of Psychiatric Epidemiology and Genetics.
[*3]Brockton/West Roxbury VA Medical Center.
[*4]Department of Epidemiology, Harvard School of Public Health.

精神病の予防に関するノルウェーの現状
Early intervention and prevention of psychosis in Norway

Tor K. Larsen*

Introduction

Early intervention is one of the new and promising strategies for treating disorders in the schizophrenia spectrum more efficiently. A number of studies around the world are now focusing on this strategy and an increasingly number of papers have been published about the subject during the last years(3). In our review in Acta Psychiatrica Scandinavica published this year, we concluded that primary prevention i.e. intervention before the onset of psychosis, is still problematic and uncertain, but ongoing studies will probably provide more solid scientific knowledge in the years to come and some of the preliminary results from these studies are very promising. At this stage we conclude that earlier intervention after the onset of psychosis, is the most promising strategy which implies no major ethical problems. This equals secondary prevention and has a number of successful parallells within the field of somatic medicine. In general there is agreement within psychiatry that people who suffer from psychotic symptoms should receive treatment with supportive psychotherapy, antipsychotic medication and family-treatment. The length of the treatment depends on the severity of the symptoms, but very few clinicians today, would argue that no treatment should be given when clear cut psychotic symptoms are present.

One of the key concepts in the field of early intervention in psychosis is Duration of Untreated Psychosis(DUP). DUP can be defined as "the time from the onset of positive psychotic symptoms to the time when the patient receives adequate treatment"(5). In order to make this definition meaningful, we also need operationalized definitions of the term "onset of positive symptoms" and "adequate treatment". In our programme we define onset of positive symptoms as ; "a score 4 or higher on PANSS positive subscale, and manifestation of psychotic symptoms such as delusions, hallucinations, thought disorder or inappropriate/bizarre behavior in which the symptoms are not apparently due to organic causes. These symptoms must have lasted throughout the day for several days or several times a week, not being limited to a few brief moments". The definition of adequate treatment was as follows ; "antipsychotic drug given in sufficient time and amount that it would lead to clinical response in the average non chronic schizophrenic patient(e.g. Haldol 5 mg a day for 3 weeks)".

A number of studies have shown that DUP in general is quite long, the mean duration beeing about 2 years and the median about 6 months. In table 1 some recent studies are reported.

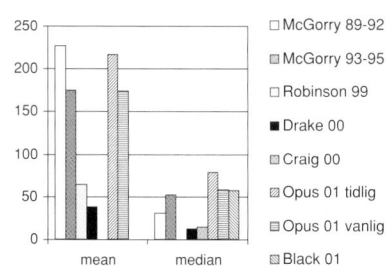

Table 1 DUP in recent international studies

The TIPS-study

Design

The study started 1/1-1997, and the inclusion phase lasted until 31/12-00. A total of 309 patients with a first-episode non-affective psychosis was included. The total population is about 630,000, and altogether we expected that about 300 patients would be included, so the final numbers came close to our initial calculations. The study aims to explore whether early identification of first-episode psychosis leads to a better long-term prognosis. Three different sites will be compared: one in Rogaland (Norway) with early identification and the two others in Oslo (Norway) and Roskilde (Denmark) with identification "as usual". A system for early detection has been be established in Rogaland county with the specific aim to reduce DUP. In addition the study explores the short and long-term outcome of optimally treated first-episode psychosis, and the problems encountered when establishing a system for early detection (ED) in a definite population. The study is a quasi-experimental comparative study with parallel control groups (main study), but also a historical control study in which we compare the early detected sample with a sample from 1993-94 (with detection as usual). The criteria for inclusion were 1) a DSM-IV-diagnosis of non-affective psychosis; 2) living in the catchment area; 3) age 15 to 55 years; 4) IQ >70; 5) suffering from a first episode of psychosis. The exclusion criterion were a history of prior first psychosis, receiving adequate prior neuroleptic treatment, organic or substance induced psychosis and inability to speak the native language.

The TIPS-education program
General population

Public education about psychosis is a tradition in Rogaland. During the last 15 years Rogaland Psychiatric Hospital has arranged the so-called Schizophrenia Days. This is a week with several programs aimed at increasing the awareness among the general population on psychiatric topics. There core elements are; 1) A political conference on psychiatry and society; 2) Art exhibition; 3) Movie with panel discussion; 4) Theatre plays; 5) Public lectures on selective psychiatric topics; 6) A professional conference on the treatment of various psychiatric disorders, especially schizophrenia.

The conference is held at the Culture House in Rogaland's main city, Stavanger. The main aim of these arrangements have been to challenge popular myths about psychiatry and to increase the knowledge about mental disorders in general. Schools have been invited to participate in art exhibitions and articles about psychosis appear in the local press.

In December 1996 all households in Rogaland County (180,000) received a 12-page brochure with information about the TIPS-project. The brochure stated; "Psychiatric disorders have at least one thing common with other diseases - the chance for a good cure is better when treatment is started as soon as possible". The brochure contained a section with general information about the early symptoms of psychosis and a symptom check-list describing different grades of severity. The psychosis Detection Teams were introduced and emphasis put on how to get in touch with them. New brochures were sent out two times more during the study periode. During the period December 1996 - February 1997 whole page advertisements were initiated in the local newspapers. The first was called "Myths and Reality" and consisted of a serie of full-page advertisements, each having a picture with a scene from the movie "One flight over the cuckoo's nest" (Myth) opposed to a picture with people working in the DT (Reality). The series of pictures used in these advertisements where the same as in the brochure sent to all households.

In the third week of January 1997 we launched a new information campaign, this time consisting of whole page newspaper advertisements, commercial radio and cinema advertisements. During the rest of 1997, on a regular basis, this was repeated. In total 10 different whole page advertisements, 3 different radio ads (where psychiatry were presented in a humorous manner) and a number of smaller newspaper ads were presented to the general population of Rogaland. Throughout the project period (3 years) these campaigns were repeated regularly.

The Schools

In co-operation with the "Pedagogic-psychological School-service" (PPT) a teaching program for all teachers at gymnasium level was developed. It was a modified version of the education program for G.P.'s. The psychologists working in PPT are also organising education-seminars in co-operation with the school-authorities (Department for Education). A video called "Something is wrong with Monica" was made by a gymnasium school-class. In the 20 minutes long video, 16 year old Monica experiences early symptoms of psychosis, withdraws from her friends and is referred to a G.P. after a consultation with the school nurse. The video is used in teaching sessions at the schools for both teachers and pupils. In January 1997 all pupils at the gymnasium level received an information brochure regarding early symptoms of psychiatric illnesses, and general information on how to seek help.

Primary health services

During the pilot-study (1993-94) we started to develop an education program for the primary health-services, especially G.P.'s and social nurses. We developed a TIPS-manual in which the nine DSM-III R prodromal-symptoms were rated on severity (0 = not present, 1 = uncertain, 2 = present) and introduced as "warning signs" of psychosis. In addition the manual contains detailed description of the 7 positive symptoms in PANSS (Positive And Negative Syndrome Scale) which are rated from 1-7. The positive symptoms are used to describe presence and severity of psychosis. A 30 minute video with a young woman suffering from emerging symptoms of psychosis, was developed. In addition several lectures on the topics of early diagnosis of psychosis and the TIPS-project, were developed. An education session lasts 3 hours and starts with the two lectures, then the TIPS-manual is introduced, the video shown and the video rated with use of the TIPS-manual. Finally, half an hour is used to discuss the scoring of the video and clinical relevance of the early detection work. All G.P.'s in Rogaland (appr. 220) have received the TIPS-manual and general information about the project. Appr. 150 other health professionals such as social nurses and school nurses have participated in the sessions. During the 6 month period preceding the start of the project, a number of educational seminars were held for different groups within the primary health services. Participants were psychiatric nurses working in the commune, social welfare professionals, teachers, school nurses etc. This work has continued as a part of the TIPS-program.

The TIPS-assessment teams

Each of the sites has a research team: The assessment teams (AT) will carry out evaluations at base-line, after 3 months, 1, 2 and 5 years. The patients has been be assessed on diagnosis, premorbid functioning, DUP, level of symptoms, social interaction, quality of life, global functioning etc. A neuropsychology group at each site have carried out testing at 3 months, 1, 2 and 5 years.

The TIPS-early detection teams

In the experiment sector (Rogaland County) early detection teams have been established. Starting 1/1-97 two Detection Teams (DT) were established, located in the north and the south sectors of the County. The DT's are clinically managed by an experienced psychologist (north) and psychiatrist (south/midth). In the north-DT one psychiatric nurse and one M.D. are employed, part-time. In the south-DT two psychiatric nurses and one social worker are working in the team, also part-time. Both teams are on call for referrals from 08.00-15.30, Monday-Friday. During week-ends the doctors in duty at the psychiatric hospitals take over the DT-function, but they only assess emergency cases. Patients or relatives who call during nights or week-ends are asked to call back on the next working day.

The DT makes a first assessment over the phone or while reading the referral, and decide whether the case is psychiatry or not. The next step is to meet with the patient or the referring persons. This can be done at the patients home, in the school, in the G.P.'s office etc. or at the DT-office. The teams are mobile and work with an active outreach attitude. They give a "24-hour guarantee", meaning that when refers a patient with probable risk of first episode psychosis, the DT should be able to offer assessment within 24 hours. In most cases the assessment is carried out within a few hours, but in some cases, especially when the patient is not motivated, longer time delays are felt to be clinically appropriate. When the DT meets the patient they carry out a PANSS-interview(2), describing actual symptoms and makes a GAF-(Global Assessment of Functioning rating scale) assessment(1). All DT-members are trained to reliability in these manuals.

Study aims

1) To test if a programme designed to reduce the duration of untreated psychosis(DUP) reduces DUP. This programme includes educational initiatives, medical/social detection networks, and early detection teams of clinicians.
2) To test in a multi-centre trial whether reducing DUP in this geographical area will improve the prognosis or long-term course and outcome of first-episode non-affective functional psychosis compared to areas without a programme for reducing DUP.

The TIPS-pilot-study

In order test out whether DUP was as long as reported in these studies in our own area at Rogaland County, Norway, we carried out a study of first episode, non-affective psychosis during the years 1993-94 (4). Patients between the ages 15-65 were included in the study. We found forty-three consecutively admitted patients and the general characteristics of the sample were; 65% males, mean age 26,3 years and mean DUP 2,1 years (median 26 weeks). We studied the pathways to care for the 34 patients in the sample who suffered from schizophrenia more closely and found that active and passive withdrawal together with poor social networks, seemed to be the main obstacles against being identified and treated earlier.

The TIPS historical control study

The results from the historical control study; Usual Detected (UD) patients from 1993-94 compared with Early Detected (ED) patients from the two first year of the TIPS-study, are to be published in a paper in the American Journal of Psychiatry November, this year. Therefore only a summary of the findings can be published here. The UD sample had 43 patients and the ED sample 66 patients. Male patients in the ED-sample were significantly younger by 3.5 years (mean age in years, UD vs ED ; 27.5 ± 7.4 vs 24.0 ± 6.2, t-test ; $t = 2.09$, $df = 65$, $p = 0.04$). There were no differences in gender distribution, age at psychosis onset or marital status. Table 2 compares premorbid functioning, GAF, DUP and diagnosis. The ED premorbid adjustment scores are significantly better. We find no differences in GAF-scores, probably reflecting active psychotic state effects at admission. DUP is significantly shorter in the ED-sample, and there is a shift to earlier forms of DSM-IV schizophrenia spectrum disorders. The PANSS symptom profiles at baseline show clear differences with the ED having less symptoms. There was an increase in substance abuse in the ED-sample, limited to drugs.

Table 2 The historical control study (modified from the American Journal of Psychiatry, November 2001, in press)

	N	UD sample 1993-94 N=43 mean SD	ED sample 1997-98 N=66 mean SD	[a]	df	p[a]
Premorbid Adjustment						
Total	42/62	2.2 0.9	1.7 0.9	2.8	105	0.007
GAF	43/65	32.3 7.7	31.9 7.9	0.1	106	0.8
DUP						
Total	43/66	114.2 173.6 (median=26)	25.3 61.7 (median=4.5)	804	107	0.0005
Diagnosis N (%)						
Schizophrenia (Sz)		32 (74)	23 (35)			
Schizophreniform d. (Sf)		3 (7)	17 (26)			
Schizoaffective (Sa)		1 (2)	12 (18)			
Delusional		5 (12)	4 (6)			
Psychosis NOS		0 (0)	6 (9)			
Brief psychosis (Brief)		2 (5)	4 (6)			
Sz+Sa / Sf+Brief		33/5	35/21	6.7	1	0.01

Conclusions

Our major finding is that an early detection system appears to have been successful in decreasing DUP in first onset non-affective psychosis. The number of schizophrenia spectrum cases increased from 43 in 1993-94 to 66 in 1997-98. The ED patient samples were younger, especially the ED males. In general ED patients had better premorbid functioning, less severe psychosis, and more frequent drug abuse.

The ED system appears to have worked in two ways, first by recruiting younger, healthier patients, largely male, with very brief symptom histories who probably would "escape" detection in the traditional system, and second by recruiting a more usual group of patients but recruiting them earlier in their course. Overall, it appears that patients are recruited to treatment when symptom levels reach a certain threshold, and the ED system significantly reduces that threshold.

A major drawback with this study is the historical control design. As outlined (6), such design cannot control for major sources of population, measurement, and treatment variance that might occur between sample time periods.

We tried to minimize these sources of variance by sampling from the same health care sector with only 4 years' difference between the comparison groups and we used the same assessment instruments in both samples. Nevertheless we cannot measure systematic rater differences between the samples because they exist in different time periods. One of the major differences was the ability to screen the outpatient clinics for first episode psychosis cases in 1997-98. Even though we assume that very few cases were treated without hospitalization in 1993-94, we do not know the exact figures. Therefore we repeated all analyses for hospitalized patients only, and found the same differences on all major variables.

A major strength of the study is the well organized, nationalized mental health care system of Rogaland County, Norway. All sector cases with any serious mental disorder receive evaluation and/or treatment from a single system. As such study case ascertainment in a defined sector over a given time provides a reasonable estimate of disorder incidence. Furthermore, given that our samples came from the same population separated by only 4 years, any differences between them are likely to reflect the influence of treatment timing rather than cohort variances.

As expected we identified a younger and less highly educated sample. But finding males younger by almost 4 years was not expected because they are traditionally the most elusive and treatment avoiding subgroup among psychotic patients. The system's ability to find them is most welcome, and suggests that early detection have considerable promise as a tool for public mental health intervention.

The ED system worked as predicted. By reducing the threshold of ascertainment it found people earlier in all phases of the course of Schizophrenia. It also found more short DUP cases with better premorbid functioning, and increased the ratio of "newer" to "established" cases of schizophrenia. We suggest the overall reduction in the incidence of schizophrenia for Rogaland in 1997 - 1998 is more apparent than real. Follow-up studies will show to what degree the "newer" cases such as schizophreniform will convert to "established" cases such as schizophrenia with time. Early detection may identify patients who are missed by usual detection systems because of their good functioning and relatively brief symptom presentations. They are, nevertheless, bonafide cases who may ultimately enter the treatment system later in more symptomatic and/or compromised states. We do not think that the ED system identified false positive cases and inflated the overall schizophrenia spectrum incidence figures. Rather, we suspect the system approximated more closely the true incidence of cases in the county.

We were surprised by the extent of substance abuse in the ED-sample. Drug abuse comorbidity, especially cannabis abuse, is typically found more frequently in psychotic people who are younger (especially males) with better premorbid social relatedness. That our ED system actively searched for first episode cases in such populations may account for the finding. Nevertheless the degree of difference remains striking, suggesting there may be additional, non study related, drug epidemic forces at work. It is difficult to assess, early in the course of illness, whether or not a psychosis is drug-induced. In this study drug-induced psychosis was an exclusion criteria, but the follow-up will teach us more about the validity of these assessments.

To conclude, our study indicates that DUP can be decreased and decreased significantly. Ambitious educational campaigns and early detection teams are capable of bringing appropriate first episode psychotic patients into treatment much earlier. Given the danger and devastation of active psychosis, we regard this as a clinically significant step forward in the treatment of schizophrenia. These findings, if replicated, should have major public health policy implications for attacking stigma and decreasing DUP through educating the public about the early signs of severe mental illness and by designing treatment centers focused on identifying and treating the early course of psychosis. We feel an important question has been answered ; it is within our power to bring effective treatment earlier to our most needy psychotic patients.

References

1) American Psychiatric Association : DSM-III-R : Diagnostic and Statistical Manual of Mental Disorders. 3rd ed., revised, vol. ed. Washington, DC, The Association, 1987.
2) Kay, S. R., Fiszbein, A., Opler, L. A. : The Positive and Negative Syndrome Scale (PANSS) for schizophrenia. Schizophrenia Bulletin, 13 ; 261-269, 1987.
3) Larsen, T. K., Friis, S., Haahr, U. et al. : Early detection and intervention in first-episode schizophrenia : a critical review. Acta Psychiatr Scand, 103 ; 323-34, 2001.
4) Larsen, T. K., McGlashan, T. H., Johannessen, J. O. et al. : First-episode schizophrenia : II. Premorbid patterns by gender. Schizophr Bull, 22 ; 257-270, 1996.
5) Larsen, T. K., McGlashan, T. H., Moe, L. C. : First-episode schizophrenia : I. Early course parameters. Schizophr Bull, 22 ; 241-256, 1996.
6) McGlashan, T. H. : Early detection and intervention of schizophrenia : rationale and research. Br. J. Psychiatry Suppl, 172 ; 3-6, 1998.

---

*Tor K. Larsen, M. D., Ph. D. : University of Oslo.

精神病の予防に関するオーストラリア・メルボルンの現状

The Early Psychosis Prevention and Intervention Centre, Melbourne, Australia : An overview, November 2001

Jane Edwards*   Meredith Harris*   Andrea Herman*

The Early Psychosis Prevention and Intervention Centre (EPPIC) is a model of early intervention that provides clinical services focused on early detection and provision of optimal treatment in psychosis *and* is engaged in substantial clinical research. This paper provides a brief description of the current status of EPPIC, having undergone significant evolution over a 15 year period. Program elements, approaches to evaluation, 'facts and figures', and the international context are outlined. It should be noted that the program is a catchment-based comprehensive community mental health service, funded by the State Government of Victoria (www.dhs.vic.gov.au/acmh/mh).

Program description

EPPIC (Edwards & McGorry, 1998 ; www.eppic.org.au) aims to reduce the level of both primary and secondary morbidity in young people experiencing early psychosis through the dual strategy of (a) identification of individuals at the earliest stage following onset of psychosis and (b) provision of intensive phase-specific treatment for up to 18 months. Historical origins lie in an inpatient ward located on the grounds of a major psychiatric hospital servicing the inner-city area of Melbourne (Edwards et al., 1994). Experience with first-episode psychosis led to increased recognition of the special needs of these patients and the limitations of an inpatient only program.

The EPPIC catchment area covers the western metropolitan region of Melbourne, a region served by four geographically-based adult mental health services. EPPIC is a specialised treatment service mandated to treat all individuals 15-29 years experiencing a first psychotic episode who present to public mental health services in the defined catchment area. Important features of the region include a high proportion of people born in other countries or with at least one parent born in another country, many people with a low fluency in English, low income, high unemployment, and a low proportion of people with university qualifications. Fewer than 20 private psychiatrists operate in the catchment area.

The service components of EPPIC include :
- prevention, promotion and primary care activities (www.getontop.org/home.htm)
- a prodrome clinic for individuals at high risk of developing psychosis (McGorry et al. 2001, in press ; www.pace-clinic.org)
- 24-hour 7 days per week mobile youth assessment and treatment team (Yung et al. 1999)
- 16-bed inpatient unit (Power et al. 1998)
- a case management team (Edwards et al. 1999 ; EPPIC 2001)
- family work (Gleeson et al. 1999)
- acute and recovery group programmes (Albiston et al. 1998 ; EPPIC 2000)
- a prolonged recovery clinic (Edwards, Maude et al. in press ; EPPIC 2002)
- an intensive mobile outreach service for youth who are difficult to engage in treatment.

Clinical research studies such as cognitively oriented therapy (Jackson et al. 2001) and interventions for problematic cannabis use (Edwards, Hinton et al. in press) contribute to the specialized early intervention approach.

Operational details including the organisational

structure, working groups, staff development and supervision arrangements are contained in the Youth Pack, reviewed twice yearly. Information on the broader youth mental health programme in which EPPIC is embedded, MH-SKY, is available at www.mhskyyouth.org. There are 108 equivalent full-time staff positions dedicated to the clinical program at MH-SKY (including management and administration) and an additional 30 full-time staff positions are employed in research, special projects, and education.

Evaluation strategies

A naturalistic effectiveness study was undertaken to evaluate the EPPIC programme, comparing 12-month outcomes among 51 patients treated under the EPPIC model in 1993 with a historical cohort of 51 patients with first-episode psychosis from the same catchment area treated under the previous generic model of care between 1989 and 1992 (McGorry et al. 1996). EPPIC patients experienced a significantly better outcome than their counterparts with regard to overall quality of life, including social and role functioning. The level of posttraumatic stress associated with hospitalisation and other elements of treatment was reduced, and the experience of psychosis itself was less traumatic. The average length of hospital stay and the mean dose of antipsychotic medication both decreased, without compromising recovery. The mean duration of untreated psychosis was reduced from 237 days to 191 days, but the difference was not statistically significant. Improved short-term outcomes were likely to result from improvements in phase-specific treatment and intensity of treatment, rather than the earlier provision of treatment. The increased costs of providing more intensive community-based care were more than compensated by the reduction in inpatient care costs (Mihalopoulos et al. 1999). A further study suggested that only patients with a mid-range duration of untreated psychosis (one to six months) experienced significantly better outcomes than patients treated in the previous model of care (Carbone et al. 1999).

Evaluation projects in progress include comparison of an EPPIC cohort with concurrent cohorts of first-episode psychosis patients from two other Melbourne catchment areas (Krstev et al. 2001) and medium-term follow up of 200 pre-EPPIC patients and 145 EPPIC patients described by McGorry et al. (1996). Planned evaluations include the extent of adherence to clinical practice guidelines, and a randomised controlled trial of the total EPPIC treatment package with a three-year follow up.

Facts and figures

An evaluation and quality officer measures performance and assesses the impact of EPPIC programmes. Clinical and service utilisation data are routinely collected and used for multiple purposes, including:

· regular monitoring of service delivery, clinical processes and patient outcomes;
· comparison with, and benchmarking against, comparable services;
· assessment of current practice against best practice recommendations and treatment guidelines; and
· application within specific evaluation projects.

EPPIC's clinical information system captures patient socio-demographic indicators, registration details and clinical review data, and has been configured to output standard reports summarising referral rates, client characteristics, registrations, discharges, and clinical caseloads. This data is used on a day-to-day basis for program management and planning purposes, for example to manage and equitably distribute caseloads and to monitor timely completion of clinical assessments and discharge procedures.

Data for evaluative purposes is also extracted from the statewide mental health information system, which captures patient socio-demographic

Table 1 EPPIC intake rates

Estimated Resident Population of catchment area (at June 1999)	Male		Female		Total	
All ages	409,823		414,163		852,417	
15-29 years	103,705		102,574		206,279	24.2%
New cases 2000 - age by gender	Male		Female		Total	
15-19 years	52	62.6%	31	37.3%	83	33.5%
20-24 years	82	73.2%	30	26.8%	112	45.2%
25-29 years	32	60.4%	21	39.6%	53	21.4%
Total	166	66.9%	82	33.1%	248	
New cases per annum 1997-2001					Total	
1997					270	
1998					211	
1999					290	
2000					248	
2001 (to end September)					218	
Mean number new cases per annum 1997-2001					260.4	
Mean number new cases per month (2001)					20.5	
Current caseload, 2/11/2001						
Current cases					396	
Average caseload per full time case manager					32.2	

characteristics, utilisation of inpatient and outpatient services, legal status, and clinical activity data. Other important sources of evaluation data include additional standalone information systems (e.g. the Critical Incidents monitoring system and database ; hospital-based information systems), clinical audits, and time-limited research projects which provide data collected using a comprehensive range of outcomes assessment instruments.

Data on Key Performance Indicators (KPIs) describing clinical outputs is collated and presented as part of a Quality Assurance programme. For example, specific inpatient KPIs include number of admissions, bed occupancy rates, length of stay, 28-day readmission rates, critical incidents and seclusions. Community-based service KPIs include occasions of service, referral rates and critical incidents. KPI data are compared across services and against benchmarks, where available.

Table 1 provides information on the number of new cases of psychosis accepted by EPPIC per year since 1997. The average number of new cases accepted for treatment per year is 260. The intake figures include individuals with both non-affective and affective psychotic disorders and need to be considered with regard to the population of catchment area. The standing case load is approximately 400 cases, reflecting the intake rates for new cases and 18-month follow-up period. Full-time case managers currently have case loads of approximately 32 patients. EPPIC operates with a 'no wait list' policy and all young people accepted into the service are assigned a case manager within 24 hours.

Table 2 provides information on diagnoses and medication for a cohort of patients studied by Power et al. (1998). In this study data describing the first three months of treatment were examined for all patients accepted into EPPIC over a 12-month period from March 1995. Approximately 2/3 of patients received a diagnosis of non-affective psychosis. Low-dose antipsychotic medications were maintained in both inpatient and outpatient set-

Table 2 DSM-IV diagnoses and prescribing patterns as assessed at the end of the initial three months of treatment, n = 231 (Power et al. 1998, cohort commencing treatment March 1995-March 1996).

Diagnosis	Male (n=167)	Female (n=64)	Total (n=231)
Non-affective psychosis			
Schizophreniform	36	9	45
Schizophrenia	65	15	80
Brief psychotic episode	3	2	5
Psychosis not otherwise stated	2	2	4
Delusional disorder	6	2	8
Total	112 (48.5%)	30 (13.0%)	142 (61.5%)
Affective psychosis			
Schizoaffective	21	4	25
Bipolar-manic	21	14	35
Bipolar-mixed	1	2	3
Major depression with psychosis	8	6	14
Total	51 (22.1%)	26 (11.3%)	77 (33.3%)
Other	4 (1.7%)	7 (3.0%)	11 (4.7%)
Antipsychotic Medication (n=230)			
Antipsychotic medication prescribed			208 (90.4%)
Mean maximum daily dose (mg Haloperidol equivalent)			
n = 230 Mean 4.1 mg per day (males 4.3 mg ; females 3.8 mg) (s.d. 25 mg per day) Range 0.5-15 mg per day			
For patients requiring admission			
n = 146 Mean 4.65 mg per day (s.d. 2.61 mg per day)			
For patients not requiring admission			
n = 84 Mean 2.97 mg per day (s.d. 1.78 mg per day)			
Benzodiazepines			
Benzodiazepines prescribed			131 (56.9%)
Mean maximum daily dose - Diazepam equivalents 11.0 mg (s.d. 7.42, range 0-50)			
Mood stabilisers			
Mood stabilisers prescribed (lithium in 91% of patients)			57 (24.7%)
Not prescribed antipsychotic medication			4/57 (7.0%)
Patients with bipolar disorder (n = 38) prescribed a mood stabiliser			30/38 (78.9%)
Antidepressants			
Antidepressants prescribed (SSRIs in 82% of patients)			39 (16.9%)
Affective psychosis			22/39 (56.4%)
Non-affective psychosis (antidepressant used in post-acute psychotic phase)			12/39 (30.7%)
Other clinical interventions			
Clozapine			3 (1.3%)
Electroconvulsive therapy			10 (4.3%)

tings.

Tables 3 and 4 summarises information on a more recent EPPIC cohort who commenced treatment over a six month period (1/9/1999-29/2/2000), obtained through examination of routinely collected service utilization data. The aim was to

Table 3 Age, sub-program utilization and discharge destinations for a six-month cohort of EPPIC patients commencing treatment at EPPIC 1/9/1999-29/2/2000 and examined over the period of care to 2/11/2001 (n = 167)

Age at entry by sex	Male		Female		Total	
15-19 years	36	59.0%	25	41.0%	61	36.5%
20-24 years	49	76.6%	15	23.4%	64	38.3%
25-29 years	26	61.9%	16	38.1%	42	25.1%
Total	111	66.5%	56	33.5%	167	
Utilisation of EPPIC subprograms	Male		Female		Total	
Recovery Group Program (outpatients)[1]	26	61.9%	16	38.1%	42	25.1%
Individual Family Work[2]	14	70.0%	6	30.0%	20	12.0%
Accommodation[3]	24	61.5%	15	38.5%	39	23.4%
Family & Friends[4]	13	61.9%	8	38.1%	21	12.6%
Treatment Resistance Early Assessment Team[5]						
Persistent positive symptoms at 9 weeks	39	67.2%	19	32.8%	58	34.7%
Persistent positive symptoms at 12 weeks	22	64.7%	12	35.3%	34	20.4%
Case presentations to TREAT panel	22	66.7%	11	33.3%	33	19.8%
TREAT Family Group[6]	3	75.0%	1	25.0%	4	2.4%
Discharge destinations					Total	
General medical practitioner					22	14.8%
Area Mental Health Service					50	33.6%
Private Psychiatrist					20	13.4%
Suicide					1	0.01%
Lost to follow-up (eg moved out of area, not able to be contacted)					26	17.4%
No discharge destination (information provided)					14	9.4%
Not stated					16	10.7%
Total (discharged patients)					149	

[1] A group program is provided for both the acute and recovery phases and all clients are invited to participate.
[2] Family work is undertaken by case managers. Families with more complex needs may be referred for Individual Family Work with a family therapist.
[3] Clients can be referred to an accommodation worker to assist in securing more stable accommodation.
[4] All families are invited to attend a multi-family psychoeducation group program which runs over 4 weekly evening sessions - sessions occur on a continuous cycle throughout the year.
[5] TREAT panel of senior clinicians meets weekly to provide consultation to EPPIC clinicians whose clients are still experiencing psychotic symptoms at 12 weeks into treatment.
[6] In cases of prolonged recovery at the 6 month point, the family is invited to participate in a multi-family group program which operates fortnightly for 26 weeks.

examine utilization of EPPIC sub-programs (Table 3) and inpatient services (Table 4). It should be pointed out that all patients receive case management services. Many patients return to school and/or work rapidly. The Group Program tends to cater for individuals with a slower recovery. Only a third of patients are referred to an adult area mental health service upon discharge, with private psychiatrists and general practitioners accepting almost 30% of the EPPIC graduates. Approximately half (78/167) of the young people avoided admission during first three months of care. Approximately 36% (60/167) avoided admission at any time during their care with EPPIC. The mean length of stay for a first admission to the inpatient service is 14 days with readmissions being somewhat

Table 4 Inpatient bed utilization for a six-month cohort of EPPIC patients commencing treatment at EPPIC 1/9/1999-29/2/2000 and examined over the period of care to 2/11/2001 (n = 167)

Rate of admission to Inpatient Unit	Male		Female		Total	
Not admitted during EPPIC treatment	36	*60.0%*	24	*40.0%*	60	*35.9%*
Admitted during EPPIC treatment	75	*70.1%*	32	*29.9%*	107	*64.1%*
Total	111	*66.5%*	56	*33.5%*	167	
First versus subsequent admissions	Male		Female		Total	
First admissions	74	*69.2%*	33	*30.8%*	107	*51.4%*
Subsequent admissions	70	*69.3%*	31	*30.7%*	101	*48.6%*
Total	144	*69.2%*	64	*30.8%*	208	
Date of first inpatient admission (cumulative)	Male		Female		Total	
Within 1 month of registration	55	*67.1%*	27	*32.9%*	82	*76.6%*
Within 3 months of registration	59	*66.3%*	30	*33.7%*	89	*83.2%*
Within 6 months of registration	63	*67.7%*	30	*32.3%*	93	*86.9%*
Within 12 months of registration	69	*69.0%*	31	*31.0%*	100	*93.5%*
Total	75	*70.1%*	32	*29.9%*	107	
Total number of admissions per patient	Male		Female		Total	
0 admissions	36	*60.0%*	24	*40.0%*	60	*35.9%*
1 admission	37	*68.5%*	17	*31.5%*	54	*32.3%*
2 admissions	24	*70.6%*	10	*29.4%*	34	*20.4%*
3 admissions	6	*66.7%*	3	*33.3%*	9	*5.4%*
> 3 admissions	8	*80.0%*	2	*20.0%*	10	*6.0%*
Total	111	*66.5%*	56	*33.5%*	167	
Readmissions	Male		Female		Total	
Within 28 days of previous admission	15	*68.2%*	7	*31.8%*	22*	*21.8%*
Not within 28 days of previous admission	55	*69.6%*	24	*30.4%*	79	*78.2%*
Total (subsequent admissions)	70	*69.3%*	31	*30.7%*	101	

*Represents 14 individuals

Length of Stay (LoS)[1]	Mean (s.d.)	Median	Range
Total LoS			
Adjusted[1]	11.13 (12.0)	7	0-65
Unadjusted	12.88 (13.3)	8	1-76
LoS for first admission			
Adjusted	13.67 (13.1)	10	0-65
Unadjusted	15.61 (14.2)	11	1-76
LoS for subsequent admission			
Adjusted	8.40 (10.1)	6	1-51
Unadjusted	9.97 (11.6)	6.5	1-54

[1] Excludes one outlier with adjusted LoS 344 days.
[2] Adjusted LoS = LoS minus leave days.

shorter.

International Context

The 1990s saw a rapid expansion of early psychosis initiatives (McGorry et al., 1999; Edwards et al.,

2000). Numerous early psychosis programs operate in Western countries and major projects are underway in Hong Kong (www.ha.org.hk/easy) and Singapore (see Edwards & McGorry, in press). Sources of information regarding four other highly regarded early psychosis services are provided in the text box. It is hoped that continued dialogue based upon experience thus far may enhance the development of early psychosis initiatives.

EXAMPLES OF MULTI-COMPONENT MODELS OF GOOD PRACTICE IN EARLY PSYCHOSIS

*Birmingham, UK
www.iris-initiative.org.uk
Spencer, Birchwood, McGovern (2001)

*Stavanger, Norway
www.tips-info.com
Johannessen et al. (2001)

*London, Ontario, Canada
www.pepp.ca
Malla et al. (2001)

*Calgary, Alberta, Canada
www.early-psychosis
Addington and Addington (2001)

Acknowledgments

We wish to thank Pip Kranz for helpful comments and Mark Henry for information regarding the current staffing profile.

References

1) Addington, J., Addington, D. : Early intervention for psychosis : The Calgary Early Psychosis Treatment and Prevention Program, Canadian Psychiatric Association Bulletin, 33 : 11-16, 2001.
2) Albiston, D. J., Francey, S. M., Harrigan, S. M. : Group programmes for recovery from early psychosis, British Journal of Psychiatry, 172 (Suppl. 33) : 117-121, 1998.
3) Carbone, S., Harrigan, S., McGorry, P. D., et al. : Duration of untreated psychosis and 12-month outcome in first-episode psychosis : The impact of treatment approach, Acta Psychiatrica Scandinavica, 100 : 96-104, 1999.
4) Edwards, J., Cocks, J., Bott, J. : Preventive case management in first-episode psychosis. In : P. D. McGorry, H.J. Jackson, eds, Recognition and Management of Early Psychosis : A Preventive Approach, (Cambridge University Press : New York) 308-337, 1999.
5) Edwards, J., Francey, S. M., McGorry, P. D. et al. : Early psychosis prevention and intervention : Evolution of a comprehensive community-based specialised service, Behaviour Change, 11 : 223-233, 1994.
6) Edwards, J., Hinton, M., Elkins, K., Athanasopoulos, O. (in press) : Cannabis and early psychosis. In : H. Graham, K. Mueser, M. Birchwood, A. Copello, eds, Substance Misuse in Psychosis : Approaches to Treatment and Service Delivery, (Wiley : Chichester, Sussex).
7) Edwards, J., Maude, D., Herrmann-Doig, T. et al. (in press) : A service response to prolonged recovery in early psychosis, Psychiatric Services.
8) Edwards, J., McGorry, P. D. : Early intervention in psychotic disorders : A critical step in the prevention of psychological morbidity. In C. Perris, P.D. McGorry, eds, Cognitive Psychotherapy of Psychotic and Personality Disorders, (Wiley : Chichester, Sussex) 167-195, 1998.
9) Edwards, J., McGorry, P. D., Pennell, K. : Models of early intervention in psychosis : An analysis of service approaches. In M. Birchwood, D. Fowler, C. Jackson eds, Early Intervention in Psychosis : A Guide to Concepts, Evidence and Intervention, (Wiley : Chichester, Sussex) 281-314, 2000.
10) Edwards, J., McGorry, P. D. (in press) : Implementing Early Intervention in Psychosis : A Guide to Establishing Early Psychosis Services. Dunitz : London.
11) EPPIC (2000) : Working with Groups in Early Psychosis : Manual 3 in a series of early psychosis manuals, (Early Psychosis Prevention and Intervention Centre : Melbourne).
12) EPPIC (2001) : Case Management in Early Psy-

chosis : A Handbook (Early Psychosis Prevention and Intervention Centre : Melbourne).

13) EPPIC (2002). Prolonged Recovery in Early Psychosis : A Treatment Manual, (Early Psychosis Prevention and Intervention Centre : Melbourne).

14) Gleeson, J., Jackson, H. J., Stavel, H. et al. : Family intervention in early psychosis. In : P.D. McGorry, H.J. Jackson, eds, Recognition and Management of Early Psychosis : A Preventive Approach, (Cambridge University Press : New York) 376-406, 1999.

15) Jackson, H. J., McGorry, P. D., Edwards, J. : Cognitively oriented psychotherapy for early psychosis (COPE) : Theory, praxis, outcome and challenges. In : P. Corrigan, D. Penn, eds, Social Cognition and Schizophrenia, (APA Press : Washington DC) 249-284, 2001.

16) Johannessen, J. O. et al. : A systematized program to reduce duration of untreated psychosis in first episode schizophrenia. In : T. Miller, S. A. Mednick, T. H. McGlashan, J. Libiger, J.O. Johannessen, eds, Early Intervention in Psychotic Disorders, (The Netherlands : Kluwer Academic Publishers) 101-122, 2001.

17) Krstev, H., McGorry, P. D., Harrigan, S. et al. : Preliminary evaluation of an early psychosis project within a mainstream setting, Manuscript submitted for publication, 2001.

18) Malla, A. K., Norman, R. M. G., McLean, T. S. et al. : Impact of phase-specific treatment of first episode of psychosis on Wisconsin Quality of Life Index (client version), Acta Psychiatrica Scandinavica, 103 : 355-361, 2001.

19) McGorry, P. D., Edwards, J., Pennell, K. : Sharpening the focus : Early intervention in the real world. In P. D. McGorry, H. J. Jackson (Eds.), Recognition and Management of Early Psychosis : A Preventive Approach, (New York : Cambridge University Press), 441-475, 1999.

20) McGorry, P. D., Edwards, J., Mihalopoulos, C. et al. : EPPIC : An evolving system of early detection and optimal management, Schizophrenia Bulletin, 22 : 305-326, 1996.

21) McGorry, P. D., Phillips, L. J., Yung, A. R. : Recognition and treatment of the pre-psychotic phase of psychotic disorders : Frontier or fantasy? In : T. Miller, S. A. Mednick, T. H. McGlashan, J. Libiger, J.O. Johannessen, eds, Early Intervention in Psychotic Disorders, (The Netherlands : Kluwer Academic Publishers), 101-122, 2001.

22) McGorry, P. D. et al. (in press) : Can first episode psychosis be delayed or prevented? A randomized controlled trial of interventions during the prepsychotic phase of schizophrenia and related psychoses. Archives of General Psychiatry.

23) Mihalopoulos, C., McGorry, P. D., Carter, R. C. : Is phase-specific community-oriented treatment of early psychosis an economically viable method of improving outcome? Acta Psychiatrica Scandinavica, 100 : 47-55, 1999.

24) Power, P., Elkins, K., Adlard, S. et al. : Analysis of the initial treatment phase in first-episode psychosis, British Journal of Psychiatry, 172 (Suppl.) : 71-76, 1998.

25) Spencer, E., Birchwood, M., McGovern, D. : Management of first-episode psychosis, Advances in Psychiatric Treatment, 7 : 133-140, 2001.

26) Yung, A. R., Phillips, L. J., Drew, L. T. : Promoting access to care in early psychosis. In P. D. McGorry, H. J. Jackson (Eds.), Recognition and Management of Early Psychosis : A Preventive Approach, (New York : Cambridge University Press), 80-114, 1999.

---

*Jane Edwards, Meredith Harris, Andrea Herman : The Early Psychosis Prevention and Intervention Centre.

精神分裂病患者に対する初期の心理社会的ならびに精神力動的治療

Early psychosocial and psychodynamic treatment of schizophrenia

西園　昌久*

I. 精神分裂病の病相，ことに初期への最近の関心

　2000年の6月，Stavanger（ノルウエー）で開催された第13回精神分裂病ならびに他の精神病の心理的治療に関する国際シンポジウムのプログラムには，歴史的に著名な学者の言葉が引用されていた。すなわち，"精神科医は精神分裂病の多くの終末状態をみていて，前精神病状態に職業的にかかわることが余りに少ない。(H. S. Sullivan, 1927)" "危機が不適切に扱われたり，かえりみられなかったりすると慢性の生活困難障害がひどく増加する。(L. B. Hill；精神分裂病の精神療法，1955)"

　精神分裂病の経過を模式化すると図1のようになる。初期あるいは早期に精神分裂病は「不安」や「体の不調」を体験する。最近では，この初期あるいは早期の考えが従来よりもっとはやい時期を想定し，引きこもりや外界の認知の変容を精神分裂病発症前段階と考え治療的介入を試みる"発症予防"策がなされつつある。しかし，わが国では精神医療態勢と認識の遅れもあって欧米におけるそのような新しい分裂病初期治療はまだ殆ど行われてはいない。「不安」や「体の不調」が体験された後に，病相がすすむと，「誤った判断」「圧倒される不安」が生じてくる。多くの患者はこの段階，あるいは次の「興奮あるいは引きこもり」の段階で医療機関を訪れ治療がはじまる。発症には，「思春期の不安とストレス」「脳の過興奮による障害」が関与する。急性期症状は治療開始とともに多くは消退しはじめるがその後の経過は図1に示すようにさまざまである。抗精神病薬と短期の入院のみの治療で十分にその能力を回復することのできるのはおそらく，10％にも満たないであろうといわれる (McGlasham, T. H. ら, 1989)[6]。多くは「誤った判断と正しい判断の混在」や「無気力／楽しめない」などの認知障害や陰性症状が残存する。それでも，慢性期病相での治療によって回復が期待されうる。しかし，初期にもっと適切な治療が行われたならばという期待は当然生じるのである。

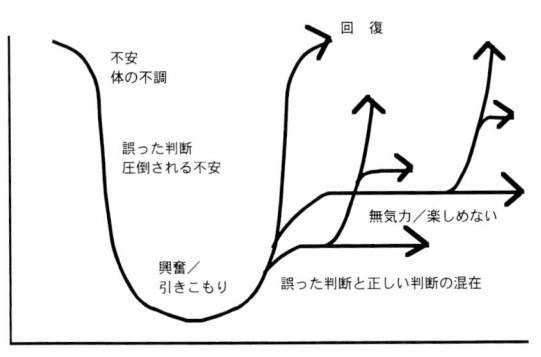

図1　精神分裂病の経過

　筆者はかねて精神分裂病の治療には次の4条件を合わせ提供することが必要であると考えている。

　1）精神症状に対する適切な薬物療法
　2）社会生活の障害に対する生活技能訓練
　3）発病による自己喪失の挫折感から救出するための精神療法
　4）家族機能・社会的支持の回復による社会的不利益の改善

　これらの関係を模式化すると図2に示す通りになる。すなわち，筆者(1999)[9]は精神分裂病の治療には，脳の機能障害によって生じた精神症状に対しては薬など医学的治療による「治す」ことの

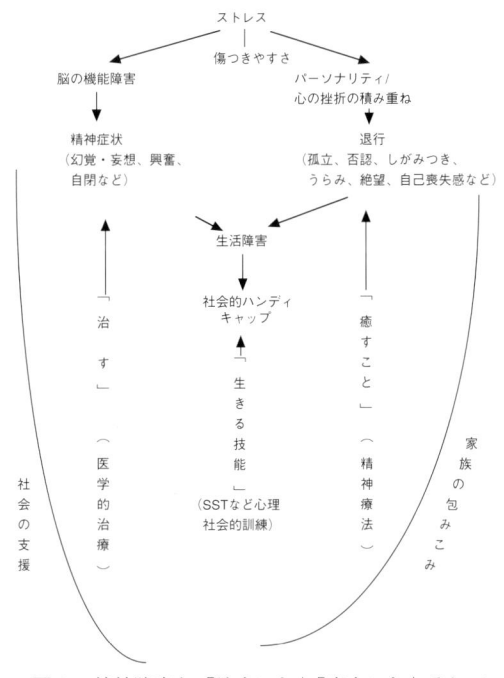

図2 精神障害と「治すこと」「癒すこと」そして「よりよく生きること」

ほかに，発病に対する人格反応として生じた退行，それは実はそれまでの人格発達上の心理的挫折の積み重ねと関連するのであるが，それらに対して「癒すこと」を目的とした精神療法，さらには生活障害—社会的ハンディキャップには，SST，心理教育などを通じて「生きる技能」の習得が必要と考えている。「家族の包み込み」機能，「社会の支援」をはかることももちろんである。そしてこれらの治療的アプローチの内容は病相によって異なるものである。ここでは，主題にそって「初期の心理社会的ならびに精神力動的治療」について述べる。

II. 外来治療を受け始めた精神分裂病患者の行動変化

今より30年ほど前のことであった。新しく医学部が開設された福岡大学に移ってのことである。新しい病院が開かれたということが関係したのか多くの患者が受診してきた。その中に年若い初発の精神分裂病患者も含まれていた。当時はまだ，精神分裂病は入院治療をするのがふつうのことであった。空床がないのと外来治療の開発とを考えてできる範囲で通院治療を行うことにした。そうなると，患者の両親はかえって不安になるのか，はじめ入院させることを強く求めてきた。しかし，やがてそのようなケースにも変化があらわれた。薬で幻聴，妄想，自閉などの症状がとれると次第に発病前よりかえって対話ができるようになったので，入院は見合わせたいと報告されることが相ついだ。これは第1回日本国際精神障害予防会議で，欧米，オーストラリアからの特別講演者たちが，精神分裂病発症ごく早期の治療的介入，すなわち，非定型抗精神病薬の少量，あるいはある種の抗不安薬(たとえばLorazepam，ワイパックス)と心理社会的治療によって病勢の進展を食いとめ，精神状態の回復をはかることができたと報告したことと共通する効果であったであろう。しかし，筆者の患者たちでは，そうした両親の喜びも長くは続かなかった。父親にいつまでも相手をさせたり，母親にしがみつかぬばかりに傍にじっと座りたがったり依存—愛着行動を起こし，そのため両親が対応するのに困りはて，入院を頼んでくるということが見られた。ところが，入院させてみると，そのような患者たちはそのような退行行動としての愛着行動を治療スタッフには決して見せないのである。筆者は共同研究者の福井(1983)[2]にHall, E.のProxemics (近接空間学)の視点からその理由を研究してもらった。それによると，入院直後の患者は一日何回となく，ナースステーションの前を往復している。しかし，そのような関心を求める行為にナースステーションの中にいる看護婦は殆ど気がつかない。そして，精神分裂病患者はまた，他者が自分の領分に近づいてきた時に緊張を感じるいわゆる個人的距離が健常者や他の障害の人よりずっと長いこともわかった。つまり，内心の愛着欲求と現実の遠ざけておかねばならない対人距離のジレンマにあるのである。この研究は筆者らのその後の治療看護や生活支援の進め方に多くの示唆を与えた。患者の個人空間を尊重して侵入不安を誘発しないように心がけるとともに，患者の同意を得て一歩踏み込んで感情的コミュニケーションが可能になる密接空間の中で治療面接や看護ができる訓練が必要なので

ある。筆者は，「精神分裂病患者は精神的無重力状態にある」と比喩している。認知障害のために空間軸でも時間軸でも対象との関係性が適切には自覚されていない。自己破滅の不安から防衛するために自閉の姿勢をとらざるを得ないのである。対象との関係に復帰するには，ちょうど宇宙飛行士がハッチを開いて宇宙に浮遊するのに命綱が必要なように，両親ことに母親に対する愛着行動が必要なのであろう。問題はこの愛着行動が対象によって現れ方が異なることと，現れた場合に対象の立場を考えない一方的なものという関係性の障害がみられることである。

III. 精神分裂病患者に対する初期の心理社会的ならびに精神力動的治療方略

ここで「初期」というのは，精神医療機関に受診してきた患者の初期病相を指すのであって，欧米・オーストラリアで今日試みられている地域でのごく早期の未受診の人びとへの支援活動で使われているのとは異なる。

1．はじめての出会い
　　―診断アセスメントと不安の収納

1）やさしい視線の接触と挨拶

やさしい視線接触は，今日では接触性を回復させる方法として広くすすめられている。コミュニケーション技能を回復させる目的のSSTの基本的技法の1つでもある。挨拶は患者の姓をよんでするのがよいとされる。それは自己破滅の不安に圧倒されている患者に自分感覚を取り戻すのに役立つからである。また，丁寧な挨拶は精神科医あるいは治療者が自分の心の窓を開き患者を受け入れ，それが患者に反映して両者の間にある安心できる雰囲気が生じ，それがその後の両者の関係に影響する。

2）オリエンテーションの回復のための構造化

患者の認知障害を考慮して，診察の理由についてたずね，あるいは説明し，関わる治療スタッフ，場所，診察時間など説明する。

3）危機介入と共感―包みこむ

誤った考えや憎しみの感情，さらにはまとまりのない考えなどは批判することなしに受けとめ，面接者が困難な状況にある患者に可能な限り協力する意志のあることを伝え，治療同盟を結ぶ道を探す。これは，一回で可能とは限らない。

4）身体状態への配慮，からだの診察

からだの診察によって異常の有無を確かめるとともに，不安をやわらげるのに努める。初期，ことに急性期症状の強い患者では，ライフスタイルの変化のために，脱水状態になっていることがある。それから脱いでもらった衣類，下着，靴下で最近のライフスタイルが一応想像できる。診察はできることなら全身，できぬでも掌，足首，皮膚を触り，発汗・乾燥を確かめる。こうした体への医師としての配慮はかつて両親に保護され抱っこされた感覚が身体記憶の中にあるのを呼び覚まし，治療者に救いが与えられる感覚を賦活するのに役立つ。

診断アセスメントはこのような不安を収納し治療同盟をつくりあげる中でなされるべきものである。

2．治療の場と方法の選択

1）治療者と患者との相互関係の重視

精神保健福祉法による入院に，任意入院，医療保護入院，措置入院，応急入院の区分があるように，患者によっては治療理解が得られず治療同盟をつくりあげることが困難な患者がいる。ただ，原則は患者の意見が精神科医にも尊重されて傾聴されたと思うことで患者の自己破滅の不安の軽減をはかる態度を示すことである。患者の意見は聴きながらも，精神科医はまた別の判断で患者を守らねばならないことのあるのを伝えることもある。患者と精神科医との間に，「あなた」と「私」の関係ができることを出発に，さらに「私たち」感覚ができることが望まれる。

2）環境の治療的要因

Gunderson, J. G. (1978)[3]は，環境の治療的5要因について見解を述べている。すなわち，①構造化(場所，時間，スタッフ，活動目標などの明示)，②収納(自己統制力をなくした場合の保護，あるいは代行)，③支持(患者のできることはなるべくやれるように支援する)，④患者の参加(スタッフの感受性と誘導技法の必要性)，⑤患者

の個別性の尊重などである。すべて人間環境に関したことでこの治療的要因論は後の治療チームの指針にもなった。治療環境に関してこれら5要因を十分に考慮することは有用なことである。さらに，初期の精神分裂病患者に愛着欲求葛藤による対人距離ジレンマがあることについて先に触れたが，プライバシイ，つまり個人空間と公共空間の両立性をどのように実現するかが問われる。外来治療では，患者の公共空間の活用が，家族による個人空間での生活支援によってすすめられることが，開放病棟入院治療では患者の病棟内公共空間活用が社会的公共空間活動へと広がることが治療スタッフによる個人空間生活支援で実現することが期待される。まずは個人空間でケアする人と共存できることが必要である。閉鎖病棟入院治療では，患者の個人空間生活での不安が治療スタッフの支援によって収納されることが期待される。わが国の精神医療では人間環境ばかりでなく，アメニティさらには自然環境，つまり，癒しの環境もまた必要で有用であろう。

3．治療技術の問題
1）薬物療法の効果とその後の心的虚脱

薬の種類と用量については今まで以上に慎重でありたい。90年代の高用量多剤併用にも拘わらず治療抵抗性障害には効果がなかったのに加え，不可逆にも近い副作用を生じたのをくりかえさないためである。

薬物療法による陽性症状の改善の後に心的虚脱状態やうつ状態が殆どの患者で見られる。今日では陰性症状と一括されるけれども中に精神病後うつ状態（McGlashamら，1976）と理解すべきものもある。陽性症状が消退した後の精神障害を患ったことを認知せざるを得ないためのとまどいと脳疲労とがうつ状態をつくりだしたといえる。

最近のSDAの治療効果の1つとして"気づきawareness"が指摘されている。精神分裂病の病識欠如は病的過程による認知障害と自己破滅の不安を防衛するための二重構造からなっていると考えられる（西園，1963）[7]。SDAの認知障害の改善作用で，その水準の病識欠如が改善し，"気づき"の二重性があらわになる。精神病後うつ状態と相まって，"気づき"は埋もれた挫折感をあらわにする。否認によってなりたっていた治療者患者関係が心理的意味のある関係へと変移しはじめるのである。

2）共感と支持

ほほえみを持って呼びかける。立ち話ではなく，時間を決め，プライバシイを守り，座って面接する。そして聴きいる。立つことは視覚優位で攻撃的姿勢ともいわれる。そのような位置関係で聴きいるのである。聴くという漢字は耳＋目＋心で構成されていることが示すように，ただ，耳できくことだけでない。目で見，心をそえてはじめてできるいわば全人間的所為なのである。

3）面接の技術／癒しの精神療法

「現在の体験が過去の記憶を書き換える」といわれる。現在の患者と精神科医あるいは治療者との関係が，患者の心に過去の困難な状況においてもベストをつくした感覚を生起し，自己評価を回復させる。筆者（1999）[9]は「癒しの精神療法」を提唱しているが，それは，1）患者が今持っている関心を取りあげ（here and now），2）断片的な思い出に共感し，3）注意ぶかく（careful），ユーモラスに（comfortable），わかるように（understanderful），イメージをふくらませるように（productive）面接を進めていくのである。

4）よりよく生きる技能の習得

精神分裂病が発病するさいの状況は人格発達途上の集団への適応をめぐってが多い。したがって，分裂病患者の治療はこの集団への参加，集団内適応などの技能習得は不可欠なことである。最近，早期退院を急ぐあまり，陽性症状がとれれば退院となる傾向が強いが，集団への参加技能の回復を無視してはならない。集団への参加には安心できる対人関係が可能になることが必要である。それに調和のとれた家族関係の回復も重要である。それには，はじめは看護者などの集団生活をイメージさせるスタッフの支援で参加し居場所を発見し，やがて役割を発揮する目標が治療チームによってつくられることが必要である。同じことは，日常生活技能や見通し技能の習得にも適用される。この時期のこれらの能力は集団適応技能が皮膚性自我（Anzieu，1985）[1]によると考えられる

のに対し，筋肉性自我(西園，1984)によると考えられスポーツ療法，作業療法がとくに有用である。工夫すればSSTもきわめて有用と考えられる。

さらに次の3つは再発を防止するために必要である。

5) 発症状況の解明
6) 家族への心理教育
7) アフターケアの約束

References

1) Anzieu, D.(1985), 福田素子(訳): 皮膚—自我. 言叢社, 1993.
2) 福井敏: 精神障害者における生活空間利用の病理性についての研究. 九州神精医, 29(2); 181-203, 1983.
3) Gunderson, J. G.: Defining the therapeutic processes in psychiatric miliew. Psychiatry, 41; 327-335, 1978.
4) International Society for the Psychological Treatments of the Schizophrenias and Other Psychoses: Final Programme of the 13th International Symposium. Stavanger, 2000.
5) McGlasham, T. H., Carpenter, W. T.: An investigation of the postpsychiatric depressive syndrome. Am. J. Psychiatry, 133; 14-19, 1976.
6) McGlasham, T. H., Keat, C. J.: Schizophrenia; Treatment Process and Outcome. APA Press, Washington D. C., 1989.
7) 西園昌久: 病識の精神力動. 精神医学, 5(2); 111-119, 1963.
8) 西園昌久: 身体的自我の構造. 九州神精医, 30(2); 200-202, 1984.
9) 西園昌久: 精神分析技法の要諦. 金剛出版, 東京, 1999.

---

*心理社会的精神医学研究所／福岡大学名誉教授
Masahisa Nishizono, M. D.: Institute for Psychosocial Psychiatry and Psychoanalysis/Fukuoka University Professor Emeritus.

胎生期・周産期のストレス指標と精神分裂病との関係
Prenatal and perinatal stress indices and schizophrenia

今村　明* 藤丸　浩輔* 辻田　高宏* 中根　允文* 浅香　昭雄** 岡崎　祐士***

I. はじめに

　胎生期・周産期の侵襲が，神経発達障害の原因となり，精神分裂病の脆弱性を生じる一因となると推測されている。我々は，胎生期・周産期の脆弱性指標と精神分裂病との関係について検討を続けている。

　今回特に2つの検討を行った。1つは皮膚紋理についてである。皮膚紋理とは，指紋や掌紋など皮膚に見られる特徴的な隆線模様の形状を言うが，胎生期の侵襲が皮膚紋理に何らかの変化をきたすことが知られている。この皮膚紋理，特に指紋の指標が分裂病の脆弱性を反映しているかどうかを検討した。もう1つは，一卵性双生児の出生順位と精神分裂病との関係についてである。後生まれは早生まれの対象者よりもより強く侵襲を受けやすく，従ってより大きな分裂病の脆弱性を有する可能性がある，という仮説を検証した。

II. 皮膚紋理の変化と精神分裂病

　指紋は胎生初期後半～中期に形成され，同じ頃に外胚葉起源の大脳皮質の基本構造も形成されると言われている。このような皮膚紋理の変化は，分裂病の原因と考えられる胎生期の障害を反映するのではないかと考えられている。

1. 対象と方法

　Inouye(1970)の精神分裂病一卵性双生児標本の指紋資料のうち，分析可能な分裂病一致31組(62人)，不一致18組(36人)を対象とした。対照群はバイアスがかかっていないと考えられる東大附属中・高校への1976～1978年応募者である健常一卵性双生児53組(106人)である。精神分裂病と診断された患者は，医師2名の診断が一致したもので

あり，ほとんどがクレペリンの症状記載に合致する慢性分裂病患者であった。また，一致群の中には分裂病様精神病一致例も含まれている。

　皮膚紋理の指標として以下の3つを用いた。

　a) 絶対隆線数(定量的指標)absolute ridge counts

　隆線数は，指紋三叉 triradius と指紋中央を結ぶ線を横切る線の数を言う。

　絶対隆線数は，指紋三叉が2個あるときに隆線を2回数えた値であり，指紋隆線数としては一般にこれが用いられる。

　b) 指紋強度(半定量的指標)pattern intensity

　指紋強度は，指紋三叉の数である。

　c) 指紋型(定性的指標)fingerprint patterns

　指紋型は，渦状紋，蹄状紋(尺側，撓側)，弓状紋の4型である。

　以下のような方法を用いて比較検討した。

　1) 双生児組内の上記各指標の差異をみた。

　2) 双生児個体内の左右差(浮動性非対称 fluctuating asymmetry：FA)を各指標で検討した。これは個体発生過程の不安定性や外的侵襲への緩衝容量の低下の指標とされている(Palmer & Strobeck, 1986)。

　3) 分裂病不一致群の罹患双生児群と非罹患双生児群との差異をみるために，一致群，不一致罹患群，不一致非罹患群，対照群の4群で各指標の比較を行った。

　統計解析の方法として多重比較を Kruscal-Wallice 検定，2標本検定を Wilcoxon 検定，多重比較を Dunett の方法を用いて行った(統計解析ソフト SPSS を使用した)。

2. 結果

　1) 双生児の各指標の差異をみたが，3群間に

有意な差はなかった(Kruscal-Wallice検定)。2群比較では，指紋型で一致群が不一致群および対照群よりも大きい傾向(Wilcoxon検定，片側でのみ危険率5％未満)，指紋強度では，一致群が不一致群よりも大きい傾向(Wilcoxon検定，片側でのみ危険率5％未満)がみられた。

2) FAについては，指紋型の左右不一致指数と絶対隆線数の第4指左右差について群間に有意差があり，一致群＞不一致群＞対照群(Kruscal-Wallice検定，$p<0.02$)であった。また，絶対隆線数の5指合計について一致群＞対照群の傾向がみられた。2群比較(Dunett，危険率5％)で一致群は他の2群より，有意に大であった。

3) 4群間比較の結果，左右第一指(拇指)の絶対隆線数について，有意な群間差を認め，不一致罹患群＞不一致非罹患群＞一致群＞対照群という値を示し，2群比較では不一致罹患群のみが対照群よりも有意に大きな値を示した(Dunett，危険率5％)。(Asaka, A., Okazaki, Y., 1994)

3．考察

指紋の形成は胎生12〜16週で，大脳皮質形成の時期と対応し，同じ外胚葉起源である。したがって，指紋形成は大脳器質形成のマーカーとみなすことができる。

本研究で見出された知見として，まず双生児組内の各指標の差異は，一致群が不一致群や対照群よりも大きかった。この結果は，不一致群の組内差異が対照群よりも大とするBrachaら(1992)の知見の不十分さを明らかにした。

また分裂病一致群は，個体発生過程における外的侵襲への緩衝容量が小さいこと，不一致群は，個体発生過程での外的侵襲への緩衝容量は小さくないが，不一致罹患群には，特に左右拇指の指紋隆線数を増加させる何らかの要因が働いている可能性が示唆された(Markow & Gottesman, I. I., 1989)。これは胎生期の環境要因が分裂病の発症に何らかの影響を及ぼしていることを示唆する。

III．双生児出生順位と分裂病重症度

産科学では，双生児出生自体がhigh-riskとされている。たとえば双生児の第2子は，出産が遅れた場合生じる低酸素状態のために周産期死亡率が高いことが報告されている(Bryan, 1983)。我々は，このような双生児の出生順位が重症度と関連がないか否かを同性双生児で検討した。

1．対象と方法

対象は，長崎県内の精神科及び精神保健施設で発見された分裂病罹患一卵性双生児19組，2卵性双生児7組である。精神分裂病の診断は，アメリカ精神医学会の「精神障害の診断と統計のための基準，第3版改訂(DSM-III-R)」を用いて，2名以上の精神科医師の診断が一致したときに行った。

卵性診断は，Torgersenら(1979，浅香ら訳1983)の「卵性診断質問紙」と末梢血の遺伝形質指標として，赤血球抗原型3項目，赤血球酵素型2項目，血清型2項目の7種類を用いた。また，DNAフィンガープリント法で出現したバンドの完全一致をもって一卵性を推定した。

重症度の指標は，DSM-III-RのGlobal Assessment of Functioning(GAF)の過去一年の最高得点を用いた。26組中女性2組が出生順位不詳か重症度の指標とした機能の全般的評価(GAF)尺度が同点であったため除外し，24組の比較を行った。分裂病不一致双生児の組では，分裂病に罹患している双生児を重症と判断した。

2．結果

一卵性双生児18組については後生まれが重症の組が15組で，有意に後生まれが重症であった($n=18$, $\chi^2=4.500$, $p=0.0339$)。一卵性双生児分裂病不一致11組では，罹患者(重症度が上であると考えられる)が後生まれである組が9組認められた。二卵性双生児6組(1組は出生順位不詳)では，後生まれが重症の組が3組であり，一卵性の結果と異なった。一卵性と二卵性を合計して解析を行っても，同様の結果であった($n=26$, $\chi^2=4.583$, $p=0.0323$) (Imamura et al.)。

3．考察

この結果は，産科合併症が分裂病発症と病態へ影響するというMcNeilら(1988)の見解に支持的

であった。これまで双生児の重症度と出生順位の関連を調査した研究はSlater(1953)の報告があるが，差は認められなかったと結論付けられている。ただしここでは重症度判定基準などは全く示されていない。

出生順位はそれに先行する諸条件の結果と思われるが，双生児出産自体が周産期異常ともとれる上，少なくとも5〜10分の分娩遅延を被る第2子の出産は，低酸素状態などの不利が加重される可能性がある。これは分裂病の発症や病態に分娩障害が関与しているという近年確認されつつある非遺伝的成因(Geddes and Lawrie, 1995)を，遺伝体質的要因をキャンセルできる双生児という対象で証明したものといえよう。なお，出生体重，頭囲，身長（あるいは頭囲／身長比）などがその後の分裂病罹患と関連するという報告もあり（否定的知見も少なくないが），今後検討する予定である。

分裂病の発症脆弱性については，我々の結果では，不一致一卵性双生児11組中9組が後生まれで，有意に後生まれが多かった。Torryらの研究(1994)では，分裂病不一致一卵性双生児群27組中12組において罹患双生児が後に生まれており，先生まれと差がなかったと報告されている。出生順位は重要な因子ではないと考察されている。このように我々の結果はこれまでの報告と一致していない部分もあるが，出生順位を分裂病の発症脆弱性を決定するいくつかの要因の一つと考えて，検討していくことは重要な意味を持つものと考える。

IV. まとめ

今回我々は2つの検討を行ったが，指紋については胎生期の侵襲が，出生順位については周産期のストレスが，分裂病の発症や重症度に何らかの影響を与えている可能性を示唆する結果となった。これらの知見は胎生期や周産期の障害が分裂病の発症や病態のリスクファクターであるという近年の仮説を支持するものである。

文献

1) Asaka, A., Okazaki, Y. : Fluctuating dermatoglyphic asymmetry in schizophrenia and control twins. Schizophr. Res. 11 ; 141, 1994 (abstract).
2) Bracha, H. S., Torrey, E. F., Gottesmann, I. I. et al. : Second-trimester markers of fetal size in schizophrenia : a study of monozygotic twins. Am. J. Psychiatry, 149 ; 1355-1361, 1992.
3) Bryan, E. M. : The Nature and Nurture of Twins. Bailliere Tindall, London, p71, 1983.
4) Geddes, J. R., Lawrie, S. M. : Obstetric complications and schizophrenia : a meta-analysis. Br. J. Psychiatry, 167 ; 786-793, 1995.
5) Imamura, A., Okazaki, Y., Tsujita, T. et al. : Is the second-born monozygotic twin more vulnerable to schizophrenia than the first-born？ (submitting)
6) Inouye, E. : Twin studies and human behavioral genetics. Jpn. J. Hum. Genet., 40 ; 307-317, 1970.
7) Markow, T. A. & Gottesman, I. I. : Fluctuating asymmetry in psychotic twins. Psychiatry Res. 29 ; 37-43, 1989.
8) McNeil, T. F. : Obstetric factors and perinatal injuries. In : (ed.)Tsuang, M.T. and Simpson, J.C. Handbook of schizophrenia vol. 3, Elsevier, New York, pp319-344, 1988.
9) Palmer, A. R., Strobeck, C. : Fluctuating asymmetry : measurement, analysis, patterns., Ann. Rev. Eco. Syst., 17 ; 391-421, 1986.
10) Slater, E. : Psychotic and neurotic illness in twins. Privy Council Medical Report Series No 278, Her majesty's Stationary Office, London, 1953.
11) Torgersen, S. : The determination of twin zigosity by means of a mailed questionnaire. Acta Genet. Med. Gemellol., 28 ; 225-236, 1976. (浅香昭雄，山田一朗訳：環境と遺伝．周産期医学, 13 ; 879-883, 1983.)
12) Torry, E. F., Bowler, A. E., Taylor, E. H. et al. : Schizophrenia and Manic-Depressive Disorder. Basic Books, New York, 62-69, 1994.

---

*長崎大学医学部精神神経科学教室
A. Imamura, K. Fujimaru, T. Tsujita, Y. Nakane : Department of Neuropsychiatry, Nagasaki University School of Medicine.
**慶友会城東病院
A. Asaka : Jo-to Hospital.
***三重大学医学部精神神経科学教室
Y. Okazaki : Department of Neuropsychiatry, Mie University School of Medicine.

通知票による病前行動特徴と成績に関する研究
Premorbid school performance and behavior of preschizophrenics

佐々木　司* 　原田　誠一** 　岡崎　祐士**

I. はじめに

1. 一次予防確立のための方略

分裂病は慢性に経過し長年障害が続く疾患であり，根本的治療の開発とともに予防策の確立が重要である。しかし予防研究，特に発病自体を防ぐ一次予防の研究は，発病の危険因子解明が不十分なこともありほぼ手付かずのままである。

分裂病に限らず疾患の予防では，対策の重点をおくべき対象を知ること，すなわちどのような人に発病危険性が高いかを知ることが，対策を講ずべき時期や年齢を明らかにし，効果的な予防策を実現する上で大切である。現時点では予防の具体的手段は確立されていないが，対策を講ずべき対象や時期を検討することはその確立の上でもヒントを与えてくれる可能性がある。

このためにはまず，発病危険性の高い人に何時どのような所見が観察されたか，それらの所見を用いて発病の判別が可能かを知る必要がある。またそれらの所見のうち，単に発病プロセスの表れとして出現する所見と，発病の原因として作用する所見を区別すること，そのような所見（特に後者）の出現を防ぐ対策と，すでに所見を示した人には発病を防ぐ対策が可能かを検討することが，基本的な筋道になると考えられる。

2. 高危険知見の応用と一般化の可能性

ちなみに分裂病罹患者の子供は非罹患者の子供に比べて発病リスクが平均10倍以上高い（＝片親が罹患者の場合，両親が罹患者なら約50倍高い）高危険児である。これらの高危険児は乳幼児期・小児期から，運動統合機能，知覚認知，言語，注意力，行動など様々な面で特徴的所見を示すことが知られている（原田・岡崎，1999）。このうち行動の特徴としては，感情抑制の悪さ，攻撃性などのほか，非社交性，孤立傾向など分裂病の陰性症状と類似した特徴も認められている。ちなみに高危険児でも過半数は分裂病の発病を免れるので，これらの特徴が実際に発病と関連するかは問題であるが，高危険児の中でも将来分裂病を発病した子供ではこれらの特徴がより強く出現することが認められている（原田・岡崎，1999）。また研究数は少ないが前方視的コホート研究でも，分裂病患者の学童期では男子では敵意や問題行動，女子では引きこもりが目立つこと（Done et al., 1994），運動統合の発達の遅れや幼児期に一人遊びを好む傾向（Jones et al., 1994）などが認められている。したがってこれらの特徴は，因果関係は別にして少なくとも分裂病発病そのものと強く関連する所見と考えられる。

このような観察を予防医学の実践に役立てるためには，いくつか解決すべき問題がある。第一は，これらの特徴からどの程度正確に将来の発病を予測できるかである。第二は，いかにして多くの子供を対象にこれらの所見の有無を観察すればよいかである。すなわち大部分の分裂病患者の両親は非罹患者であり，社会的効果のある予防策をとるには多くの一般児童を対象とした観察方法の確立が必要である。これらの観点からわれわれは，一般児童の日常的観察が行われている学校教育現場での評価が前分裂病患者の特徴把握や発病予測にどの程度役立つかを通知票により検討した。

II. 対象と方法

1. 対象と概略

DSM-IIIの基準をみたす分裂病患者と発病のない同胞の組のうち，小中学校の共通した2学年

表1　Subjects 対象

> Total subjects comprised 25 pairs of schizophrenia patients (DSM-III) and well siblings (Age: 30±8 yrs in patients and 28±9 yrs in siblings (mean±SD)).
> 分裂病患者と健康な同胞25対＝50名（行動特徴評価では21対＝42名分を使用）。年齢：患者30±8歳，同胞28±9歳（21対では，患者28±7歳，同胞26±9歳）
> Thirteen pairs among the 25 were concordant for sex.
> うち性の一致した組は13対（21対中では11対）

以上の通知票が利用できた者を対象とした。本人と家族から同意を得た後，通知票を複写・匿名化し，学業成績と行動評価の記載について患者・同胞間で比較した。対象数，年齢，患者・同胞間の性別の一致・不一致については表1にまとめた。

2．方法
1）行動評価の解析方法

全通知票の行動評価に関する記載全てから，肯定的評価44項目，否定的評価61項目を抽出した。これらの項目について明らかな肯定的または否定的評価を受けた人数を，患者・同胞群で通年および3学年毎に Fisher 直接確率法を用いて比較した。

2）学業成績の解析方法

学業成績は，各科目の総合評価と科目内小項目の評価について検討した。総合評価については，元の3，5，10段階の評価を3段階に換算し，3学年ごとに平均値を計算，患者・同胞間で対応あるT検定により比較した。科目内の小項目評価については，肯定的な評価と否定的な評価を受けた人数を Fisher 直接確率法により比較した。

III. 結　果

1．学業成績
1）総合評価

科目ごとの総合評価点では，小学校低学年で患者は図工が同胞より有意に低く（$p<0.05$），音楽・算数についても低い傾向にあった（$p<0.1$）。患者の方が優れた傾向を示す科目はなかった。高学年・中学では有意な差を示す科目はみられなかった。

2）小項目評価

各科目の小項目について記載があった少数のペアを検討した結果では，患者は小学校低学年で図工のデザインと体育の技能で，高学年では国語の読解で否定的評価を受ける傾向がみられた。

2．行動評価
1）有意差の認められた評価項目（通年での比較）

行動に関する評価項目のうち，患者・同胞間で評価を受けた人数に有意差（5％水準以上）の見られた項目を表2に示す。消極性，自信，自主性，緊張の強さ，思いやりなど対人場面・集団場面での振る舞いに関する評価で差が多くみられたほか，作業を厭う・厭わない，根気，熱心さなど思考や作業過程の特徴，責任感，規則の遵守など規範に対する態度でも差が認められた。またいずれの項目に関しても否定的項目は患者が，肯定的項目は同胞の方が多く評価を受けていた。

2）評価に差が認められた時期

患者・同胞間の行動評価の差が，いつ頃から認められるのかを知るため，小中学校3学年ごとに評価された人数の違いをまとめた（表3）。対人場面での振る舞い，作業過程の特徴のいずれについても，すでに小学校低学年から評価に差のみられることがわかる。なお中学校ではほとんど差が見られなくなるが，これは中学の通知票では小学校に比べて行動に関する評価記載が明らかに少なかったことによると思われる。

3）通知票の行動評価から将来の発病は予測できるか？

これら通知票に記載された行動評価から，将来の発病がどの程度判別できるかを検討した。行動評価項目を，対人関係・場面における振る舞い，思考や作業過程の特徴，性格・外見，基本的生活習慣，規範に対する態度の5カテゴリーに分類して得点（肯定的評価数から否定的評価数を引いたもの）を計算すると，最初の3カテゴリーで分裂病患者群は同胞群よりも有意に得点が低かった。特に，対人関係・場面での振る舞い（D3）と思考・作業過程の特徴（D4）に関する得点を用いると，患者群を同胞群から完全に区別する判別関数

表2

Negative and positive evaluations of behaviors by teachers with significant difference between patients and sibling(through 9 years of elementary and junior high schools)患者群―同胞群で教師から評価を受けた人数に差の認められた行動特徴(小中学校9年間通年での解析)

[negative evaluations] 否定的評価	(pat : sib) (人)	[positive evaluations] 肯定的評価	(pat : sib) (人)
Tense 緊張強い・溶け込めない	(8 : 1)	Lively 元気で生き生き	(0 : 12)
Withdrawn 消極的・引っ込み思案	(18 : 12)	Faithful／Loyal まじめ・誠実	(4 : 12)
Timid／nervous 自信なくおどおど	(16 : 4)	Considerate 思いやりあり人の面倒をみる	(4 : 12)
Not self-reliant 頼りがち	(13 : 4)	Respects rules 規則を守る	(4 : 11)
Not hard-working 作業を厭う	(9 : 2)	Hard-working 作業を厭わず	(2 : 11)
		Achievement striving／Industrious 根気よく努力・やりとげる	(8 : 16)

($D3+2D4 \leq 0$)が得られた。

IV. 考　察

「成績」に関しては，患者は小学校低学年で図工・音楽など技能や表現力に関連する教科と体育の技能で低い評価を受ける傾向にあった。これらは高危険児研究やコホート研究で認められた運動統合機能，知覚認知・表現機能の問題やコミュニケーション機能の問題と共通している可能性がある。

行動特徴では，対人場面での緊張の強さ，消極性，自信や自主性の欠如などが患者で多く観察された。これは高危険児の研究の一部でも観察された非社交性・孤立傾向と共通しており，分裂病の陰性症状に通ずる可能性があると考えられる。また患者は，思いやり・面倒見，真面目・誠実さ，規則の遵守，根気などの点でも低い評価を受けることが多かった。これらは，高危険児の研究で認められた集中力や感情抑制の不足と共通すると考えられるほか(原田・岡崎，1999)，内申書を用いた研究で分裂病患者(特に男子)で観察された「調和性」agreeableness(＝やさしさ・思いやり・素直さなど)の欠如とも共通した結果と考えられる(Watt, 1972)。

なお，これまで内申書や教師が記入した調査票を用いて分裂病患者の小学校から high school にかけての行動特徴を調べた研究はいくつかあるが，欧米の研究では孤立・非社交性など陰性症状に通ずる特徴は必ずしも目立たず，むしろ興奮しやすさ，乱暴さ，思いやり・やさしさや協調性のなさといった陽性特徴が強調される結果であった(特に男性で)(Watt, 1972；John and Mednick, 1982；Done et al., 1994)。これには，Watt(1972)のような古い研究では診断基準の問題も影響している可能性もあるが，むしろ文化的違いが影響しているのではないかと思われる。ちなみに我が国で分裂病患者の小学校時代の通知票を一般児童の内申書と比較した大橋ら(1976)の結果では違いがさらに大きく，我々と同様，不活発，引っ込み思案，自信のなさ，孤立傾向など陰性症状と通ずる特徴が分裂病群で明らかであったが，陽性特徴に関しては両群で差を認めなかった。ちなみに陰性特徴は男性患者で多く認められた。

今回の結果で注目すべき点の1つは，患者・同胞間で違いの目だった行動評価の得点を組み合わせることで，両群が完全に判別されたことである。このような判別可能性が，今回の対象のみでなく他の患者にも一般化できるかは検討する必要はある。しかし，これらの行動評価の差が「成績」評価の差とともに小学校低学年からはっきり認められたことと合わせて考えると，教師による学童早期の行動評価が将来の発病危険性の予測に役立つ可能性を示唆している。

教育現場での観察を精神疾患の発病予防に活用するには，観察者ごとの評価基準の違いや精度の問題のほかに，親や教師の不安への対応，具体的

表3

Behavioral evaluations in every 3 grades with significant difference between patients and siblings($*$: p<.05, $**$: p<.01) 患者−同胞の群間で教師から評価を受けた人数に差の見られた行動特徴（3学年ごとの比較）

	Grade 学年		
[Negative evaluations] 否定的評価項目	1−3 低学年	4−6 高学年	7−9 中学
Timid　自信なくおどおど	**		
Not self-reliant　頼りがち	*		
Tense　緊張強い・場に溶け込めない		**	
Lacking leadership　指導性に欠く		*	
Withdrawn／Unsociable　消極的・引っ込み思案			*
[Positive evaluations] 肯定的評価項目	1−3 低学年	4−6 高学年	7−9 中学
Faithful／Loyal　まじめ・誠実	*		
Cheerful(Lively)　明るい・明朗	**		
Achievement striving／Industrious　根気・やり遂げる	*		
Considerate　思いやりあり，面倒みる	*	**	
Sense of responsibility　責任感あり		**	
Having leadership　指導力あり・ムードメーカー		**	
Hard-working　作業を厭わず進んでする		**	
Careful／Conscientious　作業が丁寧・丹念・着実		*	

にどのような働きかけを児童に行うべきか（あるいは止めるべきか）など，現時点では検討すべき問題がきわめて多い。しかし，今回の報告でみられた結果は，それらの問題が解決されるならば教育現場での観察や働きかけが予防医学の実践における重要なポイントとなり得ることを示唆している。今後，対象数の増加，同胞のみでなく一般児童との比較などの検討を重ねることが，実際の発病予防への応用のために重要である。

参考文献

1) Done, D. J. et al.: Br. J. Med, 309; 699-703, 1994.
2) 原田誠一，岡崎祐士：精神分裂病ハイリスク児研究と病前特徴の研究．中根允文，小山司，丹羽真一，中安信夫編：臨床精神医学講座 2. 精神分裂病Ⅰ，中山書店，東京，pp97-115, 1999.
3) John, R. S., Mednick, S. A.: J. Abnorm Psychol. 91; 399-413, 1982.
4) Jones, P., et al.: Lancet, 344; 1398-403, 1994.
5) 大橋秀夫ほか：精神分裂病の病前性格．臨床精神医学，5; 15-24, 1976.
6) Watt, N. F.: J. Nerv. Ment. Dis., 155; 42-54, 1972.

---

*東京大学保健管理センター
Tsukasa Sasaki, M. D.: Health Service Center, University of Tokyo.
**三重大学医学部精神神経科
Seiichi Harada, M. D., Yuji Okazaki, M. D.: Department of Neuropsychiatry, Mie University.

脳画像による早期診断

Possibility of early diagnosis of schizophrenia by three-dimensional magnetic resonance imaging

川崎　康弘*　　中村　主計*　　野原　茂*　　萩野　宏文*
松井　三枝**　鈴木　道雄*　　倉知　正佳*

Introduction

The concept of prevention has not yet received wide acceptance in the treatment field of psychiatric disorder, particularly in regard to schizophrenia. One of the reasons for the present unfavorable status is that the neurobiological basis of clinical diagnosis is still undefined. It is urgently necessary to improve diagnostic methods together with more detailed understanding of the neurobiology of schizophrenia. If the disease can be detected in its earliest stages, future nosology will allow early intervention and prevention by more rational approaches.

During the past decade serial morphological neuroimaging studies of schizophrenia have provided valid evidence of the structural abnormalities in this disorder (Shenton et al., 2001). Researchers are only now beginning to assess the possibility of applying neuroimaging to the early diagnosis of schizophrenia. We describe our three recent studies using high-resolution magnetic resonance imaging (MRI) and discuss the issues mentioned above.

Frontal cortex in schizophrenia evaluated by visual inspection and symptoms

The notion that structural and functional deficits in the frontal region underlie schizophrenia has received support from recent neuroimaging studies. We have evaluated frontal cortical morphology and their association with symptoms.

Frontal cortical morphology was evaluated by visual inspection of two consecutive 5-mm-thick

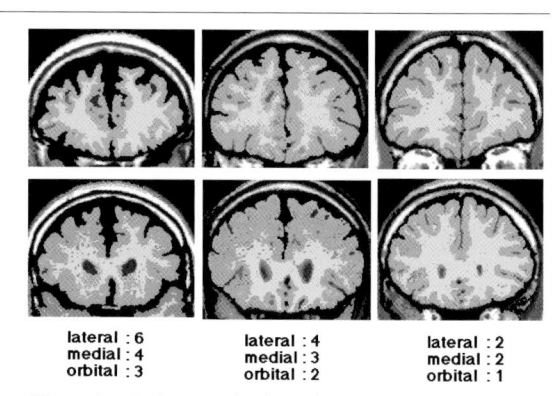

Figure 1　Rating standards of the frontal regions with 7-point scales.

coronal T1 MRI images located anterior to the slice through the genu of the corpus callosum. Figure 1 shows the 7-point rating standards for the lateral, medial, and orbital frontal regions. Clinical symptoms were also evaluated using the Positive and Negative Syndrome Scale (PANSS ; Kay et al., 1987). The subjects consisted of 48 male and 17 female patients with schizophrenia diagnosed by DSM-IV (APA, 1994). All of the subjects were informed of the study and consented to participate. Their mean age was 26.6 ± 5.7 (S.D.) years, their age at the onset of psychotic illness was 21.5 ± 4.0 years, and their education level was 13.3 ± 2.0 years. The subjects were treated with typical neuroleptic medication (mean chlorpromazine equivalent, 646.9 ± 538.9 mg/day).

Principal component analysis disclosed orthogonal 5 factors structure from 30 symptoms of the PANSS. The symptom factors represented the hostility-excitement, negative symptoms, thought disorder, depression, and delusion-hallucination. These constructed symptom items resembled those in our previous report (Kawasaki et al, 1994), and their factor scores were computed. Pearson's product-moment correlation coefficients were calculated to evaluate linear correlations between cortical morphology and the symptom factors. There were correlations between morphological deflection in the medial frontal region and negative symptoms severity (Lt.; $r=0.27$, $p=0.034$. Rt.; $r=0.30$, $p=0.017$) and inverse correlation between that in the lateral frontal region and the hostile-excitement (Lt.; $r=-0.36$, $p=0.004$. Rt.; $r=-0.38$, $p=0.002$). Because our previous study demonstrated an inverse correlation between hostility-excitement and negative symptoms to some degree, these results supported previous assumption that negative symptoms are associated with the morphological abnormalities in the frontal regions.

Structural brain differences in patients with schizotypal disorder and schizophrenia using the voxel-based morphometry

Schizotypal disorder is thought to be genetically and biologically related to schizophrenia. It is particularly noteworthy that schizotypal disorder presents with prodromal symptoms alone, whereas schizophrenia is accompanied by additional florid psychotic episodes. The aim of the second study was to identify morphological characteristics associated with prodromal and florid psychotic symptoms.

Novel technique of the voxel-based morphometry (Ashburner & Friston, 2000) applied to assess differences in gray matter concentrations of high-resolution three-dimensional MRI among each 21 patients group with schizotypal disorder and schizophrenia of ICD-10 (WHO, 1993) and 42 control subjects group. The mean age of schizotypal disorder, schizophrenia, and control was 24.2 ± 6.0 (SD) years, 25.0 ± 4.9 years, and 25.5 ± 6.8 years, respectively. The schizophrenia patients could be classified as being in relatively early stage of their illness, because their mean duration of illness was 1.2 ± 1.1 years. All of the patients except 2 schizotypal subjects were on neuroleptic medication (mean haloperidol equivalent neuroleptic dose, 4.1 ± 5.1 mg/day in schizotypal disorder and 9.7 ± 8.6 mg/day in schizophrenia). Among the 19 patients with schizotypal disorder 13 patients were treated with typical neuroleptics, and the other 6 patients were receiving the atypical neuroleptica of risperidone. The control subjects matched the schizotypal and schizophrenic patients in terms of age, but had relatively higher educational achievement (schizotypal disorder, 12.8 ± 2.4 years; schizophrenia, 13.9 ± 2.0 years; healthy control, 15.1 ± 2.0 years). After the purpose and procedures of the present study were fully explained, definite informed consent was individually obtained from all of the subjects.

As compared with the controls, statistical parametric mapping (SPM) 99 using a 1 x 1 x 1 mm voxel size demonstrated that schizotypal disorder had significant reduced gray matter concentration in the medial temporal region, and the periventricular region, and that schizophrenia had significant reductions in the medial, lateral and orbital fontal regions, the medial temporal region, and the periventricular region as well as a significant increase in the basal ganglia. An absence of any change in the medial frontal gray matter was found in schizotypal disorder by applying the SPM99 post-hoc statistic to schizotypal disorder and schizophrenia. Observed findings are summarized in Table 1.

A comprehensive assessment throughout the brain clearly confirmed the previous conclusion that schizotypal disorder is associated with morphological abnormalities that are similar to but less extensive than in schizophrenia. Observed commonalities of gray matter concentrations in the medial temporal region could be associated with the fundamental neurobiology of schizophrenia-related disorders. Moreover, additional involvement of the medial frontal region can be postulated as a pathognomonic factor in the genesis of the florid psychotic symptoms in schizophrenia.

Table 1 Changes in the regional gray matter concentrations of patients compared to the controls

Anatomical region	Schizotypal disorder	Schizophrenia
Medial frontal region	→	↓↓
Lateral frontal region	↓	↓↓
Orbital frontal region	↓	↓↓
Medial temporal region	↓↓	↓↓
Periventricular region	↓↓	↓↓
Basal ganglia	↑	↑↑

Abbreviations: ↓, trend toward decreased ; ↑, trend toward increased
↓↓, significantly decreased ; ↑↑, significantly increased
→, no statistical significance

Discriminant analysis for the diagnostic value of structural data in schizophrenia

Several neuroimaging reports have indicated structural abnormalities in the brain of schizophrenia. Even the most consistent finding of the ventricular enlargement could not be of diagnostic value with greater regional specificity (Daniel et al., 1991). The diagnostic ability of a single anatomical variable may be quite limited, but its sensitivity should improve when combined with other brain regional variables.

The subjects consisted of 57 patients with schizophrenia (30 males and 27 females) diagnosed by ICD-10 (WHO, 1993). The mean ages were 26.2 ± 5.6 years for male and 29.3 ± 7.6 years for female patients. The mean ages at the onset of psychotic illness were 21.2 ± 4.5 years for male and 23.1 ± 5.5 years for female patients. The mean education levels were 13.8 ± 2.0 years for male and 13.6 ± 2.1 years for female patients. They were treated with typical neuroleptic medication (mean chlorpromazine equivalent, 409.3 ± 314.8 mg/day for male and 599.3 ± 563.9 mg/day for female). The control subjects consisted of 47 healthy volunteers (25 males and 22 females). The mean ages were 25.1 ± 5.5 years for male and 26.3 ± 7.1 years for female. The mean education levels were 17.4 ± 3.5 years for male and 14.7 ± 1.0 years for female. The purpose and procedures of the present study were explained to all the subjects, and informed consent was obtained.

The three contiguous 1-mm-thick coronal slices in which the mammillary body was most clearly visible were adopted for the measurements. The following region of interest (ROI) were evaluated for regional volume : the body and inferior horn of the lateral ventricle, the third ventricle, the Sylvian fissure, the inter-hemispheric fissure, the temporal lobe, the gray and white matters of the superior temporal gyrus. Average ROI volume was calculated from 3 consecutive slices. With regard to the correction for individual brain size, the relative ROI volume was obtained by dividing the absolute ROI volume by the cerebral hemispheric volume.

Following a significant diagnosis effect of the ANCOVA (covariate with age), the post-hoc comparisons pointed to regional volume differences between schizophrenia and control. In the left and right bodies of the lateral ventricle the male patients, but not female patients, had larger ventricle than the controls (diagnosis effect of ANOVA : $F = 7.52$; $df = 1,99$; $p = 0.007$. post-hoc Sheffe's test : left, $p < 0.001$; right, $p < 0.001$). In the left Sylvian fissure, but not in the right one, male and female schizophrenia subjects revealed larger volume compare to the controls (diagnosis effect of ANOVA : $F = 14.66$; $df = 1,99$; $p < 0.001$. post-hoc Sheffe's test : male, $p = 0.005$; female, $p < 0.001$). An enlarged third ventricle was observed in the male patients alone in comparison with the controls (diagnosis effect of ANOVA : $F = 15.00$; $df = 1,99$; $p < 0.001$. post-hoc Sheffe's test ; $p = 0.006$).

The discriminant functional analysis combined with the stepwise procedure correctly classified 62.5% of subjects into 2 diagnostic groups (i.e., schizophrenia and control). In the case of the separate assessment of the male or female subjects, sensitivities (male, 72.7% ; female, 81.6%) were improved. Elicited variables following the stepwise procedure were shown in Table 2. There were differences in variables entered into the discriminant equations for the male and female subjects. Irrespective of gender, the Sylvian fissure seemed to be the most common denominator of morphologi-

Table 2 Adopted valuables of the discriminant analysis between schizophrenia and control

Anatomical region		Combined gender	Male	Female
Body of lateral ventricle	Left	O	O	
	Right	O	O	
Inferior horn of lateral ventricle	Left	O		O
	Right			
Sylvian fissure	Left	O	O	O
	Right		O	
Temporal lobe	Left	O		O
	Right	O		O
Superior temporal gyrus Gray matter	Left			O
	Right			
Superior temporal gyrus White matter	Left	O	O	O
	Right	O	O	
Interhemispheric fissure		O	O	
Third ventricle		O	O	

cal abnormalities. It can be assumed that selected variables of male subjects consist of ventricular systems, while variables belong to temporal region in female subjects. Further question arises whether the observed differences are the result of gender-specific pathological nature.

In the obtained discriminant function of diagnosis by sex groups, subsequent canonical analysis disclosed 2 orthogonal axes. The first axis can be regarded as a discriminator of gender, and the second axis can be postulated as the diagnostic axis. The average values of each axis in the 4 groups were plotted into the 4 rational domains with a fair degree of certainty : schizophrenia male, $x = -1.02$, $y = 0.31$; schizophrenia female, $x = 0.64$, $y = 0.62$; control male, $x = -0.34$, $y = -0.74$; control female, $x = 0.98$, $y = -0.35$. There was no evidence for an additional axis that could distinguish schizophrenia male from female. These results could be interpreted as indicating that the gender differences in morphological characteristics in schizophrenia never exceed those in the healthy control. In other words, the gender differences as a general rule may be considerably responsible for the gender-related heterogeneity in schizophrenia.

Conclusion

Our studies have provided several findings with respect to the neurobiology of schizophrenia. The first study underscored the relationship between the frontal region and negative symptoms. The second study emphasized antecedent pathology of the prodromal symptoms and additional involvement in the genesis of the florid psychotic symptoms. The third study stressed the possibility that structural data may be of diagnostic value, and that gender differences as a general rule may be responsible for gender-related findings. More data will be needed to clarify the clinical implications of these findings. With further refinements in neuroimaging technique, there will be a definite possibility to make an early diagnosis of schizophrenia.

References

1) Ashburner. J., Friston, K. J. : Voxel-based morphometry–the methods. Neuroimage, 11 ; 805-821, 2000.
2) Daniel, D. G., Goldberg, T. E., Gibbons, R. D., Weinberger, D. R. : Lack of a bimodal distribution of ventricular size in schizophrenia. Biol. Psychiatry 30 ; 887-903, 1991.
3) Kawasaki, Y., Maeda, Y., Sakai, N., Higashima, M., Urata, K., Yamaguchi, N., Kurachi, M. : Evaluation and interpretation of symptom structures in patients with schizophrenia. Acta Psychiatr. Scand. 89 ; 399-404, 1994.
4) Kay, S. R., Fiszbein, A., Opler, L. A. : The positive and negative syndrome scale (PANSS) for schizophrenia. Schizophr. Bull. 13 ; 261-276, 1987.
5) Shenton, M. E., Dickey, C. C., Frumin, M., McCarley, R. W. : A review of MRI findings in schizophrenia. Schizophr. Res., 49 ; 1-52, 2001.

---

*富山医科薬科大学精神神経医学教室
Yasuhiro Kawasaki, Kazue Nakamura, Shigeru Nohara, Hirofumi Hagino, Michio Suzuki, Masayoshi Kurachi : Department of Neuropsychiatry, Toyama Medical and Pharmaceutical University.

**富山医科薬科大学心理学教室
Mie Matsui : Department of Psychology, Toyama Medical and Pharmaceutical University.

高危険児研究の結果と早期介入プログラム

The results of our schizophrenic high-risk follow-up study and a new psychoeducational approach to the primary and secondary prevention of schizophrenia

原田　誠一* 　岡崎　祐士* 　佐々木　司**

I. はじめに

本論で、筆者らが行ってきた分裂病患者の子弟（＝高危険児）の追跡研究の結果を報告する。さらに、「分裂病予防への寄与を目指す疾患教育プログラム」を紹介する。

II. 筆者らの高危険児研究の主な結果

筆者らは、岡崎が中心となり、現在のところ我が国唯一の分裂病ハイリスク研究を遂行中である[5-7]。我々の研究結果の概要を、表1に示す。現在、本研究の対象者は分裂病者（DSM-III診断）32名（母親26名、父親6名）を片親に持つ子供62名（男性32名、女性30名）であり、2000年末における平均追跡期間は21年となった[5]。

2000年末までに分裂病圏障害を呈した対象者は7名（男性3名、女性4名）存在し、全対象者の11.3％を占めた。発症者のDSM-III-Rによる診断は、分裂病6名、特定不能の精神病性障害1名であった。

分裂病発症者と非発症者を比較すると、発症群で以下の事項が多く認められた[5]。

①親の分裂病が比較的重症（転帰不良者が多い）。②配偶者に分裂病の遺伝負因がある。③配偶者が、分裂病以外の精神障害に罹患。④胎生期から周産期にかけての異常（妊娠中毒、過期産、切迫流産など）。⑤乳幼児期の養育環境の重大な問題（施設での養育、両親間の強い葛藤・不和など）。⑥小児期の顕著な陰性行動特徴（内気、消極的、非社交的、神経質など）。⑦WISCで言語性IQと動作性IQの差が10以上（学童期の言語発達と非言語面の発達に不均衡が存在する可能性）。⑧MMPIでの異常所見（発症した1名で、顕在発症の2年前の検査で「F値が高値、追加尺度の抑圧尺度、敵意の過剰統制尺度が低値」という異常所見）。⑨対象者が、発症に先行して強いストレス因となるライフイベントを体験し、家庭内に葛藤・混乱が出現。

分裂病発症者で認められるこれらの事項は、他の高危険児研究の知見と共通するところが多く、分裂病発症に促進的に働く危険因子の候補と考えられよう。

表1　わが国のハイリスク児研究の概要（岡崎らによる）

・前向きのダイナミックコホート法による調査
〈調査対象〉分裂病ハイリスク児62名
〈追跡開始〉1976年
〈追跡期間〉平均21年（2000年）
〈主な結果〉
・分裂病が6名、その他の精神病が1名（DSM-III-R）
・精神病を発症したハイリスク児で多く認められた特徴
　①親の分裂病が比較的重症
　②配偶者に分裂病の遺伝負因がある
　③配偶者が、分裂病以外の精神障害に罹患
　④胎生期から周産期にかけての異常
　⑤乳幼児期の養育環境の重大な問題
　⑥小児期の顕著な陰性行動特徴
　⑦WISCで言語性IQと動作性IQの差が10以上
　⑧MMPIでの異常所見
　⑨発症に先行するストレス因となるライフイベント体験、それに伴う家庭内葛藤
・発症者の早期発見・早期治療は実現でき、経過も比較的良好（2次予防の実践）
・一部の対象者は精神病状態に陥ったが、危機介入によりごく短期間で改善し、その後の経過も現在までのところ順調（顕在発症を頓挫できる可能性）

（文献6）より引用）

表2　分裂病の1次・2次予防実現のための3つのポイント

(1) 病前特徴への働きかけ
　　対人関係能力
　　問題処理技能
　　自己評価，など
(2) ライフイベントに関する心理教育
(3) 1次予防実現の困難さ
　　→2次予防実現のために役立つ可能性がある情報を提供
　　精神病理現象（前駆症状，初期症状，精神病症状），精神科の治療の内容，早期治療の必要性・有効性，利用できる社会資源，など

(文献6)より引用)

表3　心の病を予防するためのパンフレット
　　―心の健康を守り育てるための9項目の説明―

(1) 心の病について知っておく利点
(2) 心の病とは？
　　―代表的な心の病「分裂病」のアウトライン―
(3) 分裂病でよくみられる「空耳」について
(4) 分裂病でよくみられる「空耳」の内容と影響力
(5) 分裂病でよくみられる「勘繰り」について
(6) 分裂病が起こるきっかけになりやすい生活環境
　　―ストレスによるピンチ―
(7) ピンチに陥った時の上手な対応法
　　―逆境の受け止め方，しのぎ方―
(8) ピンチに陥らないために役立つこと
　　―「転ばぬ先の杖」になりうる事柄―
(9) 心の病が出てきた時の対処法と精神科の治療の説明
　　―利用できる社会資源の紹介―

Ⅲ．高危険児研究からみた分裂病の予防

　筆者らは，高危険児の追跡研究を遂行しながら，分裂病の1次・2次予防の実現を目指して実践活動を行ってきた[5-7]。具体的には，①精神科医が随時本人や家族の相談にのり，②危機状況では迅速に対応し，③必要時には治療的介入を実施した。しかし上述のように，分裂病の1次予防の困難さが示された。

　現在筆者らは，分裂病の1次・2次予防の実現のためには3つのポイントがあると考えている（表2）。すなわち「病前特徴への働きかけ」「ライフイベントに関する心理教育」「2次予防実現に役立ちうる情報提供」である。

　1つ目のポイントは，病前特徴への働きかけである。筆者らの病前特徴研究の結果[1]から，分裂病患者は発症前から「消極的，自信がない，対人緊張が強い，非社交的で孤立しがち」などの性格・行動上の特徴を示す場合が多く，発症しない人は「自己肯定的で自己評価が安定，積極的で自主性がある，対人関係が円満」などの対照的な特徴を示す場合が多いと明らかになった。発症者で乏しく発症しない人で認められやすい「対人関係能力，問題処理技能，自己評価」は，分裂病発症に対して防御的に働く抗罹病効果をもつ可能性がある。そこで予防のポイントの1つ目は，これらの特性を自分の個性にあった方法で学習し獲得する大切さを本人，家族，教師などに伝え，習得方法の例を紹介することである。

　予防の2つ目のポイントは，ライフイベントに関する心理教育である。従来から，分裂病発症前に様々なライフイベントがみられる場合が多いと知られていたが，筆者らの高危険児研究でもあらためて示された。そこで，ライフイベントに関する説明を行い，困難に陥った際の対処法を伝える心理教育が予防に役立つ可能性がある。

　3つ目のポイントは，逆説的であるが，1次予防実現の困難さである。高危険児研究を通して，親の精神状態が比較的安定していて，精神科医が相談にのっても，1次予防が容易には実現できないと明らかになった。そこで，2次予防の重要性があらためてクローズアップされる。その実現には，「精神病体験の実際の現れ方や悪影響，精神科の治療の内容と必要性・有効性，相談・治療で利用できる社会資源」などの情報伝達が役立つ可能性がある。

　筆者らは，以上の「3つのポイント」の内容をわかりやすく解説したパンフレットを作成した。次節で，パンフレット9項目の表題と内容の概要を紹介する。

Ⅳ．予防教育の教材用パンフレット[3]

　パンフレット全体の表題は，「心の病を予防するためのパンフレット―心の健康を守り育てるた

表4 疾患教育の聴講者を対象として行ったアンケート調査の結果

質問内容	結果
（1）講義内容への興味・関心の有無	「大変興味を持った」または「少し興味を持った」＝88%
（2）パンフレット内容の理解の可否	「よく理解できる」または「一部理解できる」＝81%（第9項目）〜97%（第1項目）
（3）講義内容の有用性の有無	「有用性を感じた」＝80%
（4）講義内容を一般教育の場で扱う必要	「もっと早く知っておいた方がよい」＝70%「今頃でちょうどよい」＝14%

（文献6）より引用）

めの9項目―」で，9項目の説明事項からなる。表3に，9項目の表題を示した。

第1項目の表題は，「心の病について知っておく利点」である。ここでは，分裂病についての正しい知識を身につけると「1次，2次予防」「偏見や誤解の払拭」「心に関する理解を深める」などの利点が生じると伝える。

第2項目の表題は，「心の病とは？―代表的な心の病「分裂病」のアウトライン―」である。本項目では「好発年齢，有病率，主な症状，発症状況，経過，早期発見の必要性と有効性」などの一般的な情報を提供する。

第3項目は，「分裂病でよくみられる空耳について」，第4項目は「分裂病でよくみられる空耳の内容と影響力」，第5項目は「分裂病でよくみられる勘繰りについて」である。この3項目では，分裂病の代表的症状である幻覚妄想体験を詳しく説明し，これらが実際にどのように現れ，様々な混乱，誤解，悪影響を生むかを理解してもらう。こうした知識を身につけることで，自分あるいは周囲の人が幻聴や妄想を体験した際に，早目に病的体験と認識して受診行動をとれるよう意図している。なおこの説明内容は，筆者らが考案した幻覚妄想への認知療法[2]を参考に作成した。

第6項目の表題は「分裂病がおこるきっかけになりやすい生活環境―ストレスによるピンチ―」，第7項目の表題は，「ピンチに陥った時の上手な対応法―逆境の受け止め方，しのぎ方―」，第8項目の表題は，「ピンチに陥らないために役立つこと―転ばぬ先の杖になりうる事柄―」である。第6，7項目では，発症の誘因となりうるライフイベントを具体的に説明し，有効と思われる対処法を紹介する。第8項目では，抗罹病因子である可能性がある「基本的な生活技能」「肯定的自己評価」「対人葛藤の乗り越え方」を紹介し，その習得法の一例を伝える。以上の3項目は，分裂病の1次予防への寄与を目指す内容である。

第9項目の表題は，「心の病が出てきた時の対処法と精神科の治療の説明―利用できる社会資源の紹介―」である。最後の項目では，分裂病の前駆症状，初期症状を紹介した上で，精神科関連の社会資源と精神科の治療内容を説明し，2次予防への寄与を目指している。

V．予防教育受講者を対象とするアンケート調査の結果

筆者らは，このパンフレットを用いて青年期の一般者を対象とした予防教育を実践し始めた。その際，受講者の関心の度合や理解の程度などを調べるために，講義終了時に無記名でアンケート調査を行った[4]。対象者は，大学や専門学校の入学生320名である。

表4に結果の概要を示したが，この結果から予防教育がある程度受講者の興味・関心を引き，内容の一部を伝達でき，有用性も一定程度感じとってもらえたとみなせるであろう。

筆者らの方法は，分裂病の予防実現のために必要な様々なアプローチ法の一つに過ぎず，本方法だけで分裂病の予防という重大で困難なテーマに対して，大きな貢献ができるとは考えていない。しかし，現在実施可能で，実施方法にもよるが危険性・副作用が比較的少ない方法であると思われるため，今後ともささやかな努力を続けて行きたいと考えている。

文　献

1) 原田誠一, 岡崎祐士, 増井寛治ほか：精神分裂病患者の病前行動特徴. 精神医学, 29；705-715, 1987.
2) 原田誠一, 吉川武彦, 岡崎祐士ほか：幻聴に対する認知療法的接近法(第1報). 精神医学, 39；363-370, 1997.
3) 原田誠一, 岡崎祐士, 増井寛治ほか：一般者を対象とした精神分裂病に関する疾患教育プログラムの作成(第1報)―分裂病の1次・2次予防への寄与を目指す疾患教育パンフレットの紹介. 精神医学, 41；811-819, 1999.
4) 原田誠一, 岡崎祐士, 増井寛治ほか：一般者を対象とした精神分裂病に関する疾患教育プログラムの作成(第2報)―疾患教育の受講者を対象にしたアンケート調査の結果. 精神医学, 41；937-945, 1999.
5) 原田誠一, 佐々木司, 福田正人ほか：精神分裂病の「病前特徴と発症予防」及び「発症後の認知療法」の研究(2). 分裂病患者を片親に持つ子どもの20年転帰. 厚生省精神・神経疾患研究委託費「精神分裂病の病態, 治療, リハビリテーションに関する研究」(主任研究者：浦田重治郎)平成11年度報告書, 2000.
6) 原田誠一, 岡崎祐士：ハイリスク児研究からみた分裂病の病因と予防. 臨床精神医学, 29；367-374, 2000.
7) 岡崎祐士：精神分裂病ハイリスク児. 精神医学, 39；346-362, 1997.

---

*三重大学医学部精神神経科学教室
Seiichi Harada, Yuji Okazaki : Department of Neuropsychiatry, Mie University School of Medicine.
**東京大学健康管理センター
Tsukasa Sasaki : Health Service Center, University of Tokyo.

学校精神保健システムにおける予防的介入

Early intervention and prevention in psychiatric disorders at the university health center

福治　康秀* 　平松　謙一* 　小椋　力*

I. はじめに

　大学生は精神分裂病の好発年齢であり，現に在学中の学生が精神分裂病に罹患し当科で診療を受ける学生が少なからずいる。演者らは，1994年4月より，当大学保健管理センターと協力して，精神障害の早期発見・早期対応プロジェクトを実施してきた。今年度で8年目になる。この7年間を振り返り，その概略と今後の課題などについて報告する。本プロジェクトの目的は，当大学の学生に対して，精神障害，特に精神分裂病の早期発見・早期対応を行うことであり，対象者は，琉球大学学生である。

II. 方　法

　方法は，1994年から1996年までと1997年から2001年までが一部異なるので，それぞれを分けて示した（図）。まず，1994年から1996年までについては，一次スクリーニングを，毎年5月に保健管理センターで行われる全学生を対象にした定期健康診断のときに，新入生を対象に実施した。スクリーニング検査としては，Chapmanら（文献1980，1987）が開発したPsychosis Proneness Scales (Chapman's Scales)を用いた。本スケールにはMagical Ideation Scale, Perceptual Aberration Scale, Social Anhedonia Scaleの3スケールが含まれ，全質問項目数は105である。この検査において，全対象者の2 SD以上の学生に対し，面接の必要性を記載した文書を郵送し，同意の得られた学生に対して診断的面接を行った。また，補助検査として事象関連電位（ERPs）と心理テストとしてロールシャッハテストを行った。そのうち，介入が必要と判断された学生のうち同意の得られた者に対して，面接や必要に応じて与薬，病院受診などの継続した介入を行った。

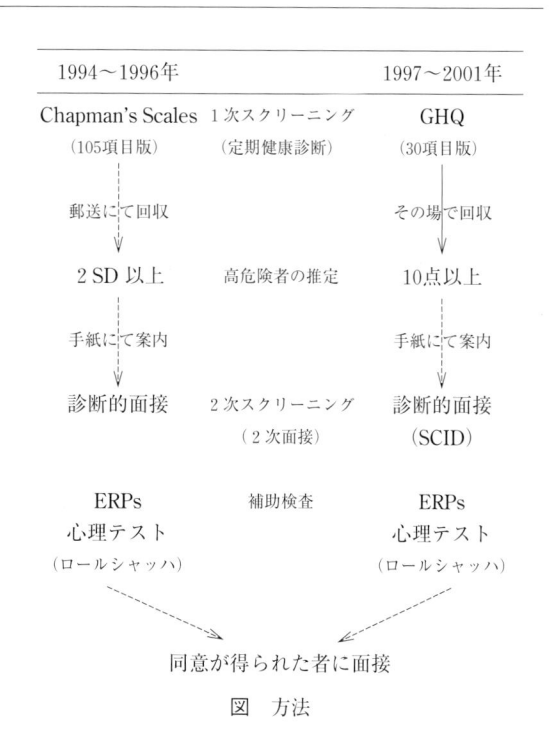

　1997年から2001年までについては，一次スクリーニングとして，一般健康調査質問紙General Health Questionnare (GHQ)の30項目版を用いた。Chapman's ScalesからGHQに変えた理由は，一次スクリーニングの回収率を上げるためである。Chapman's Scalesの場合，105項目と質問数が多いため，健康診断を受けている間の約30分間にすべてを回答するのは困難であり，全問について回答した後，郵送による回収が必要であった。しかし，そのために，回収率は約35～60％と低くなってしまった。そこで，他科の検査などの健康診断を受けている間にすべての項目が記入でき，その場で回収できる自己記入式テストとして，GHQの30項目版に変更した。得点が10点以

1994～1996年		1997～2001年
Chapman's Scales (105項目版)	1次スクリーニング (定期健康診断)	GHQ (30項目版)
↓郵送にて回収		↓その場で回収
2 SD 以上	高危険者の推定	10点以上
↓手紙にて案内		↓手紙にて案内
診断的面接	2次スクリーニング (2次面接)	診断的面接 (SCID)
ERPs 心理テスト (ロールシャッハ)	補助検査	ERPs 心理テスト (ロールシャッハ)
	同意が得られた者に面接	

図　方法

表1 精神障害の早期発見・早期対応プロジェクトの年次推移の概略

年度	新入生数	健康診断を受けた者	スクリーニングテストを受けた者	高得点者	面接を受けた者	継続的に面接を受けた者
1994	1,839	1,416(77.0)	830(58.6)	31(3.7)	27(87.1)	
1995	1,812	1,449(79.6)	555(38.3)	32(5.8)	19(59.4)	5
1996	1,842	1,481(80.4)	519(35.0)	26(5.0)	19(73.1)	7
1997	1,868	1,495(79.9)	1,493(100.0)	199(13.3)	20(10.1)	18
1998	1,764	1,181(70.0)	1,168(98.9)	213(18.2)	13(6.1)	8
1999	1,642	1,214(73.9)	1,201(98.9)	217(18.1)	9(4.1)	5
2000	1,589	1,044(65.7)	863(82.7)	171(19.8)	11(6.4)	4
計	12,365	9,278(75.0)	6,629(71.4)	889(13.4)	118(13.3)	47

単位は人で括弧内は%を示す

上の学生に，面接の必要性を記載した文書を郵送した。GHQでは，カットオフポイントは4点とされているが，4点とすると，かなり多数の学生が面接診断の必要性ありと判定される。しかし，限られた期間に多数の学生に診断面接を実施することは，マンパワーのことも含めて困難であったため，10点をカットオフポイントにした。

診断的面接には，DSM-III-Rの構造化面接であるSCID-IIを用いた。人格障害，特に，クラスターAの分裂病型人格障害，分裂病質人格障害，妄想性人格障害を中心に診断面接を行った。また，補助検査としてERPsとロールシャッハテストも施行した。そして，介入が必要と判断され，同意の得られた学生に対して，面接や必要に応じて与薬，病院受診などの継続した介入を行った。

III. 結 果

本プロジェクトの対象者数などの概略を年次別に示した(表1)。新入生数は，単年度で1,589から1,868人で，7年間の合計では12,365人であった。そのうち1,044から1,495人(65.7から80.4%)の学生が健康診断を受けている。その全員にスクリーニングテストをその場で手渡している。Chapman's Scalesを用いた1994年から1996年においては，先ほども述べたように回収を郵送にしたため，35から58.6%の回収率となっている。1997年以降GHQに変えてからは82.7から100%と回収率が上がっている。高得点者は，Chapman's Scalesにおいては，26から32人(3.7%から5.8%)，GHQにおいては171から217人(13.3から19.8%)となっている。その全員に面接の案内を郵送し，実際に面接を受けに来た学生は，9から27人であった。そのうち，継続して面接を行った学生は，4から18人であった。7年間の合計では，新入生は12,365人，健康診断を受けた者9,278人，スクリーニングテストを受けた者6,629人，そのうち，高得点者は889人，面接を受けた者は118人，継続的に面接を受けた者は47人であった。

面接を受けた118人のうち精神医学的に問題を持つ者は24人(20.3%)であった。

表2に診断の内訳を示した。分裂病の前駆期(DSM-III-R)が12人，境界性人格障害が4人，分裂病型人格障害が3人，強迫性障害が2人，社会恐怖，性同一性障害，解離性障害がそれぞれ1人であった。なお，在学中に精神分裂病が発症した学生はいなかった。

IV. 考 察

この7年間の結果をもとに，本プロジェクトにおける問題点と今後の展望について考察した。

まず，GHQの得点が全体的に高い結果となり，カットオフポイントを上げざるを得なかった点についてであるが，それは，おそらく健康診断の時期の影響ではないかと考えられた。つまり，健康診断を行う5月は，新入生にとって，まだ慣れない状況であり，それが，GHQの結果にも反映していると考えられた。

次に，回収率と面接を受けた人数についてであるが，1997より一次スクリーニングをChapman's

表2 精神医学的に問題をもつ者の主な診断

診断	人数
DSM-Ⅲ-R	
分裂病の前駆期	12
DSM-Ⅳ	
境界性人格障害	4
分裂病型人格障害	3
強迫性障害	2
社会恐怖	1
性同一性障害	1
解離性障害	1
計	24

ScalesからGHQに変更し，その場で回収する方法にしたため，スクリーニングテストの回収率は上昇した。しかし，高得点者で面接を受けた人数は，Chapman's Scalesで19～27人，GHQで9～20人であり，一次スクリーニング法を変更する前後であまり変化しなかった。今後，高得点者で面接を受ける人数を増やすにはどうするか，工夫が必要と考えられた。また，一次スクリーニングとして，GHQで妥当かどうか。さらに妥当なスクリーニング検査はないか，今後検討してゆく必要があると考えられた。

次に，大学を卒業した後のFollow-upの問題がある。卒業後は，保健管理センターでのFollow-upができないため，大学病院精神科や近くのクリニック，または病院に紹介をしているが，十分ではなく中断してしまう者が多い。卒業後の相談や治療のFollow-upの体制をどのようにしてゆくかが今後の課題である。

つぎに，本プロジェクトの有用性の検証についてであるが，現在のところそれができない。個々のケースにおいて，本プロジェクトを通して早めの相談につながったり，治療開始が早くなったりと，本プロジェクトが有用であったと考えられるケースを認めた。しかし，本プロジェクトの有用性を検証するためには疫学調査が必要であり，今後の課題である。

要　約

1．1994年度から琉球大学学生を対象に，精神分裂病など精神障害の早期発見・早期対応を目的としたプロジェクトを開始し7年が経過した。

2．新入生12,365名中健康診断を受けた者は9,278名（75％）であり，そのうち精神医学的スクリーニングテストを受けた者は6,629名（71.4％）であった。そのうち高得点者は889名（13.4％）であり，そのうち面接を受けた者は118名（13.3％）であった。

3．精神医学的に問題を持つ者を診断別にみると，分裂病の前駆期（DSM-Ⅲ-R）が12人で最も多く，次いで境界性人格障害（DSM-Ⅳ）の4人，分裂病型人格障害3人，強迫性障害2人などであった。当大学保健管理センターに継続して面接を受けた者は47人であった。これらの学生に対して発症予防，早期発見，早期治療の目的で介入した。対象者の中には在学中に精神分裂病が発症した学生はいなかった。

4．今後の課題として，有用性の検証のための疫学調査が必要なこと，面接を受ける学生数を増やすこと，より合理的な一次スクリーニングの使用，卒業後の治療の継続，追跡調査，Follow-up等がある。

文　献

1) Chapman, L. J., Chapman, J. P. : Scale for rating psychotic and psychotic-like experiences as continua. Schizophrenia Bulletin, 6 ; 476-489, 1980.
2) Chapman, L. J., Chapman, J. P. : The search for symptoms predictive of schizophrenia. Schizophrenia Bulletin, 13 ; 497-503, 1987.

---

*琉球大学医学部精神神経科学講座
Yasuhide Fukuji, Ken-ichi Hiramatsu, Chikara Ogura : Department of Neuropsychiatry, University of the Ryukyus.

精神分裂病の脆弱性指標としての探索眼球運動
—臨床への応用—

Exploratory eye movements as a vulnerability marker of schizophrenia
—Application to the clinical practice—

松島　英介* 　大林　滋** 　太田　克也*,** 　高橋　栄*** 　小島　卓也***

Introduction

Many investigators have proposed impairment in a fundamental cognitive process that could explain the clinical diversity of schizophrenia. Andreasen (1999) also proposed in her perspectives that an abnormality in brain development of schizophrenic patients leads to some impairment in cognitive process. At present we do not have a well-defined and agree-on cognitive marker, but we have been studying cognitive function in schizophrenia using exploratory eye movements in the S-shaped figure test (Kojima et al., 1990, 1992).

Methods

1. Examination procedure

The subject is fitted with a nac the seventh type eye mark recorder, and shown S-shaped figures, which consist of the target figure (at the top of the Figure 1) and two figures partially different from the target; one has a bump in a different place and the other has no bumps (at the bottom of the Figure 1), on a screen. The eye movements of the subject are recorded on a videotape as he or she looks at the S-shaped figures. The examination procedure is as follows:

Step 1) The target figure is shown for fifteen seconds.【memory task】

Step 2) Immediately afterwards, the subject is asked to draw the target figure from memory.【reproduction task】

Step 3) Each of the two figures partially different from the target is shown for fifteen seconds. After fifteen seconds have passed, and with the figure still showing, the subject is asked if it differs from the target figure and, if different, how it differs. After the subject finishes replying, he or she is asked: "Are there any other differences?"【comparison task】

2. Measurements

In memory task, two indicators of exploratory eye movements, that is, the number of eye fixations (NEF) and the mean eye scanning length (MESL) were analyzed for fifteen seconds. In comparison task, the responsive eye movements which occurred in the five seconds following the question: "Are there any other differences?" were analyzed, and counted of the two figures partially different from the target as a responsive search score (RSS).

Discriminant analysis

Using the number of eye fixations (NEF) and responsive search score (RSS), schizophrenics could be discriminated from non-schizophrenics such as patients with depression, amphetamine psychosis, alcohol psychosis, anxiety disorder, frontal lobe lesions, temporal lobe epilepsy and healthy normal controls, with a sensitivity of 76.7% and a specificity of 81.4% (Matsushima et al., 1998). This finding indicates that exploratory eye movements (NEF and RSS) can be a specific marker for schizophrenia.

Family and twin studies

1. Healthy siblings and parents of schizophrenics

Takahashi et al. (1999) compared the RSSs among 3 subject groups, 23 proband-sibling pairs in which were included 23 schizophrenic probands and 23 their healthy siblings, and 43 unrelated normal controls which had no history of psychotic illness in their first-degree family members. Not only the schizophrenic probands but also their siblings had significantly fewer NEF and lower RSS than the normal controls.

Also, the healthy parents of schizophrenic patients had a few NEF and a low RSS, falling into values that lie between those of the patients and the normal controls (Moriya, 1979; Kojima et al., 1996).

The family studies suggest that few NEFs and low RSSs shown in schizophrenics and their family members can be a trait marker for schizophrenia.

2. Twins

Matsushima et al. (1997, 1999) examined the RSSs in 28 monozygotic twin pairs, which consist of 12 pairs discordant and 8 pairs concordant for schizophrenia, and 8 normal control pairs. There was a significant relationship between each twin pair in the RSS, even including discordant twins. The result suggests that a low RSS shown in schizophrenics may be a trait marker for schizophrenia. Furthermore, they compared the RSSs among these 3 groups. The RSS of discordant twin group was higher than that of concordant twin group but was lower than that of normal twin group. The result suggests that concordant twins are more strongly related to genetic factors of developing schizophrenia than discordant twins.

First-episode of schizophrenia

Obayashi et al. (2001) investigated 28 schizophrenic patients in repeat eye movement test design over a certain period (the average duration be-

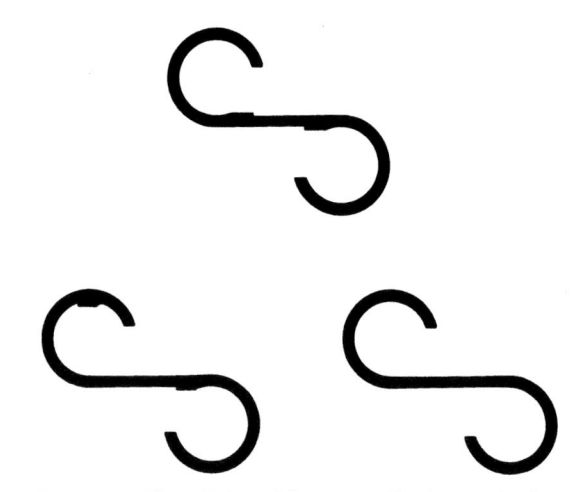

Figure 1 Three S-shaped figures used in the examination
The two at the bottom are partially different from the target figure at the top.

tween both tests was 8.3 months). All patients were first-medicated schizophrenics that were consisted of 24 first-episode schizophrenics and 4 second-episode ones. According to whether their symptoms evaluated by Brief Psychiatric Rating Scale (BPRS) improved or not, patients were divided into two groups, 15 improved group and 13 unchanged group. Mean eye scanning length (MESL) value differed significantly between the first and second test only in unchanged group. This unchanged group, whose BPRS score remained unchanged over an approximate 8-month period, was regarded as the model of chronicity, because this group showed no improvement during various therapies, including neuroleptic medication. Kojima et al. (1990) previously reported exploratory eye movements of schizophrenics in three clinical stages, chronic, acute and remitted of schizophrenia and healthy controls. As for the MESL, only chronic schizophrenics had small values compared to other three groups. These results suggest that shorter MESL values are linked to a chronic process of schizophrenia.

Conclusion

The above results suggest that (1) NEF and RSS

values can be a vulnerability marker of schizophrenia and that (2) MESL value may be a sensitive indicator in the development of chronicity in schizophrenia. Therefore, NEF and RSS can be applied to prevention and early detection of developing schizophrenia and MESL can be applied to grasp of chronic process of schizophrenia in our daily clinical practice.

References

1) Andreasen, N. C. : A unitary model of schizophrenia. Arch. Gen. Psychiatry, 56 ; 781-787, 1999.
2) Kojima, T., Matsushima, E., Nakajima, K. et al. : Eye movement in acute, chronic and remitted schizophrenics. Biol. Psychiatry, 27 ; 975-989, 1990.
3) Kojima, T., Matsushima, E., Ando, K. et al. : Exploratory eye movements and neuropsychological tests in schizophrenic patients. Schizophr Bull, 18 ; 85-94, 1992.
4) Kojima, T., Takahashi, S., Tanabe, E. et al. : Eye Movements in family of schizophrenia. In : Annual Report '90 of the National Project Team (Basic and Clinical Studies on the Onset Mechanism and Pathophysiology of Schizophrenia) (ed. Toru, M.), pp.5-8, 1996.
5) Matsushima, E., Ohta, K., Obayashi, S. et al. : Exploratory eye movements in patients with schizophrenia : A monozygotic twin study, 2nd report. Psychiat. Clin. Neurosci., 51 ; S84, 1997.
6) Matsushima, E., Kojima, T., Ohta, K. et al. : Exploratory eye movement dysfunctions in patients with schizophrenia : possibility as a discriminator for schizophrenia. J. Psychiat. Res, 32 ; 289-295, 1998.
7) Matsushima, E., Kubo, H., Kojima, T. et al. : Exploratory eye movements in patients with schizophrenia - a monozygotic twins study. In : Abstracts II of the XI World Congress of Psychiatry, Hamburg, p.11, 1999.
8) Moriya, H. : A study of eye movement in patients with chronic schizophrenia and in their relatives, using an eye-mark recorder. Psychiat. Neurol. Jap., 81 ; 523-558, 1979.
9) Obayashi, S., Matsushima, E., Okubo, Y. et al. : Relationship of exploratory eye movements with clinical course in schizophrenic patients. Eur. Arch. Psychiat. Clin. Neurosci. (in press)
10) Takahashi, S., Tanabe, E., Kojima, T. et al. : Exploratory eye movement dysfunctions in schizophrenic patients and their siblings. In : Abstracts II of the XI World Congress of Psychiatry, Hamburg, p.15, 1999.

---

*東京医科歯科大学大学院心療・ターミナル医学分野
Eisuke Matsushima, Katsuya Ohta : Section of Liaison Psychiatry & Palliative Medicine, Graduate School of Tokyo Medical & Dental Univesity.

**東京医科歯科大学大学院精神行動医学分野
Shigeru Obayashi, Katsuya Ohta : Section of Psychiatry & Behavioral Science, Graduate School of Tokyo Medical & Dental University.

***日本大学医学部精神神経科学教室
Sakae Takahashi, Takuya Kojima : Department of Neuropsychiatry, Nihon University School of Medicine.

日本における初回エピソード精神病患者への治療戦略
Treatment strategies for patients with first-episode psychosis in Japan

嶋田　博之[*]

I. はじめに

近年，精神病の早期介入に対する関心が世界的に高まっている。特に精神病を発症してからの数年間は，その後の予後に大きく影響する決定的時期だと言われており，集中的な介入が必要とされる。こうした早期介入の重要性をふまえた精神保健サービスが各国でも発展しつつある。

オーストラリアのメルボルン市には，McGorryらのグループによって1992年から運営されているEPPIC (Early Psychosis Prevention and Intervention Centre) があり，ここでは初回エピソード精神病患者に特別に焦点をあてた包括的プログラムが行われている。その成果についても多くの報告がなされ，世界的な注目を集めている。筆者は2000年9月にEPPICを訪問し，その臨床を目の当たりにする機会に恵まれ，EPPICが精神病の初回エピソードに対する早期介入の理想的なモデルの1つであろうと改めて感じた。

一方，本邦ではEPPICのようなプログラムは存在せず，日本はこうした世界の流れから取り遅れている感がある。現在，筆者は，公立単科精神科病院である山梨県立北病院を受診した分裂病圏の初回エピソード患者をリスペリドンを第1選択薬として治療し，48週間にわたり経過を追跡する研究[*]を行っている。この研究結果には，日本の初回エピソード精神病患者に対する介入の現状が反映されていると思われる。今回筆者はEPPICとの比較を用いながら，民間病院主体で地域での責任ある経過追跡が難しい日本特有の状況において，初回エピソード治療戦略を発展させていくために我々が行うべきことを考察することとした。

II. 北病院における初回エピソード患者への介入の現状と問題点 : EPPICとの比較から

北病院とEPPICは，ともに公的な精神科サービスであるという点では共通しているものの，表1に示したように多くの相違点が存在する。

初回エピソード患者への介入は，薬物治療から治療教育にわたるまで慢性患者のそれとは異なる特殊なものである。スタッフから医療施設にいたるまで，初回エピソード患者には慢性患者とは異なる治療環境が望ましい。そのためEPPICでは対象となる患者群を15～30歳の初回エピソード精神病患者とかなり限定している。また初期1～2年の治療内容がその後の予後に大きな影響を与えるとの認識から，18カ月という期間を限定した集中的な介入プログラムを提供している。

一方，北病院ではあらゆる精神疾患から癲癇などの神経疾患にいたるまでの幅広い患者を対象としている。特にその中でも中心となっている患者群は，慢性のエピソードを繰り返している分裂病圏の精神病患者である。北病院では多くのスタッフや時間は慢性患者に費やされており，それと比較すると初回エピソード患者に対する介入にはさほど重点が置かれていない。

この違いが端的に現われているのが治療の継続率である。今回の北病院の初回エピソード研究では17例中6例 (35.3％) が48週以内に治療を中断していた。一方EPPICにおいて経過追跡が中断されるのは，患者が転居する場合以外はほとんどない。北病院の施設中心型のサービスに対して，EPPICでは初期のアセスメントから，その後の治療にいたるまで，積極的に訪問を行う地域中心型のサービスが提供されている。EPPICでは，

表1　北病院とEPPICの比較

	北病院	EPPIC
対象患者群	精神疾患患者	15～30歳の初回エピソード精神病患者
治療期間	制限なし	18カ月の期間限定プログラム
サービスの提供方法	施設中心型サービス	地域中心型サービス
治療の中心となるスタッフ	精神科医	ケース・マネージャー（多職種チーム）
地域責任制	不明瞭	明瞭
医療費	5～30％負担	無料

たとえ患者が受診を拒否したとしても、ケースマネージャーが訪問を行うし、もし訪問も拒否したとしても家族とのコンタクトは継続し、治療教育などを行いながら、介入のチャンスを探っていくアプローチをとる。

北病院における治療中断の理由は、（通常の北病院での診療と同じように）訪問や電話による追跡を行っていないので明らかとなっていないが、仮に症状が消退したから中断したのだとしても、その後のフォローアップが不要ということにはならない。初回エピソードにおける治療目標には症状の速やかな消退だけでなく、その後の再発の予防や社会生活への復帰を目的とした治療教育や精神療法の提供など多くの課題がある。北病院の初回エピソード研究で治療を中断した6例のうち2例は初診のみ、もう2例は3回の受診のみで通院を中断しており、こうした課題の多くが未達成のままに終わっている可能性が大きい。現在の北病院の介入のように、「去る者は追わず、問題が大きくなってから、あるいは再発を繰り返してからようやく本腰を入れる」といった介入では、常に後手にまわるばかりで精一杯となろう。

初回エピソード患者に限らない日本の精神科医療全体の特徴として、患者のケアを継続する責任を誰が負うのかが不明瞭なことがある。その原因としては、日本では民間病院が主体となっていることや、マンパワー不足などが挙げられるかもしれない。マンパワー不足を助長する要因として、医師の裁量権や負担が大きすぎることが挙げられる。日本では診断から治療計画の策定、そして治療の実践にいたるまで医師が中心となっている。一方、EPPICを含めオーストラリアでは、多職種からなるケース・マネージメント・チームによってケアが提供されている。この多職種チームは精神科医の他、精神科看護、ソーシャルワーカー、臨床心理士、作業療法士などからなるが、こうした医師ではないスタッフたちが診断や薬物治療を含めた治療計画の策定に中心となって関わっているのである。

EPPICでは各患者に対して担当となるケースマネージャーと精神科医が割り当てられ、担当患者数はそれぞれ30～40、70～80となっている。北病院では9人の精神科医が約300人の入院患者と1日平均144人の外来患者の診療にあたっている。精神科医1人あたりの担当患者数は200に達しており、初回エピソード患者に十分な時間をあてるのが困難な状況にある。

医師を中心とした外来診療と入院治療以外にも、北病院にはデイケア、作業療法、訪問看護、家族教室などのサブプログラムが存在する。今回の初回エピソード研究における各プログラムの利用頻度をみると、治療を中断した患者群では、入院治療を受けた1例以外の全例が医師による外来診療のみであった。しかしこれらサブプログラムの利用率は、（治療を継続した患者群を含め）初回エピソード患者全体において低い傾向が認められた。その主たる理由として考えられるのは、こうしたサブプログラムが元来、慢性患者のニーズに合わせて発足しており、初回エピソード患者が利用するには適していないことである。

入院治療は17例中7例(42.2％)が経験し，平均入院期間は8.9週であった。北病院は施設中心型のサービスであり，初回エピソード患者にとっても入院治療は比較的利用頻度の高かったプログラムといえる。しかし，この入院治療といえども基本的には慢性患者のためのプログラムであって，初回エピソード患者には相応しくないことは明らかである。初回エピソードでは，治療による心理的外傷を最小限にして，その後の治療関係を安定させることが重要であるが，現在の北病院の入院治療はそれに見合ったものではない。多くの慢性患者が入院する騒がしい病棟，あるいは欠陥状態や薬物による過鎮静で異常に静かな病棟にいきなり閉じこめられるのは恐ろしい体験となりえることは想像に難くない。EPPICの入院施設は16の個室からなる開放病棟であり，患者は初回エピソード患者のみである。入院期間も平均で約2週間と短く，4週間を越える場合はほとんどない。

北病院の入院治療が初回エピソード患者に適していないことは，薬物治療に関する結果にも現われている。本研究における薬物治療を入院群と外来群に分けて比較してみると，リスペリドンの初回投与量の平均が入院群で3.2mg，外来群で1.3mgと2倍以上の差が認められた。また薬物の増量や切り替えも，入院群では明らかに急速に行われる傾向が認められた。EPPICにおける抗精神病薬治療は，長期的コンプライアンスに対する影響を考慮して，副作用を避けつつ，少量から開始し，緩徐に増量させていくという「low and slow principle」を採用している。本研究の外来群ではEPPICに似通った薬物治療ができているが，入院群では「low and slow」とは逆の「せっかちな」処方が行われている傾向がある。その理由として，入院群では病状自体が重いことや，入院治療では頻回に診察をして処方変更が速やかにできることが第一に考えられるが，初回エピソードに相応しくない病棟に入院することで逆に不穏となることや，初回エピソードの特性などに対する理解が不十分な病棟スタッフによって安易な薬物の増量が助長されること，薬物治療以外に介入する術や時間のない病棟スタッフなどもその一因となっているかもしれない。

III．日本における初回エピソード精神病患者への治療戦略の発展

上述した問題点を克服していくための道筋を考察する。

初回エピソード患者だけの入院施設やスタッフがあれば理想的だが，それだけの予算を確保するのは容易ではない。実験的なモデル地域を設定し，費用対効果の面まで含めた評価を行うことも日本においては困難に思われる。現時点で実行可能と思われる方策は，先ず初回エピソード精神病や早期介入を専門とする多職種チームを立ち上げることである。

このチームの負うべき役割には，院内スタッフに対する教育やスーパービジョン，患者や家族に対する介入，一般市民に対する教育や広報活動などが考えられる。具体的には，新患をチェックし初回エピソード患者を(出来れば前駆段階にある患者も)選定すること，定期的に症例カンファレンスを開いて，治療の進行状況などを確認し，必要なアドバイスを担当医に対して行っていくこと，初回エピソード患者に焦点をあてた家族教室，初回エピソード患者のためのグループ・プログラム，初回エピソード患者に対する訪問活動など様々なものが含まれるが，最初から全ての役割をこなすのは不可能である。チームメンバーの増員や成長に伴い，少しずつ手を広げていくのが良いだろう。

初回エピソードを専門とする病棟，または病棟の中の1ユニット(病室やエリア)が設定できれば，こうした動きも促進されるであろう。また初回エピソードに限らず，施設中心型のサービスからの脱却や多職種によるチーム医療も促進していかなければ，こういった方策も計画倒れに終わる可能性がある。

最後に一番重要と思われるのは，こうしたチームを立ち上げて，維持し，発展させていくために不可欠なチームメンバーおよび院内スタッフ全体の士気である。先ず，初回エピソードからの予防的アプローチが重要であるとの認識を深めるための教育的活動を院内スタッフ全員に対して行い，共鳴するスタッフを選出してチームを立ち上げる

ことがスタートラインとなるかもしれない。北病院もようやくスタートラインに立つための準備体操が整ったところであろうか。今後，日本の多くの医療機関でも早期介入に向けた取り組みが始まり，新たな希望の時代の幕開けとなることを願っている。

*この研究は(財)井之頭病院研究基金の助成を受けています。

参考文献

1) Aitchison, K. J., Meehan, K., Murray, R. M. : First episode psychosis. Martin Dunitz, London, 1999.(嶋田博之, 藤井康男訳：初回エピソード精神病. 星和書店, 東京, 2000.)
2) McGorry, P. D., Edwards, J. : Early psychosis training pack. Gardiner-Caldwell Communications Ltd, 1997.
3) McGorry, P. D., Jackson, H. J., ed. : The recognition and management of early psychosis. Cambridge University Press, Cambridge, 1999.(鹿島晴雄監修, 水野雅文, 村上雅昭, 藤井康男監訳：精神疾患の早期発見・早期治療. 金剛出版, 東京, 2001.)

---

*山梨県立北病院
Hiroyuki Shimada : Yamanashi Prefectural Kita Hospital.

長期転帰から見た初回エピソードに対する治療戦略

Treatment in the first episode of schizophrenia
—A strategy based on a long-term follow-up study—

小川　一夫*

The aim of this paper is to present a strategy of treatment in the first episode of schizophrenia based on a long-term follow-up study of schizophrenic patients consecutively discharged from Gunma University Hospital.

First of all, the outline of the long-term follow-up study is described, and then the findings concerning the strategy is presented.

A long-term follow-up study

The subjects of the follow-up study were 140 schizophrenic patients consecutively discharged from Gunma University hospital between 1958 and 1962. In 1958, a five-year project aimed at preventing the relapse of schizophrenic patients was initiated at the Department of Neuropsychiatry, Gunma University Hospital. The project was carried out until 1967, and the subjects were subsequently followed up. Of the 140 subjects, 79% were first admissions, 81% were under 30 years old and the average was 24.4 years old at the time of discharge. Most of the subjects were in the early stages of schizophrenia.

The long-term follow-up of the subjects was completed as shown in Table 1. In the study in 1979 (Miya et al., 1984), the follow-up was completed in 130 (93%) of the 140 patients. Of the 130 patients, 109 were alive at the time of the study, and in 102 of these living patients, the longitudinal courses were fully observed. The investigations were subsequently carried out in 1984 and 1996 (Ogawa et al., 1987; Ogawa et al., 1997). The last follow-up in this study covered the period up to the end of January 1996. The follow-up was completed in 127 patients, and 86 patients were still alive. In 83 of these patients, the longitudinal courses were fully observed. The observation period for the 86 living patients ranged from 33.1 to 39.2 years, with an average of 35.6 years. The mean age of the patients was 60 years (range 48-82) at the end of the follow-up period.

The investigation of the course and outcome of the subjects was concentrated mainly on the aspect of social adjustment. For the assessment of social adjustment, Eguma's Social Adjustment Scale (ESAS) was used, which consists of five grades: 'self-supportive,' 'semi-self-supportive,' 'socially adjusted to family or community,' 'maladjusted,' and 'hospitalized.' The longitudinal courses were assessed and illustrated month by month using the five ESAS grades.

Long-term course and outcome

The social outcome of living subjects in 1979, as assessed on ESAS, is shown in Table 2. The outcome was regarded as favourable in 'self-supportive' cases, which constituted 49% of the 109 living subjects, and unfavourable in 'hospitalized' and 'maladjusted' cases, which totalled 34%. The cases in the middle grades of ESAS, namely 'semi-self-supportive' and 'socially adjusted to family or community,' amounted 17%.

Table 3 shows a series of social outcomes in 1979, 1984 and 1996. The percentages of social adjustment at the each point of assessment are similar, and more than 50% of living patients were 'self-

Table 1 Follow-up of 140 subjects

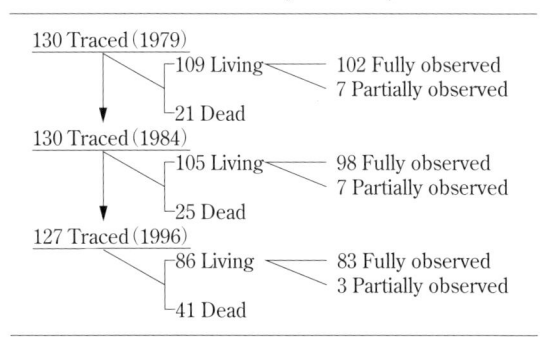

```
130 Traced (1979)
       ├─ 109 Living ─┬─ 102 Fully observed
       │              └─ 7 Partially observed
       └─ 21 Dead
130 Traced (1984)
       ├─ 105 Living ─┬─ 98 Fully observed
       │              └─ 7 Partially observed
       └─ 25 Dead
127 Traced (1996)
       ├─ 86 Living ─┬─ 83 Fully observed
       │             └─ 3 Partially observed
       └─ 41 Dead
```

Table 2 Social outcome (1979)

Social adjustment	Male	Female	Total	(%)
Self-supportive	27	26	53	(49)
Semi-self-supportive	5	6	11	(10)
Socially adjusted to family or community	3	5	8	(7)
Maladjusted	0	3	3	(3)
Hospitalized	15	19	34	(31)
Total	50	59	109	(100)

Table 3 A series of social outcomes

	Year		
	1979	1984	1996
Number of living subjects	109	105	86
Social adjustment (%)			
Self-supportive	49	47	43
Semi-self-supportive	10	8	8
Socially adjusted to family or community	7	11	13
Maladjusted	3	3	1
Hospitalized	31	31	35

supportive' or 'semi-self-supportive' state at every point of assessment.

In the study of longitudinal courses of the patients, fluctuating courses of social adjustment were the most numerous in the early stages, whereas in the later stages many of the patients showed differentiation in one of two directions, namely the 'stable self-supportive' state and the 'chronic institutionalized' state (Figure 1).

Social task at onset

This differentiation occurred in relation to the various conditions of life, such as the change of position in work, the change of family living together, or an encounter with a key person, and not infrequently, did dramatically by chance. However, in any case, it was common that forming the basis of life was a necessary requirement for attaining the 'stable self-supportive' state. Unfortunately, most of patients generally get ill at the crucial time to perform the basis of life, and are then faced with an important social task to affect their whole life. So we called this task 'social task at onset,' and examined the achievement of the task and its correlation with the long-term outcome.

Social task at onset was identified based on the viewpoint as follows. Firstly, it is what is generally expected from each patient's age, sex, and social status. Secondly, each patient wishes to achieve it to a certain extent. Finally, it is closely related to the development of subsequent social life. To be concrete, if a patient becomes ill while he is a high school student, the social task at onset is usually identified as going back to school or graduation from school. If a patient falls ill shortly after getting a job, the social task is mostly identified as being reinstated in his former position.

As to the achievement of social task at onset, we assessed it based on the following views. When the social task is completed as generally expected and as suiting patient's wish, it is obviously regarded as a successful achievement. Even if the social task is dealt with in a different way from the original one, when it is settled for the second best in the context of social life development, it is also regarded as a successful achievement. For example, in case of going back to work, when the patient can return to the place of work, if not the same as former position, it is regarded as a successful achievement.

Table 4 shows the occupational status of the subjects at onset. It can be seen that the proportion of the patients who were in work (including housewife) amounted to 54%. The proportion of students were 41%. In 101 (78%) of the 130 patients who

Table 4 Occupational status at onset

Occupation	Male	Female	Total
Teacher, Profession	8	3	11
General office work, Engineer	4	12	16
Farmer	4	0	4
Factory worker, Workman	18	19	37
Housewife	0	7	7
Assistant housekeeper, Unemployed	2	6	8
Student	31	26	57
Total	67	73	140

Table 5 Social task at onset and social outcome

	Social adjustment (1979)				
	A B	C	D E	F	Total
Social task at onset					
Achievement	36	4	14	8	62
Failure	12	2	18	7	39
Total	48	6	32	15	101

A : Self-supportive   B : Semi-self-supportive   ($P<0.05$)
C : Socially adjusted to family or community
D : Maladjusted   E : Hospitalized   F : Death

were followed up in 1979, the social task at onset was identified. Of these 101 social tasks, 55 were related to schoolwork or student affairs, 22 were related to work, 21 were related to marriage or family, and 3 were others.

Table 5 shows the correlation between the achievement of social task at onset and the long-term social outcome in 101 patients. Sixty two of 101 patients successfully achieved their social task at onset and the remaining 39 patients failed to achieve. Among the former patients, 36 (58%) were 'self-supportive' or 'semi-self-supportive' in long-term social outcome. On the other hand, only 12 (31%) of the latter patients were 'self-supportive' or 'semi-self-supportive.'

A strategy of treatment in the early stages of schizophrenia

From these results, it is found that there is a close correlation between the achievement of social task at onset and long-term social outcome. Of course, the achievement of social task at onset does not have direct effect on the long-term outcome. However, it must be an important step to built up the foundation of social life. It should also give opportunities to pursue subsequent developmental task achievement and enlarge possibilities to attain the favourable long-term outcome. From this perspective, the psychosocial treatment, which promotes the achievement of social task at onset, ought to be placed as a strategy of management of the early stages of schizophrenia.

Although it is getting more complicated to identify the social task at onset because life style has become diversified, social resources available for the achievement of social task are also increasing. So it is becoming possible to achieve the task in various ways once the task is identified.

As the findings concerning the strategy presented in this paper are based on the retrospective study of the long-term outcome, they have some limitation. To make them sure, it is expected to investigate prospectively the correlation between the achievement social task at onset and long-term outcome.

References

1) Miya, M., Watarai, A., Ogawa, K., & Nakazawa, M. : Course of the social life of discherged schizophrenic patients : catamnestic results of long-term study (in Japanese). Psychiatria et Neurologia Japonica, 86 ; 736-767, 1984.
2) Ogawa, K., Miya, M., Watarai, A., Nakazawa, M., Yuasa, S., & Utena, H. : A long-term follow-up study of schizophrenia in Japan -with special reference to the course of social adjustment. The British Journal of Psychiatry, 151 ; 758-765, 1987.
3) Ogawa, K., Watarai, A., Miya, M. & Nakazawa, M. : Trente-cinq annees de suivi de patients schizophrenes au Japon. L'Information Psychiatique, 73 ; 792-796, 1997.

---

*東京都立中部総合精神保健福祉センター
Kazuo Ogawa : Tokyo Metropolitan Chubu Center for Mental Health.

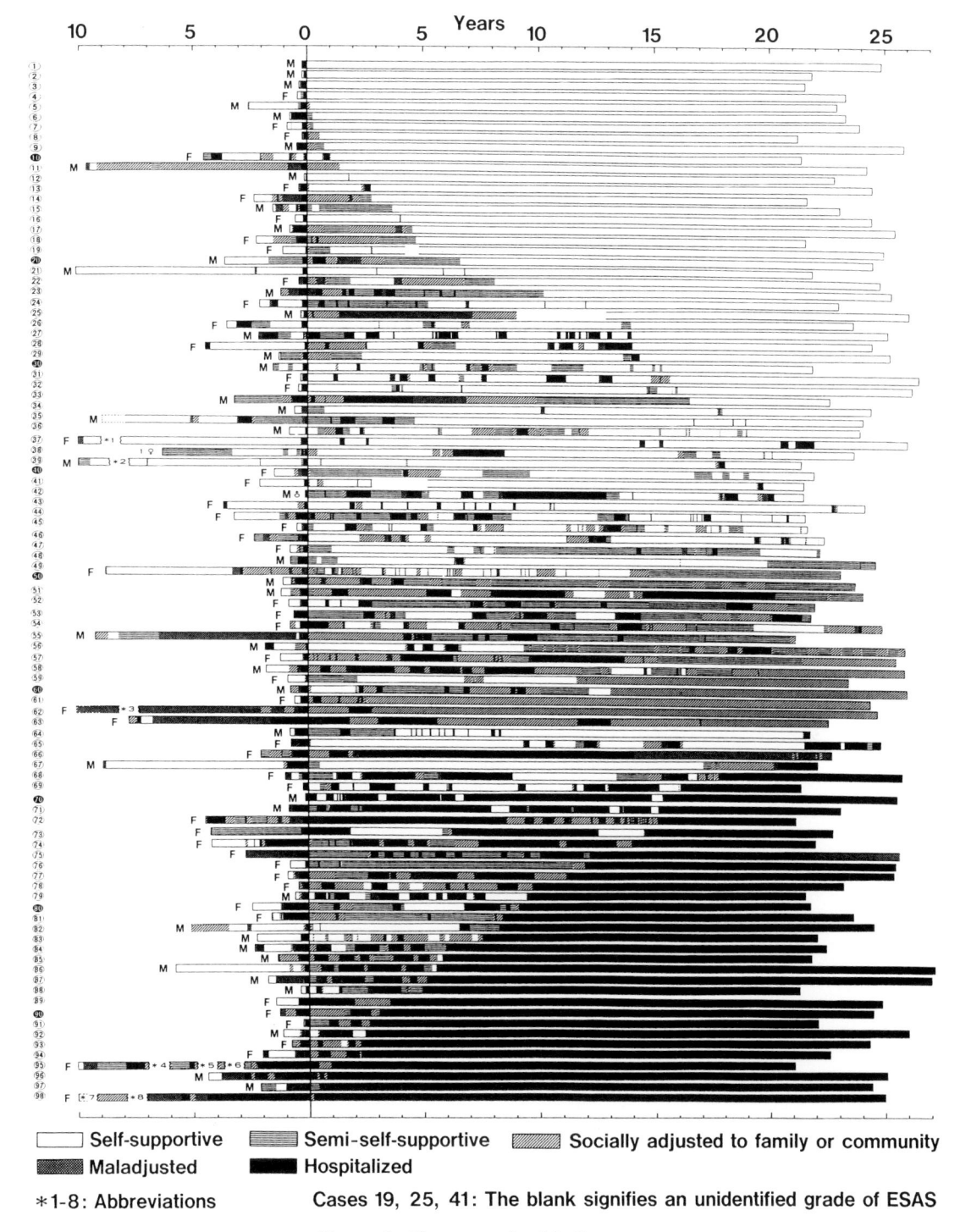

Figure 1 The course of social adjustment

精神障害者の権利と予防
―当事者の立場から精神障害の予防への期待―

Patients' right and prevention of psychiatric disorders

大島アヤノ*

　私は，今年，2001年の1月から，障害を持ちながらも自立と納得のいく社会参加を目指す『ふれあいセンター』の所長になりました。

　『ふれあいセンター』は精神科に通院する仲間が中心となって運営する活動センターで有限会社『ふれあい工場』と精神障害者小規模作業所『ふれあい広場』，グループホーム『ふれあい』を併せ持っています。有限会社『ふれあい工場』の取締役社長も精神科に通院する仲間です。精神科に通院しながらも，安心して働ける場と安らぎの場，生活の場が保障されることで再発予防の可能性が広がるのではないかと思います。

　第1回日本国際精神障害予防会議が開催された6月23日は，沖縄戦の終った日の『慰霊の日』ですが，私にとっても，この6月は10年前に発病した頃の時期で，この壇上に立っていることじたい複雑な心境でした。

　しかし，この壇上に立てるようになるまでに至る経験と当事者の立場から精神障害の予防への期待を述べさせていただきたいと思います。

　私は10年前の20歳のときに発病しました。私には知的障害を持つ兄と妹がいますが，母は私が小学校の頃に亡くなりました。男手一つで苦労しながら育ててきた父にとって，私の発病は大変なショックだったかと思います。

　でも発病した当時は自分のことで精一杯で，父の苦労を受け止める余裕はありませんでした。その頃は，落ち着きが無く不安定な毎日を過ごしていました。昼間でも何の目的もなく家の近所を行ったり来たりして，目はうつろで，話もしないという状態だったので，周囲の人からは，いかにも気ちがいになっていると思われ，子どもたちは，石を投げたりしてからかうか，すぐ逃げ出していくか，という状態でした。

　周囲からのそんな目が続いているうちにも，私が自分の方からあいさつをするようになれば，周りの人の私を見る目は変わってくるだろうと思って，自分から，あいさつをするようにしました。そんな私を見て，最初はみんなびっくりしていたけど，毎日それをやっていくうちに，みんなも私に対し理解を示してくれるようになり，私もだんだんと会話ができるようになっていきました。

　しかし，そうしているのもつかの間，私が23歳～25歳にかけて，よく眠れるから，調子がいいから，ということで，自分の勝手な判断で薬を飲むのをやめてしまいました。再び調子を崩してしまったのは，それからです。25歳のときには，誇大妄想や幻聴に惑わされて深夜徘徊をしたり，高価な車を買おうとしたり，気分はハイテンションになってしまいました。それを心配した私の家族がいろいろな医療機関を一緒にたずね歩き，現在通院しているクリニックから『ふれあいセンター』を紹介されました。

　父に連れられて初めて参加したのは『ふれあいセンター』が運営する『那覇のつどい』でした。その日の『那覇のつどい』が現在の夫・清正との初めての出会いでした。

　その日の出会いをきっかけに親しくなり，お互いの悩みや夢を語り合い，励まし合うようになりました。

　『ふれあいセンター』に通い始めた最初の頃の私は落ち着きがなくて，みんなに迷惑をかけていました。そんな私をなんとか落ち着かせようと，話し相手になってくれたのも清正でした。彼は，休みの日なども一緒に遊びに行ったりしてくれました。彼とそんなお付き合いをしているうちに，

私たちは結婚を考えるようになりました。「結婚」というと，とても大変なことなので，家族や医療機関の職員などから猛反対をされました。

しかし，私たちの結婚について話し合う家族会議が開かれた結果，私たちは結婚し，子どもを産んで育てることになりました。『ふれあいセンター』のなかにグループホームもあって，皆の支えがあったことも決心させた要因でした。『ふれあいセンター』のグループホームには1996年の10月に入居しました。いつでも周りに仲間がいることはとても安心でした。

しかしそれでも，私の中には子どもを産みたいという気持ちがある一方で，産んで育てることができるかな，という不安な気持ちも続いていて，妊娠期間は時々調子をくずして変な行動をとったりしたこともありましたが，夫の清正や仲間たちに励まされ，薬も飲みつづけながら，出産までなんとかがんばることができました。

そして，1997年の3月14日，長男の清隆を出産しました。出産のときは陣痛が痛くて耐えきれなくて泣きわめいていたけれど，産まれてきた我が子を見ると，ホッとしました。

『ふれあいセンター』はお互いの必要性でいろんな役割を生み出しますが，清隆の誕生で，「乳児保育班」も出来ました。子育てを体験した仲間たちや将来の勉強にと赤ちゃんの好きな仲間たちが率先して「乳児保育班」に加わりました。

私自身は子育てが初めてなので，息子が産まれたばかりの頃は育児の不安などが重なり，幾度か調子をくずして泣いたり，自分が子どものようになって幼児返りをしたり，急に遠いところへでかけて行方不明になったりすることもありました。それでも『ふれあいセンター』の乳児保育班の仲間や清正や父の手を借りながら，四苦八苦しながらもなんとか育児を続けることができ，息子の清隆もすくすくと育ち，4歳になりました。今は『ふれあいセンター』の「保育園送迎班」の協力で保育園に通うようになりました。保育園に通うようになってからの清隆は，大変なおしゃべりやさんで，『ふれあいセンター』のなかでも，ムードメーカーとなっています。

また，子どもの成長と共に私自身も成長したようで，最近では毎日の夕食も自分で作れるようになりました。今は，子どもとの会話の中で「今日のごはんなに？」と聞かれるのが何より嬉しく思います。息子もだんだんとしっかりしてくれて，母親である私に「くすりのんだ？」と聞いたりするときには，私も「あー，そうだった，飲み忘れていた」ということもでてきました。子育てや結婚となると大変な事もいろいろありますが，私にとっては，生きがいとなっています。これからも，家族のためにも，再発予防のためにも，『ふれあいセンター』での活動を大切にしたいと思います。仲間たちとの貴重な語り合いの場である『つどい』への参加を大切にして行きたいと思います。所長としての力量も，生まれたばかりの赤ちゃんのようなもので，不安だらけではありますが，息子の成長と共に，私自身も成長していきたいと願っています。

これまで『ふれあいセンター』と共に歩んできての私の感想ですが，たとえ障害を持っていても，お互いにはげまし合える仲間がいて，少し支えてくれる伴走者がいてくれれば，自立と納得のいく社会参加は可能だと思います。

---

*ふれあいセンター所長
　Ayano Oshima : Fureai Center.

精神障害者地域生活支援と予防
―作業所，グループホームでの再発予防と地域づくり―

Support for patients' daily life in workshops and group homes

石川英五郎*

　グループ・オアシスは東京・江東区にあり，5つの作業所と2つのグループホームで構成され約100名の精神障害をもつ人たちが利用している。またソーシャルクラブ(「就労」と「生活」の2グループ)やクラブハウスを夕方，休日に開催し，OB等や作業所の利用を中断している者への対応も行っている。(表1を参照)

　作業所やグループホームは精神障害者の地域生活の重要な場の一つである。利用者の生活支援を進めるうえで，再発予防は大切な課題である。しかし再発を恐れるあまり，リスクを避け，失敗しないように狭く判で押したような生活を彼らに求めることはどうであろうか。人生には目標や夢が必要であり，自分が役に立つこと，達成できること，生きがいがあることなどが大切である。私たちは，利用者が抱える様々なストレスをただ排除するよりも，利用者のストレスを受けとめ，乗り越えるための手段をともに検討することを重視し，利用者が困難に立ち向かえるよう生活全般を支援してきた。

　また作業所やグループホームは，利用者にとって安心して「失敗できる場」「失敗を語れる場」としての機能があり，私たちはこれを重要と考えている。利用者はここでの失敗の体験を通して，失敗を最小限にすること，失敗したときの乗り越え方などを個人的に経験学習することに留まらず，利用者集団にとって「仲間の経験」として普遍化され教訓化されることにもなっている。

　2つのソーシャルクラブは「就労」と「生活」の二部門で運営され，作業所OBを含む企業就労者と就労希望者(求職者)，単身生活者等が参加している。ここでも失敗経験の交流が行われ，そのなかから「成功」を指向しようとしている。それ

表1　グループ・オアシスの事業と設立年

〈共同作業所〉	
オアシス第2	(1983-)
リサイクルショップ・オアシス	(1986-)
オアシス第4	(1988-)
オアシス・プランニング	(1993-)
オアシス第3	(1998-)
〈グループホーム〉	
クローバーハウス	(1996-)
第2クローバーハウス	(1998-)
〈ソーシャルクラブ〉	
「就労」グループ	(1986-)
「生活」グループ	(1989-)
クラブハウス	(1999-)

ぞれのグループは機関紙をもち，就労や生活の実際，困難の乗り越え方，危機回避の方法，ちょっとしたつまづきや大失敗の体験を朗々と伝えている。表2に示したものは，2つのグループが参加者の失敗の体験から導き出したもので，「就労」「生活」するための3原則である。

　5つの作業所での労働活動だが，下請け受注作業のほか，木工玩具製作，ステンドグラスやビーズを使ったアクセサリー製作，ステンシル染めの袋物製作，パソコンによるデータ入力と軽印刷，宅配便の配達代行，昼食づくりなど多岐にわたっている。利用者は作業所と労働活動の選択が可能である。なかには工作機械を使用したり，接客技術が必要とされるものもあり，多くの作業所にとって敬遠されるような種目が見あたるかも知れない。しかし当グループの場合，利用者に仕事をあわせるようにして少しずつ種目を広げてきたというのが実際のところである。労働活動のなかには困難が多い仕事もある。また納期に迫られ猛烈に手指を動かさなければならない時もある。利用者には役割と責任が強調されることがありストレス

表2

「就労」するための3原則
①誰にでも，気軽に，無理なく，少しだけ背伸びをして可能となる就労を
②入院覚悟の就労ではなく，悪化する前にいさぎよく離職を
③離職しても胸を張って作業所に戻れるようなゆたかな就労を

「生活」するための3原則
①誰にでも，気軽に，無理なく，少しだけ背伸びして可能となる生活を
②すべてにおいて，いまより悪くならないという生活のペースを築く
③出来ないことにも胸を張り，ときにうそぶいて，くよくよしない生活を

表3

5作業所合同自治会活動
● リーダー（自治会長）会
● 作業主任会
● 工賃会計センター（専従配置）
● スポーツ担当者会
● 行事レク担当者会
● ボーナス捻出活動実行委員会
● 夏季旅行実行委員会
● バレーボール大会実行委員会

も生じやすい。しかし，それだけではない。こうした労働活動を通して，良質の製品を完成させたこと，協力しあい目標を達成できたこと，あるいは励ましあい助けあって困難を乗り越えたことなど，このような体験の蓄積は，利用者の健康を支えるための大切な要素と考えている。

自治活動は労働活動と同様に大切な利用者の活動である。5つの作業所には表3のような活動・組織があり，各作業所から選ばれた利用者で構成されている。自治活動は労働活動以上に役割や責任が伴う。例えば，工賃（時給）額の決定や管理。ボーナス捻出活動においては年2回300～400万円の財源を物品販売の売り上げなどから捻出しなければならない。また行事の企画立案なども大変にストレスフルなものである。しかし作業所の主体は何よりも利用者である。そのためには彼らが思考し判断すること，そして行動し自ら困難を切りひらいていかなければならないと考える。私たちは利用者とともに悩み，ともに考え，ともに歩むようにして，これら自治的活動への支援を行なっている。

一方，地域に対しては，職親の開拓や集団アルバイト等の雇用の実現，リサイクルショップの運営やボーナス資金捻出のための活動等，利用者と地域住民や企業との接点を広げる活動を行なってきた。これらの活動もまた利用者とスタッフが中心となって実施している。このような地域に向けられた活動は市民との協力共同で実現し，地域における利用者の可能性を広げ社会参加を具体化するものである。利用者が「ごく普通に地域で働き暮らしていける」には，地域市民との接点がなくては実現しないものである。私たちは利用者が困難に立ち向かえるように生活全般を支援し，そんな利用者の社会参加を一市民として受けとめる地域づくりを重視し活動してきた。

支援の実際について4事例を以下に紹介する。

事例A：男性　43歳　（クラブハウス）

最初の就労先での人間関係でつまずき発症に至る。以後，些細なことで傷つき，人との接触を断ち自宅に引きこもる。その結果，再発再入院を長く繰り返していた。30代後半より作業所の利用を開始するが利用者との人間関係で悩み利用を中断。援助者は「週に1度，短時間のクラブハウス利用」を提案。「これ以上人間関係で傷つき自信を失いたくない」と言いながらも「入院するよりはいい」とクラブハウスの利用を選択する。

クラブハウスでは他の利用者の言動に怯えている様子も見られ，また作業所利用時よりもさらに苦手なタイプの利用者がいると利用継続に不安をのぞかせていた。援助者は「たくさん傷ついてもいい。傷つくことに慣れよう。傷ついてもなるべく速く回復しよう」と提案。その後も人間関係での緊張は強く，傷つきながらも援助者と相談しながら利用を継続。次第に他の利用者との会話も多くなり，苦手とされた利用者には自ら進んで声をかけるようになった。同時に訴えも「傷つけられた」から「（自分の言動が他者を）傷つけてしまったのではないか」に変化していった。また「入退院を繰り返すだけの人生にしたくない」と言い，

援助者はこの言葉を支持し「まず簡単に出来ることで有意義なことを目標に置こう」と提案した。その後，目標を作業所復帰に具体化。「仕事が忙しいときは役に立たないかも知れないが遠慮なく声をかけてほしい」と話してくれたことから作業所復帰が実現。現在は"ピンチヒッター"として通所日数は少ないながらも存在感があり，作業所利用者との交流も徐々に深まっている。

　　事例B：女性　50歳　（グループホーム）
　事務職をしていた20代に発症。以後，数カ所の企業で働くがいずれも疲労をつのらせ退職と同時に入院。家庭では家族への依存が強く，家庭での役割はまったくなかった。困難を目前にしたり，あるいは軽い失敗を重々しくとらえて状態悪化，入院を繰り返していた。両親亡き後の生活を考慮し45歳でグループホームに入居となった。
　ホーム入居後は，他の女性入居者を意識し，調理，洗濯，清掃などを負けずに行おうとするが，気持ちだけが空回りして混迷。入院や退居を希望し床に伏すこととなった。援助者は「周りを気にせず自分のペースで疲れないように生活する」ことを提案するが，他者の評価が気になり，必要以上に頑張り過ぎて疲れ果ててしまうことが度々あった。そんなときホームのミーティングで男性入居者から「自分は何一つ満足な料理が作れない」と話しかけられ，「私だって満足な料理は一つも作れない」と応答したことから「気持ちがすごく楽になった」という。その後，「これまで何もしてこなかった。だから上手くいかなくて当たり前」と割り切り，こつこつと様々なことにチャレンジすることになった。ときには大きな失敗もあり落ち込みもするが，入院や退居を口にすることはなくなった。小さな失敗は笑い話にして入居者同士の「失敗経験交流」に活かされ，現在もホームでの生活を継続している。

　　事例C：男性　45歳　（ソーシャルクラブ／「生活」グループ）
　20年間の入院を経て，退院後は単身アパート生活，次いで作業所利用となった。新たな生活への適応は難しく，入院生活とのギャップに苦しんでいた。とくにアパート生活では近隣住民との間に様々なトラブルを抱え，なかでも訪問販売，勧誘などは生活を脅かす敵としてとらえるあまり，トラブルに発展した際には警察の介入が必要とされることもあった。そのため援助者は生活上の困難を語り合える場としてのソーシャルクラブ「生活」部門への参加を勧め，これに本人は同意した。
　ソーシャルクラブでの話し合いでは「もう二度と入院したくない」と発言する一方，他の参加者の提案や助言を受け入れず「自分は何も困っていない」と言い続けた。他者からの提案や助言は自分を否定するものととらえ頑なであった。その後数カ月間グループでの話し合いは平行線をたどるが，生活面はグループでの提案や助言を少しずつ生活に取り入れはじめ，穏やかでトラブルのないものに変わっていった。現在は生活を安定させ，逆に困っていること，悩みや不安を積極的にグループに相談している。またグループに参加した当初のことを振り返り次のように話している。
　……20年間も入院して，病気だから仕方がないと言われたことはあったけど，あなたの健康を信じて言うんだよと言われたことはなかった。グループに参加していなかったら病気のままで生きていくしかなかった。

　　事例D：男性　58歳　（作業所・自治会長）
　家庭での本人への評価は極めて低く，作業所利用についても，企業への就労についても否定的であった。家族に対しては何も言えず従うだけ，ダメな人間と言われ続け，八方ふさがりで，何をやっても変わらないというあきらめの態度が強く，目的なく作業所を利用していた。しかし作業所への通所は安定し，もともと真面目な性格であったこともあり，他の利用者の信望を集め2年前の作業所自治会役員改選の際には自治会長に選出された。
　当初は自治会長という役割が重く，また自信もなく投げやりであった。5つの作業所の自治会長が集う会議では「話しあうだけ無駄。作業所に戻って下請け仕事をしている方がみんなのためになる」と発言していた。しかし他の作業所の自治会

長と交流するうちに,自分の所属する作業所の自治システムに疑問を抱き,少しずつ意見を示すようになった。その後,それらの意見が支持されて,行事を実施するための財源の確保,利用者に支払われる工賃の時給額の改定,年2回の利用者ボーナスに家族手当等を付加することなどが次々と検討されることになった。いずれも全利用者にアンケート等で意見を求めるなど困難な作業ではあったが,そのときの彼は「自分が何か言えば仕事が湧いて出てくる。少し発言をひかえた方がいいかも」と言いながらも楽しそうであった。

そうして自分の発言をきっかけに自治会運営が改善。これを機に作業所生活は意欲的になった。

58歳という年齢からも,すべての場面でリーダーシップを発揮できるわけではないが,周囲の利用者には「みんなが発言し行動すれば作業所は変わる」と呼びかける。そのときの利用者の反応はそれに響き応えるものでなく,沈黙も多い。このことに彼はしばしば落胆するが,そんなときは他の作業所の自治会長たちが彼を支えている。これにより彼は自らの役割を忘れることなく,さらに機能しようと努力を続けることができる。

---

*東京江東区グループオアシス
　Eigoro Ishikawa : Group Oasis（Koto-ku, Tokyo）

医療機関と地域の連携
―地域における精神障害の予防と医療の役割―
Dynamism between mental hospitals and community

蟻塚　亮二*

I. はじめに

　近年精神科リハビリテーションの進歩には目覚ましいものがあるが，大局的には未だ地域ケアシステムは貧困であり，精神疾患をかかえた人々の多くが地域福祉の対象ではなく医療の枠内つまり長期入院という形で処遇されている。言うまでもなく，日本の精神病床は34万床と，人口対比でも絶対数でも世界最大であり，人口が5,500万の英国の精神病床がおよそ3万程度であることを考えると，日本の精神医療システムは明らかに「グローバル・スタンダード」から逸脱している。日本の社会がかかえるこの隔離収容政策を欧州並のものに変えることこそが，精神疾患に対する社会的偏見を減らし，発病後の早期受診や早期治療を促進し，この会議の目的を達成することに寄与するのではないか。

　また国際的な視点から精神分裂病の予後を比較すると，発展途上国の方が先進国つまり高度工業化社会よりも回復の予後が良い。英国の精神医療の歴史をみても工業化が進む時に精神病床が増大した。つまり高度工業化社会は，精神障害をもつ人にとって特有の「生きにくさ」をもっている。この点からも日本の精神医療や福祉をグローバル・スタンダードに則して変革することは21世紀日本社会の課題の一つであろう。

　さて，病院は地域資源の中で精神障害をもつ人々を支える社会資源の一つでしかなく，当事者のニーズのごく一部に応えているにすぎない。決して，医療を提供することにより当事者のニーズの多くを満たしていると思ってはいけない。むしろ医療関係者は，地域で生活する当事者の視点でニーズを総合的に把握し，あるいはライフサイクルに応じて変動する当事者のニーズや主観的満足度を正確に把握して病院の役割を考える必要がある。そして作業所や保健所，家族会などの地域資源を支援しなければならない。

II. 病院と医療に求められるもの

　1）地域ケアシステムが成立するために病院の果たす役割をあげると，救急，再発を防ぐ外来診療，デイケアなどのリハビリテーション，長期入院患者の退院促進，短期間で質の良い入院医療の提供，他の地域資源との連携や可能な限りの支援などであろう。そして精神科病院の役割をこのようにコンパクトな内容に限定するとおのずから病院の規模は小さくなるであろう。

　2）まず精神科救急システムであるが，これは地域ケアシステムを支える必要条件である。これは精神科救急輪番病院制度により一定度解決されつつある。しかしその制度により入院したとしてもその病院の医療の質により，あるいは地域の支援システムの水準によっては入院が長期化する可能性もあるのが問題である。英国では救急による入院期間は4日ないし1週間程度と聞いたが，地域システムが整備されていればこその話であろう。あるいは南ストックホルムのある地域では人口30万のキャッチメント・エリアを6つに分けてそれぞれの地域に外来診療所を設け，そこに7床程度のベッドをおいて再発時の入院治療に対応していたが，ここも入院期間は1週間程度と短かった。以上のように日本の救急システムはまだまだ改善の余地があると思われる。繰り返しになるが，地域ケアシステムの水準と入院期間とは密接に関連している。

　3）退院した人の再発を防止する点について言

うと，まず発病後10年以内の再発率が高いこと，そして10年以内の再発の80％が発病後5年以内に集中することを念頭におく必要がある。再発したことにより逆にその経験を学習の機会として生かし，それ以後定期的な服薬を順守する態度に変わられる人もおられるので，一概に再発を悪いとは考えないが，薬についての情報を十分伝え，薬をのむ当事者と相談しながら最適な処方内容を作るという共同作業は不可欠の課題である。またデポ剤を使いこなす技術も医療側には欠かせない。ただしいわゆる維持薬物療法に関して言うと，まだ未開拓の分野であると言える。急性期に用いる向精神薬の標的は症状の鎮静である。これに対して外来での投薬つまり維持薬物療法の目標は再発の防止であり，急性期と再発防止目的とでは同じ薬物療法でもその目的あるいはコンセプトは全く異なる。しかし再発防止のためにはどの薬がいいのか，どの程度の量が最低必要であるかといった研究は全くなされていない。米国のある研究ではクロルプロマジン50mgを最低維持量としていた。しかしそれぞれの患者さんを取り巻く環境によってストレスの強さが異なり，かつストレス脆弱性にも個人差がある以上，一律に最低薬物量を決めることは出来ない。臺弘先生によると，再発は病的条件反射であり，従って条件反射回避作用の強いハロペリドールが再発防止に向いているとのことであるが，最近市販された非定型抗精神病薬も含めて維持薬物療法については急性期対応とは別の角度から検討されねばならない。また米国で論議を呼んでいるように抗精神病薬と耐糖能低下との関係や，長期使用による遅発性ジスキネジアとの関係についても考慮が必要である。

4）次に，デイケアは明らかに再発率を低下させ障害の度合いを軽減させる効果はあるが，デイケアをやめると再発率が元に戻るというのが今後の問題であろう。これをデイケアの問題と考えるか，それともデイケア以後の地域生活支援システムの問題と考えるか。筆者としては地域システムの問題と考え，その充実が必要だと考える。また，かつて英国で1960年代の初めに全国のデイケアの必要数を算出した試みがあったが，我が国でも一定人口あたりに必要な数のデイケアを計画配置する必要があろう。精神保健福祉法はそのような政策的な側面に欠けていると言わねばならない。また僻地などにおいてはケンブリッジで行っていたと聞いたが，自動車に必要な道具を乗せて出掛ける「移動デイケア」のような試みも我が国で試されていいと思う。

5）長期入院患者の退院促進について言うと，新たな長期入院者を作らないことと，既に長期入院している人の退院を目指す活動がある。最近筆者は複数の病院を渡り歩いて合計43年間もの長きにわたり入院を続けていた男性を援護寮に退院させた。あるいは19年間入院していた女性を昨年退院させたが，いずれの場合もいったん援護寮に入所という形で退院となっている。もしも援護寮という中間的な住居がなかったならばそれらは不可能であっただろう。因に援護寮開設と同時に退院・入所した2年以上の長期入院患者8名のうち6名が円満に退所してグループホームもしくは市内のアパートで生活している。

また退院に向けて準備する際には，地域で生活するために必要なスキルを出来るだけ具体的に絞り込んで，退院へのハードルを低くする必要がある。つまり「目標限定的アプローチ」が有効である。例えば，服薬通院が出来，電気釜でご飯を炊け，洗濯機を回すことができて，いざという時にSOSを出す能力があり，自分の症状を一定度セルフコントロール出来る人なら，たとえ幻聴があろうが妄想があろうがそれらによる行動化さえなければ退院とするべきである。症状いかんでなく生活能力が問題であり，かつ生活能力も具体的な内容で絞り込んだものを獲得目標とするなら，退院は難しくない。問題は患者と治療者のやる気である。

6）最後に，地域資源及び草の根運動への支援と自発的な参加は病院関係者の無条件の義務だと思う。もう十数年前に私は授産施設設立の運動に参加したことがある。その時に福祉の心というのは医療と違うと思った。医療は一定の基準をクリアーする事を求められる。従ってある程度の資金がないと新しい施設などは作れない。たとえ民間病院であるにしても病院職員の考えはいささか硬直的・官僚的にならざるをえない。これに対し福

祉というものは資金があろうがなかろうが「必要だから作る」のだと思った。核になって先頭を走る人がいれば金は後からついてくるものである。働く場所を作る運動に参加してもう一つの収穫は私のそれまでの医師としての姿勢が全く一人相撲でしかないと痛感させられたことである。授産施設という新しい環境を得て，患者さんたちは表情も症状もみるみる変わり，つくづく「参加する場面」を彼らに提供しないで，病院という場面だけで働きかけていたことが間違いだった事を知った。いま人口17万の私たちの地域には，授産施設が2つ，福祉工場が1つ，作業所が3つ，グループホームが4つ，援護寮と福祉ホームが1つ，そして高齢者を含む単身生活者のための宅配弁当屋が1つ，地域生活支援センターが2つ，雇用支援センターが1つと社会資源が増えた。つまり地域で利用出来る社会資源とその選択肢が増えた。すると病院における医療内容も変わる。病院スタッフの考え方も無理のないものに変わる。つまり，社会資源が乏しい状況で患者さんを退院させようとすると，必然的に患者さんに高い水準の生活能力を求めざるをえなくなる。地域に利用出来る資源が増えれば，患者さんに求められる生活能力，つまり患者さんへの要求は無理のないものになり退院へのハードルは低くなる。病院が病院らしくなれるのは，地域ケアシステムの整備による。医療関係者はすべからく，地域草の根運動に支援もしくは参加することにより，自分と病院とを変えることが出来るのである。従ってそれは医療関係者の義務である。

III. 最後に

最近大阪でおきた多数の小学生への殺人という悲惨な事件にひどい衝撃を受け，英国における「犯罪を犯した精神障害者のリハビリテーション」について読み直した。英国の制度がすべて良いとは思わなかったが，一人の女性が犯罪を繰り返したあげく，持続的な支援のもとで地域に帰り，結婚し，子供ができ，しかし母として悩み，それをまた援助し続けるというケース記録を読んでいたく感動した。そして，いわゆる「触法精神障害者」と言われる人たちへの対応が氷山の一角だとすれば，氷山の目に見えない水面下の部分での対応，つまり犯罪と何の関係もない人達への地域ケアシステムの充実があってこそ，そのような対応が可能なのだろうと思った。従って「触法精神障害者」への「対策」は決して氷山の目に見える部分だけへの小手先の問題として扱われるべきではなく，精神障害を抱えつつ地域で生きるすべての人達への地域ケアシステムの整備充実を基本目標に据えて，考えられるべきであろう。そのためにも単なる「入院手続き法」の色彩の強い精神保健福祉法ではなく，もっと政策的な内容を充実させ，もはや国際的にも主流となっているキャッチメント・エリア方式を基本とし，必要な社会資源を計画的に配置するべきだと思う。

財政の視点から見ると，ドイツのデータでは入院している人が地域に必要な住居などの社会資源を作って退院した時に，地域で生活する時の費用は入院に比べてその43％に低下するという。例えば青森県と宮城県の精神科入院医療費を比較すると，精神分裂病で外来通院している人の割合は宮城県が70％強，青森県が58％程度なので，人口が青森県の1.5倍の宮城県の方が青森県よりも入院医療費の絶対額が少ない。つまり作業所やグループホームなどを自治体が率先して作り，長期入院の人達を退院させた方が国民健康保険財政は好転するのである。また平成12年度版の厚生白書によると，それぞれの産業の二次的経済的波及効果は，農業が1.3倍，建設業が1.9倍であるのに対し，福祉や社会保障の場合には2.3倍に上るとされている。以上のような点からも，地域ケアシステムを整備充実したほうが良い社会を作ることができる。

障害をもつ人達が安心して生きることができる社会は障害のない人にも優しい社会であり，犯罪の少ない社会であろう。障害に伴う社会的不利の少ない社会を作ることができれば，障害への偏見の少ない社会を作ることができる。

＊藤代健生病院
　Ryoji Aritsuka, M. D. : Fujishiro-Kensei Hospital.

日本における精神障害に対する早期介入と予防

Early intervention and prevention of psychiatric disorders in Japan

山本　和儀*

I. Characteristics of mental health and psychiatric care in Japan

Historically, legal protection of persons with psychiatric disorders in Japan was started by the Mentally Ill Custody Act in 1900. However, developments of mental health services has been slow and insufficient. Recent frequent amendments of the Mental Health and Welfare Act have encouraged the protection of human rights of persons with mental disorders and disabilities, and integration of persons into the community. Incline from hospitalization to community based care has been seen for a few decades but it is still hospital-centered. Long-term hospitalization (average length of stay was 406.4 days in 1998) and abundant beds at private mental hospitals are one of the characteristics of mental health and psychiatric care in Japan.

Currently, there are 358,609 psychiatric beds served by 1,670 mental hospitals for 126,487,000 inhabitants in Japan (Ministry of Health and Welfare, 2000). The ratio of psychiatric beds per 10,000 people was 28.4 in 1999 and the figure is ten to hundreds of times bigger than other countries in Asia. However, psychiatric beds in general hospital settings are scarce, and training of physicians in the detection and treatments of psychiatric disorders are also insufficient. There are also a variety of needs in mental health and welfare services according to social changes, and mental health promotion is encouraged generally, but preventative approaches in clinical settings are scarce, though lengthy in-patient treatment and rehabilitation have been insisted.

II. Preventative approach in psychiatry and mental health services in Japan

The concept of primary, secondary and tertiary prevention proposed by G. Caplan was spread among Japanese mental health professionals in the late 1960's and early 70's. However, the majority of academic research and clinical efforts for major psychiatric disorders have been focused on relapse prevention and rehabilitation (Tertiary Prevention). Few pioneers explored the possibilities of primary prevention and early intervention into schizophrenia in the 1970's and 80's. As one of the challenges for the primary prevention and early intervention into schizophrenia by the pioneers in Japan, Nakai described symptomatology of pre-morbid and acute phases of schizophrenia and raised arguments and warnings of the possibility of prevention (Nikai, 1974, 1979). Nakayasu proposed a new clinical entity, Early schizophrenia. He described four principle symptoms and research on treatment (Nakayasu, 1986, 1990). Okazaki et al. studied high risk persons for schizophrenia and discussed the strategies for primary prevention of schizophrenia (Okazaki, 1990). Systematic clinical trials for primary prevention and early intervention of psychosis were commenced by a few pioneer groups from several years ago in Japan.

Early detection of pre-psychotic university students and follow ups for indicated prevention and secondary prevention were started at the health administrative center of the University of the Ryukyus in 1995 (Nakamoto, 1997; Ogura, 1998). The methodology adopted by the group includes:

screening using questionnaires which include GHQ-30, the Chapman's Psychosis Proneness scale, SPQ (Schizotypal Personality Questionnaire) and structured interviews with SCID-II for schizotypal personality disorders (DSM-III-R), Brief Psychiatric Rating Scale and Event-Related Potentials Recording (Nakamoto, 1997 ; Ogura, 1998, 2000). Another clinical trial using MMPI was started at Toyama medical pharmaceutical college in 1997. These activities brought the first step in development of academic enthusiasm in prevention and early Intervention in psychiatric disorders.

III. Establishment of academic field of prevention in psychiatric disorders in Japan

A symposium chaired by Ogura and Kato, on the possibility of primary prevention of schizophrenia was held at the 18th annual conference of Japanese Society of Social Psychiatry in Okinawa in 1996. Among four contributors, Niwa reviewed the stand point of prevention, on the mechanism of cognitive-behavioral disorders leading to schizophrenia and neurophysiological findings indicating cognitive disorders (impairments) in schizophrenia (Niwa, 1997). Okazaki discussed the feasibility of primary prevention of schizophrenia implied by high-risk and related epidemiological studies (Okazaki, 1997). Nakamoto introduced their clinical research trial for early intervention and prevention of psychiatric disorders among students at the University of the Ryukyus (Nakamoto, 1997). As the only foreign guest speaker, McGorry from the University of Melbourne, Australia proposed a framework and strategies for prevention in Early psychosis (McGorry, 1997). He also introduced the positive outcome of the early intervention project at the EPPIC, Melbourne which was started in the public sector and spread state-wide and interstate.

A preparatory meeting of the Japanese Society of Prevention of Psychiatric Disorders (JSPPD) was held just after the closing of the symposium on the same premises and the 1st academic meeting of the JSPPD was held during the 19th annual conference of the Japanese Society of Social Psychiatry in Tokyo in 1997 (Figure). The 2nd, 3rd and 4th academic meetings were held in Takamatsu, 1998, Fukushima, 1999, and Tokyo, 2000 respectively. The 5th academic meeting of JSPPD was held as the First Japan International Conference on Early Intervention and Prevention in Psychiatric Disorders in Okinawa in 2001 for the first time in Asia. Before the conference, a publication of a special volume on Prevention of Psychiatric disorders in the Encyclopedia of Clinical Psychiatry series was launched in 2000. The book, edited by Ogura and Kurachi is comprehensive and contains four chapters for general remarks and eighteen chapters for itemized particular discussions by 52 contributers, from prevention of Alzheimer's disease to prevention of school bullying.

Figure   News letter for JSPPD

Conclusion

Japan started the studies on primary prevention

of psychiatric disorders 3 decades ago and leads this area in Asia. However, it practically remains as academic research trials. In order for Japanese psychiatry to change to the early intervention and prevention model, from the rehabilitation model, there needs to be a strong commitment from psychiatric hospitals because these hospitals are currently seen as the center for psychiatric resource and services. The primary care psychiatry models which were adopted by developing and developed countries, for detecting psychiatric disorders in primary health care settings is also considered relevant in Japan due to the high prevalence of psychiatric disorders among patients with physical disorders.

References

1) Ministry of Health and Welfare : Handbook of Mental Health and Welfare Japan 2000, Kouken Shuppan, Tokyo, 2000 (in Japanese)
2) Nakai, H. : The process of onset and distraction thereafter. B. Kimura ed. Psychopathplogy of schizophrenia Vol. 3., Tokyo University Press, Tokyo, 1974 (in Japanese)
3) Nakai, H. : Strange murmur and jostle - on the specific term directory prior to clinical onset. H. Nakai ed. Psychopathology of schizophrenia-Vol.8., Tokyo University Press, Tokyo, 1979 (in Japanese)
4) Nakayasu, N. : Early symptoms of schzophrenic Schub -on the easily over-looked fine symptoms. Psychiatric therapeutics, 1 ; 545-546, 1986 (in Japanese)
5) Nakayasu, N. : Early schizophrenia. Seiwa Shoten, Tokyo, 1990 (in Japanese)
6) Niwa, S. : A view on the mechanism leading to schzophrenia from the stand point of prevention.Japanese Bulletin of Social Psychiatry, 5 ; 224-227, 1997 (in Japanese)
7) Ogura, C. : Prevention in schizophrenia - from a dream to practicable planning. Psychiatria et neurologia japonica, 100(8) ; 501-506, 1998 (in Japanese)
8) Ogura C. : Prevention of psychiatric disorders. C. Ogura & M.Kurach eds. Prevention of Psychiatric disorders in the Encyclopedia of Clinical Psychiatry series special issue No. 3 ; 3-11, Nakayama shoten, Tokyo, 2000 (in Japanese)
9) Okazaki, Y. : Research on persons with the high-risk for schizophrenia. Encyclopedia of Modern Psychiatry Year Book 89-A, Nakayama shoten, Tokyo, 1990 (in Japanese)
10) Okazaki, Y. : The feasibility of primary prevention of schizophrenia implied by high-risk and related epidemiological studies. Japanese Bulletin of Social Psychiatry, 5 ; 228-237, 1997 (in Japanese)
11) McGorry P. : Strategies for prevention in early psychosis : A framework and strategies. Japanese Bulletin of Social Psychiatry, 5 ; 242-247, 1997 (in Japanese)
12) Nakamoto, H. & Arakaki, H. : Clinical research on early intervention in students vulnerable for schizophrenia. Japanese Bulletin of Social Psychiatry, 5 ; 238-241, 1997 (in Japanese)

---

*琉球大学医学部精神神経学講座
Kazuyoshi Yamamoto : Department of Neuropsychiatry, University of the Ryukyus.

学生の精神保健：台湾における精神障害に対する早期介入と予防
Students' mental health : The early intervention and prevention of mental disorders in Taiwan

Eng-Kung Yeh*

College students are a highly selected group of the society. The study of mental health problems of students in terms of early intervention and prevention of mental disorders has thus been the subject of study with increasing attention in recent years. Two studies conducted by Yeh and his colleagues during the 1960s and 70s in Taiwan are reported in this conference.

Study I : "An epidemiological study of students' mental health"

This is a longitudinal study conducted in an university in Taipei City during 1963-1967 (1).

Background

Under the National Joint Examination System (NJES) all universities and colleges in Taiwan cannot enroll their own freshmen independently. All the freshmen are assigned by the committee under the Ministry of Education to the particular department or school according to the students' order or preference and the records they made in the 2-day nationwide joint examination. The higher the record they achieved in the examination the greater the opportunity they are admitted to the school they applied with higher priority. Thus, the mental health problems of the newly enrolled students are totally unknown to every university health authorities.

Specific aims of study

To find out : (1) psychiatric morbidity among freshmen, (2) validity of case-finding and case-predicting tools, (3) factors related with high risk of psychiatric morbidity, (4) relationship between academic achievement and psychiatric morbidity, and (5) the changes of psychiatric morbidity during 4 years of college experiences.

Methods

All the 1,137 newly enrolled students were studied by means of specifically designed mental health questionnaires and individual clinical interview at the time of entrance in 1963, and were regularly followed up every year until the time of graduation in 1967. The study was designed to estimate the proportion of psychiatric "caseness" who were in need of psychiatric care among the students rather than to make diagnosis on individual students.

Major findings

(1) Nearly one third (30.7%) of freshmen were raterable as "definite" (5.1%) and "highly probable" (25.6%) psychiatric cases according to the criteria defined by psychogeneicity, degree of impairment, and need for treatment. (2) A great majority of symptoms were psychophysiologic reaction, anxiety, depression, and much less frequently personality disorders with differences in prevalence of symptoms between sexes and domicile of origin. Female students from overseas were more venerable to environmental changes with higher rates of psychophysiologic reactions than male's students, and "Taiwanese" and "mainlanders" students. There were two psychotic cases during the freshman year. One was the relapsed case of schizophrenia, and finally dropped out in sophomore year. The other one was a paranoid disorder

of acute onset, but showed complete remission after short-term treatment. (3) Though statistically insignificant, several social and environmental variables seemed to be related to high risk of psychiatric morbidity. (4) Among the "definite" and "highly probable" psychiatric cases, 62.5% had onset of symptoms before entrance to college, out of which 16.7% was over 5 years. This meant high school years were a critical time for those psychiatric cases. (5) Prevalence rates in the freshman year did not show significant changes during the 3 later years. There were changes in manifested symptoms, namely, more psychophysiologic symptoms in the freshman year compared to more psychological, neurotic, anxiety or depressive symptoms in the senior year. This seemed to imply that four years of college experiences affected the students' coping mechanism of life events and stress. Emotional problems had seemed to become less somatized, and more expressed in psychological and neurotic terms. (6) There were favorable changes in the students' perception of their own health, physical as well as mental. Significantly more senior students rated their health to be "beyond average", and "better than in the freshman year". This was more obvious in male students than in female students. (7) There was a general trend of negative correlation between the academic achievement and psychiatric morbidity through all 8 semesters. (8) The scores of Neurotism of Maudsley Personality Inventory and Mental Health Questionnaire showed good validity in both psychiatric case-finding and case prediction. (9) The increased awareness of the importance of mental health of the students by university authority together with the increased utilization of the university health center during and after this research contributed to the development of better mental health service for the students.

Study II: "Cross-cultural adaptation of taiwanese students in the United States"

This is a series of studies conducted during the late 1960s through early 70s, a part of which was in collaboration with the Wisconsin Psychiatric Institute of the University of Wisconsin.[2-9]

Background

As overseas study became a more common experience for university graduates, stress aspects of cross-cultural adaptation, and its effects on mental health of the students during and after sojourn had received rapidly increasing attention for study.

Aims of study

To find out (1) the psychosocial background of Taiwanese students who applied for overseas study; (2) typical and unique style of their adaptation with the host and co-nationals; (3) unique features of psychiatric symptoms if any; (4) factors related with high risk for psychiatric morbidity; (5) the attitude of psychiatric help-seeking; (6) the strategies in predicting high risk students before sojourn.

Methods

All the students applied to the University of Wisconsin (UW) as well as to other universities in the US. Whoever possible were studied by means of specifically designed schedules and clinical interview before sojourn. Those who were accepted for admission to UW were regularly and intensively followed-up at the UW. All the repatriated students from UW as well as from other universities because of psychiatric illness during sojourn were examined and treated by Yeh in Taipei systematically.

Major findings

(1) Compared to graduate students at home, Taiwanese students in the US during the 60s and 70s

when these studies were carried out were the better selected group in terms of ① higher socioeconomic status of family, ② more family members and close relatives in overseas study, ③ more confident in own health and academic achievement, ④ more open to new experiences, ⑤ greater appreciation of and identification with positive aspects of American people. (2) Like most of the Asian students, social isolation from host nationals was a fact of life for Taiwanese students. They formed a strong subculture group within a university subculture. They even resisted change. These unique features of adaptation style may be understood as "*psychoeconomicis* of the adaptation of these highly task-oriented Taiwanese students in foreign cultural environment". These phenomena, which are quite opposite to what is expected of international students, may come as a surprise. (3) Furthermore, those most motivated to reach out to Americans were the most vulnerable. They expected more adaptation problems, and scored low on personality measures of adaptive capacity. Conversely, this suggested that students with favorable adaptive potential were less interested in contact with Americans. (4) There was a seasonal difference in the incident of health problems. They were predictable from the anticipated amount and nature of stresses. (5) Out of 580 students from 35 countries in the U.W. during 1966-1969, over 40 foreign students had received psychiatric treatment including hospitalization. Te diagnoses ranged from severe depression, paranoid psychoses, to milder anxiety and neurotic state. In addition to the students' personality problems, situational factors seemed to play important roles in psychotic break down. Stresses varied at difference phases in the sojourn. There was no single case of aggressive acting out and substance use disorder. (6) Once language and problems of communication were solved, there seemed to be nothing unique about psychiatric illness in foreign student population. (7) Like other Asian students, Taiwanese students came to psychiatric facilities as a desperate last resort. They were usually sent by friends involuntarily or referred by school authority. They were prone to experience psychological problems in physical terms, and expected medications, advice, and change in the environment. They were not open to verbal insight-oriented psychotherapy. Thus, more flexible methods, such as irregular attendance, short-term supportive therapy, and parrying threat to dropout, had to be adopted. (8) The importance of pr-departure study to find out high-risk students was demonstrated. Eight students out of 54 repatriated paranoid cases treated by Yeh had previous paranoid break down, and 12 other cases had disturbed behavior suggestive of paranoid or personality disorder prior to sojourn. (9) The study on returnee students from overseas study revealed that the life experiences during sojourn made the students more confident in their mental health and career development, though there were pain and loss during the time of overseas study.

Overall concluding remarks

These two studies present very similar features which are crucial in terms of early intervention and prevention of mental disorders of the university students, undergraduate at home as well as graduate students studying abroad. For the undergraduate students, mental health problems are in the "problems of the illness-prone individuals" who happen to be students, and not in the university environment. In the similar way, the mental health problems of the students in overseas study are more in the problems of the students themselves who are in cross-cultural adaptation than in the different cultural environment during sojourn. It is concluded, therefore, that the risk for mental health problem of these students can be reliably predicted from the study on the students' socioeconomic background, developmental and psychiatric history, particularly the skills and efficacy in coping with past stress.

References

1) Yeh, E. K., Chu, H. M., Ko, Y. H. et al. : Student Mental Health : An Epidemiological Study in Taiwan. Acta Psychologica Taiwanica, 14 ; 1-26, 1972.
2) Yeh, E. K. & Chu, H. M. : Who go and Who Stay : Psychosocial Background of Taiwanese Students Going For Overseas Study. Presented at the Annual Meeting of Formosan Medical Association, Nov. 1969.
3) Chu, H. M., Yeh, E. K., Klein, M. H. et al. : A study of Chinese Students' Adjustment in the USA. Acta Psychologica Taiwanica, 13 ; 206-218, 1971.
4) Klein, M. H., Alexander, A. A., Tseng, K. H. et al. : Far Eastern Students in a Big University : Subcultures within a Subculture, Bulletin of the Atomic Scientists, 27 ; 10-19, 1971.
5) Yeh, E. K. : Paranoid Manifestations Among Chinese Students Studying Abroad : Some Preliminary Findings. In W.P. Lebra (Ed.), Transcultural Research in Mental Health. Volume II of Mental Health Research in Asia and Pacific, University Press of Hawaii, pp.326-340,1972.
6) Yeh, E. K., Miller, M. H., Alexand, A. A. et al. : The American Students in Taiwan. International Study Quarterly, 17 ; 359-372, 1973.
7) Yeh, E. K. & Chu, H. M. : The Images of Chinese and American Character : Cross-cultural Adaptation by Chinese Students. In W.P. Lekra (Ed.), Youth, Socialization, and Mental Health. Volume III of Mental Health Research in Asia and Pacific, University Press of Hawaii, 1974.
8) Yeh, E. K. : Cross-cultural Adaptation and Personal Growth : the Case of Chinese Students. Acta Psychologica Taiwanica, 18 ; 95-104, 1976.
9) Yeh, E. K., Chu, H. M., Klein, M. E. et al. : Psychiatric Implications of Cross-cultural Education : Chinese Students in the United States. In S. Bochner (Ed.). The Mediating Person : Bridge Between Cultures. G.K. Hall and Co. Boston, Massachusetts, pp.136-168, 1981.

---

*Eng-Kung Yeh, M. D. : Professor Emeritus of Psychiatry, Taipei Medical University.

インドネシアにおける精神障害に対する早期介入と予防
―歴史的概観―

Eearly intervention and prevention of psychiatric disorders in Indonesia (Historical review)

Sasanto Wibisono*

Introduction

Early intervention and prevention of Psychiatric Disorders in Indonesia were reviewed from a historical and situational perspective. Early intervention and prevention are universal public health strategies suitable for most ill-health problems, but when it comes to psychiatric disorders, a different kind of nuance stands out distinctly with respect to prevention, especially where the basic needs of social-economic survival is still the priority. The complexity of the problems and dimensions of factors being involved, made the preventive aspect of psychiatric disorders very challenging and difficult to define.

The modern concept of 'mental health' does not seem to represent the true nature or condition of what should be perceived as 'Mental health problems' in daily life. In particular, with respect to living conditions in under-developed countries as compared to developed countries.

This presentation is an inference based on review of past experiences in Indonesia, a country of complex geographic situation, ethnological and social-cultural diversities. We need to know the whole country profile before we can foresee the extent and complexity of the Mental health problems.

Geographic & demographic profile

Indonesia is a tropical volcanic archipelago in South East Asia Region, consisting of 17,000 islands (13,000 inhabited - the largest archipelago in the world).

The population exceeds 210 million, 70% live in the island of Java, which covers only 7% of the country's land area - very crowded. There are more than 300 diverse ethnic groups known in the country with different cultural and traditional background and speak different languages (with more than 600 dialects). More than 95% are Moslems, the largest Moslem population in the world, and yet Indonesia is not a Moslem country.

Its social-economic status is poorest among the ASEAN countries. During the last 3 years it had been in a critical social, economic and political situation.

That gives an idea of the complexity of the situation and inherent problems.

The past experience

Despite the fact that intervention and preventive strategies had been worked-out extensively through government national mental health policies and supported by private sectors for many decades (since early 1960's), in fact the attainment of such activities were difficult to assess.

Some studies[1,2] revealed that 40% - 70% of psychiatric patients did not go initially to medical or psychiatric facilities. There are various intricate factors that should be considered if we sincerely want to be realistic in the preventive efforts, it is not just a matter of overcoming the stigma.

Intervention and prevention with respect to 'hard core' psychiatric disorders had become stereotyped strategy, but if we consider Mental Health problems in a broader perspective, we might need stratified strategies to cope. Unlike preventive measures adopted for infectious diseases or other tropical diseases, most psychiatric disorders are virtually not preventable with almost the same incidence rate throughout time (i.e., schizophrenia, MDD, ADHD, etc.).

Historical background

Historically psychiatric intervention in Indonesia started when the first mental hospital was built in 1882 (Bogor). Consequently, 12 large custodial type mental hospitals were built by 1935.

In 1928, the first neuropsychiatric unit in general hospital was established. It was only after 1960 that psychiatry was separated from neurology.

The 1st establishment of a private mental health foundation and hospital was in 1961, right in the center of housing quarters, marking community acceptance of psychiatric service (Dharmawangsa mental health foundation & clinic). This private foundation also started public mental health educational campaign in 1968 by promoting mental Health courses and one-day symposia for laymen as well as medical practitioners. The first issue of the Indonesian psychiatric quarterly ("JIWA") was also published in 1968 in Indonesian language.

In 1966, a Mental health law was amended separate from the Health Law, maybe the first among Asian countries followed by the establishment of a National Mental Health Delivery System (1969). Compared to other medical specialties, it was a major lead. All mental hospitals were assigned responsibility to be the Mental Health Center to provide consultation and supervision to the neighboring Primary Health Care Centers.

1969 - Saw the first officially alerted Drug Abuse problems, which lead to the establishment of a Drug Dependence Unit (now a hospital) in 1972.

In 1970, the 1st SEA Regional Seminar on Psychotropic Medication was held in Jakarta) / also the ASEAN Federation for Child and Adolescent Psychiatry (AFCAP). Followed by the establishment of the ASEAN Federation for Psychiatry and Mental Health (AFPMH) in 1972 (proposed by Prof. Kusumanto Setyonegoro, as also most of the other activities).

The Society for Neurology-Psychiatry-Neurosurgery was founded in 1971, and in 1974 each specialties established their own Society. For psychiatry, it was the Indonesian Psychiatric Association.

Community Psychiatry was started in 1971. The BPKJM was founded (Coordinating Body for Community Mental Health Activities) : a collaborating body under the provincial governor, consisting of various Mental Health and Social Welfare agencies, especially geared to community participation in the preventive and rehabilitative activities. It was set up in every province (26 provinces).

An innovative activity was inaugurated in 1972 : The Dharmawangsa MH Radio Broadcasting Station (maybe the first and the only one in the world), dedicated to public Mental Health education. Unfortunately it had to be closed down in 1980 because of a shortage in financial support. This program was then done in collaboration with other commercial radio and television program.

During the period between 1973 to 1988, 22 new Mental Hospitals were built throughout 25 provinces (out of 27 provinces), in addition to the existing 12 old Mental Hospitals. Because of the active performance and program development in the field of Mental Health, the Directorate of Mental Health in Jakarta was appointed to become WHO Collaborative Center for SEA (1971 - 1980?). However, closing the XXth Century, a major drawback happened in Indonesian Psychiatry.

In 1993 - Mental Health Law was withdrawn and integrated into the General Health Law. By the year 2000, the Directorate of Mental Health was dissolved to be the Directorate of Community Mental Health under the Directorate General of Community Health.

In the aspect of intervention and prevention of Mental Disorders, in fact Indonesia had started early (1966), compared to the other ASEAN country, but progressed very slowly. So after about 15 years or so, were left behind.

It seems that we had neglected the most essential part in developing the National Mental Health strategic plan during the past, which is not to put the priority on the basic infrastructure development to ensure continuity of program implementation. Instead, developing too much over-ambitious program which proved to be short lived because of lack of basic support for long-term implementation of the program.

Even though in public MH education topics such as family life, childhood development, personality development and other MH aspects were touched upon, too much attention was posed toward the narrow concept of MH in Health Services.

Early intervention

Despite the intensive public MH education, early intervention and treatment are still facing a dilemma in its reality. Most people still (40% - 70%) have the preference to go first to the traditional healers. The conventional intervention and secondary preventive approaches that has been done during the past mostly consist of: isolation, ICT (until 1961), ECT, psychopharmacological treatment, supportive type of psychotherapeutic measures, family involvement and social participation to various extend. After 1965, intensive psychotherapy, cognitive and behavioral approaches, group therapy and group-psychotherapy, were also done. Many of the Mental Hospitals provide simple facilities for rehabilitation activities and also rehabilitative program involving the patient's families.

To encourage family inherent resources and participation, short-term hospitalization policy (3 months at the most) was implemented in the State Mental Hospitals, except for three larger State Mental Hospitals (Bogor, Magelang and Lawang).

Despite the economic crisis of the country, almost all psychopharmacological drugs existing in the world market are available in the Indonesian market (including atypical antipsychotics such as: clozapine, risperidone, olanzapine, quetiapine, and the new generation antidepressants such as: fluoxetine, sertraline, fluvoxamine, paroxetine, citalporam, tianeptine, mirtazapine).

Manpower and MH services facilities

In 1960, the number of licensed psychiatrists was only less than 30 for 160 million population. By 1970 there were about 80 psychiatrists, and in year 2001 - 430 psychiatrists. It is still very low (1 psychiatrist to 500,000 people).

Up to early 70th, certification for a psychiatrist was based on unstructured internship. In 1973, a more structured system of Postgraduate Psychiatric Teaching was instituted (oriented toward the American model because many of the older generation psychiatrists had their additional training in the USA). Emphasis was also directed to undergraduate Psychiatric teaching to give the coming GP generation the skill to cope with commonly encountered psychiatric problems, and to be more receptive toward psychiatry.

There are at present 8 psychiatric training centers (out of 18 medical schools providing undergraduate psychiatric teaching).

As far as MH Service Facilities are concerned, aside from the 34 State Mental Hospitals there are 17 Private Mental Hospitals. The total number of psychiatric beds is only close to 9000 beds. There are more than 33,000 Primary Health Centers and close to 800 General Hospitals. Not even 50 General Hospitals have a psychiatrist. Posting of a psychiatrist in General Hospitals should become priority.

After observing the impact of our three year social-economic and political crisis, we are more convinced that the future indicator of MH problems should not be on the classical mental disorders, but to other aspects of the broader concepts of MH. Those are aspects such as: violence, criminality, suicides, abusive behavior, street children, declining norms and values, urban mental health, acculturation, etc. With the present critical condition in Indonesia, we should envision the future of preventive efforts in different, long-term perspectives.

Treatment and re-socialization has become some kind of standard procedures, but to achieve those objectives in relation to relieving the above problems, we should be focused on long-term preventive measures based on broader MH concepts. As such, involvement and contribution of psychiatric and MH expertise in various educational, disciplinary, social-environmental and mass movement policy should be emphasized.

In setting the priorities of future programs of early intervention and prevention, we should review realistically the availability of resources. The 'inherent preventive role' of cultural/traditional resources should also be better accounted.

The realistic thing is that we do not have a dependable infrastructure and lacking many of the basic supporting prerequisites (manpower, financial support, social security and welfare system, epidemiological and basic logistic data).

Summary

Considering the social and economic condition of the people (in Indonesia) a more realistic early intervention and prevention of psychiatric disorders should be considered. With the present escalation of more relevant psychosocial problems (violence, abusive behavior, criminality, other urban MH problems, acculturation-related problems, etc.) which are basically MH problems, priorities of preventive efforts need to be shared with those problems. There is also the need to improve other basic requirements such as the infrastructure, system supports, epidemiological data, etc.

Important as it should, early intervention and prevention of psychiatric disorders are subject to other important basic considerations, such as social-economics, cultural (ethnic/tradition) and political aspects.

---

*Sasanto Wibisono, M. D. : Department of Psychiatry, Faculty of Medicine University of Indonesia.

韓国における精神障害に対する早期介入と予防
Early intervention and prevention of psychiatric disorders in Korea

Sung Kil Min*

1. Introduction

Issues of early intervention and prevention of mental disorders have been one of the important subjects for study since Caplan (1964) had described primary, secondary and tertiary prevention. Recently, the Institute of Medicine, Committee on Prevention of Mental Disorders of USA, defined prevention as intervention before the on set of disorders and differentiated it into selective preventive intervention, indicated preventive intervention, and universal intervention. Universal interventions are targeted to the general public, independent to risk factors. Selective interventions are targeted to individuals and groups thought to have a higher-than-average risk of developing mental illnesses. Indicated interventions are targeted to risk-high individuals with biological markers or early signs of illness who do not yet meet the 4th edition of DSM-IV diagnostic criteria (Elpers 2000).

2. Current status in Korea

In Korea, the concept of early intervention and prevention of mental illnesses have not widely understood by the general public. The concept of early intervention is not familiar to psychiatrists, too. Though national mental health policy and mental health law in Korea refer to early detection and prevention, they are focused on rehabilitation of chronic schizophrenic patients. Even the community services are provided only in limited numbers of model community mental health centers. Only recently, researches on community psychiatry and rehabilitation have started because of limited research fund.

There are many obstacles in promoting preventive activities in Korea. First is stigma relating to mental disorders. Public concern for the mentally ill is not sufficient. People do not care about mental health so much as physical health. Also lack of information on mental health, lack of experiences of practice and lack of researches have also been obstacles for those people who have concerns for mental health. Insufficient and poorly systematized national mental health policy is delaying development of preventive activities. Public investment for mental health is in low rank in the order of priority. Somatization tendency of Koreans, traditional beliefs about health, folk medicine and flourishing religions are also obstacles preventing activities for mental illnesses. These lead people to consider psychiatric disorders to be either physical problems or spiritual problems.

The difficulties in practice of intervention and prevention in Korea are evidenced by difficulties in conducting a school mental health service (Min et al. 1997, a, b), in which subjects were 3,021 students in a rural area and 2,899 students in a metropolitan city of Seoul. The main difficulty was failure to get cooperation of family and teachers. Family, due to ignorance and stigma of mental disorders, did not cooperate with activities and even protested against mental health workers due to fear of their family problems being exposed. Teachers, due to lack of moral and enthusiasm, were "already too busy" to help students with problems. Even principals had frequently complained that it was a burden and irksome. All these obstacles reflect the general attitude of Koreans.

Stigma, ignorance and lack of interest

The general public as well as patients do not want to be seen as crazy "psychiatric" patients because of the stigma and prejudice related to psychiatric disorders. Non-psychiatric physicians and other health professionals are also failing in early detection and prevention of mental disorders because of limited knowledge, skills and indifference. Even physicians sometimes project their prejudice to stigma which patients have. They used to explain that, though they have tried to refer their patients with mental health problems to a psychiatrist, they could not persuade patients to go to psychiatrists because patients do not want to be seen by psychiatrists. Health policy makers in government, due to lack of interest, lack of funds, and bureaucratic attitude, have contributed partly to delaying early intervention and prevention for mental disorders in Korea.

Somatization tendency

Koreans are known to have high tendency to somatize their emotional problems (Kim 1998). One example is hwabyung, an anger syndrome. The Korean word for anger is hwa. Main symptoms of hwabyung are somatization symptoms of chronic suppressed anger, which include a hot feeling in the body, pushing-up sensation in the chest, epigastric mass, pains, chest oppression, sigh, and weakness as well as depression, mortification and angry mood (Min and Kim 1998). Because of these somatic symptoms, patients with hwabyung frequently visit herb physicians to control "fire" or other specialists such as cardiologists to treat their somatic symptoms (heart pounding) caused by anger. And health professionals used to give patients physical explanations of their symptoms, ignoring their emotional or psychological problems, thus patients miss the opportunity to have proper early psychiatric care.

Influences of traditional thoughts

It has been known that Koreans have some difficulties to accept western medicine because of old traditional thoughts of Korea (Rhi 1972). The traditional Chinese medicine has well-systematized knowledge for the somatic symptoms in relation with emotions, which are familiar to Koreans for a long time. Besides folk Medicine, old traditional philosophical ideas like Shamanism, poong-ryu thoughts, Taoism, Buddhism, Confucianism, and poong-su theory are all influencing the concepts of mental health, mental disorders and help seeking in Koreans (see table 1). All these beliefs and thoughts have their own explanation on life and health and, therefore, seem to interfere with learning modern scientific medical knowledge on mental health and visiting psychiatrists for professional help.

National health policy in Korea

National health policy in Korea is now moving toward a "managed care system", but it is neither well developed nor yet systematized. Naturally it has not include any guideline for early detection or prevention of mental disorders. At the present time, the government seems to have an interest only in controlling cost. Furthermore, physicians have to see as many patients as possible to ensure the same income as before. Naturally, they would not try to refer their patients to psychiatrists, unless they are severely psychotic. These interfere with early detection and intervention by psychiatrists in Korea.

Help seeking behaviors

Because of various reasons, Koreans are said to have confusion in help-seeking behavior for their mental health problems. Kim (1998) had characterized these behaviors as multiple visiting (doctor shopping), non-compliance, preferring physically oriented treatment, shamanism incantation, health food, consulting non-professionals, everybody try-

Table 1 Visiting of patients with depression before coming to psychiatrists at a tertiary care hospital (Min 2000)

	no. of patients (N = 82)	
	First visiting	All visiting
psychiatrists	60	68
herb doctors	8	32
internist		12
other specialists		10
primary care physicians	10	10
neurosurgeons	2	2
Christian priests	2	12
Shaman		4
others (Buddhist temple, drug store, folk medicine and acupuncture)		8

Table 2 Diagnosis patients had labeled for their depression

	No. of patients (N = 82)
Terms	
depression from the onset of illness	42
"nervous"	42
stress	22
hwabyung	12
schizophrenia	6
manic-depressive disorder	4
"psycho"	4
"don't know"	12

(Min 2000)

ing to give advice and syncretism.

For this presentation, the author conducted a small survey to see what kind of help people with depression are seeking these days (Min 2001). The results reflect confusion of Koreans in help-seeking (table 1). This confusion is also delaying early detection and proper intervention.

Diagnosis by patients themselves is also important in help seeking behavior, because patients decide where to go for help according to this knowledge. In Korea, terms for mental health problems and psychiatric diagnosis are diverse and confusing, too. This confusion is leading people to visit wrong places for help. In case of depression, for example, terms for their conditions are various and confusing (table 2), reflecting ignorance and misunderstanding for mental disorders (Min 2001).

3. Efforts of psychiatrists in Korea

Anti-stigma campaign

Psychiatrists in Korea and the Korean Neuropsychiatric Association have made efforts for long time to improve knowledge and to increase concerns for mental health among people. These days, one of the most significant activities is anti-stigma campaign for mental disorders, which has been done jointly with other mental health professional organizations including family organization.

For example, in 2001 mental health day (April 4), public education was done on the burden of mental disorders (Murray and Lopez 1996) and stigma, and how to detect early signs of mental problems. Education was given to special groups of patients, family and students at schools. The education was conducted through lectures, exhibitions, dramas, music concerts T.V., newspapers and other media. This event was highlighted by a street campaign with distributing screening check list for depression and alcoholism in the middle of cities including Seoul. Beside this mental health day activities, the Association advised its members to serve our society with school visiting and consulting, invited public lectures and other voluntary activities to advance knowledge for mental health among people.

Researches

Researches on early intervention and prevention are yet to be developed in Korea. Many psychiatrists have tried to obtain funds for researches on this subject. But funding for these researches are in low rank in the order of priority in general. To share research findings, the Korean Society of Social Psychiatry and the Korean Association of Psychiatric Rehabilitation were founded. However their academic activities are still limited compared to what is expected.

Organizations

The Korean Neuropsychiatric Association has encouraged its member to cooperate with other mental health workers as a team at community mental health centers. Following are organization with which psychiatrists are expected to cooperate for early intervention and prevention in Korea : public organizations including community mental health centers and district welfare centers, school health services, self-help groups including alcoholic anonymous (AA) and family mental health organization, religious organizations including education program for Christian counseling and public health education programs including TV, newspaper and magazines. Especially the Association have supported the foundation and activities of the Korean Family Mental Health Association.

4. Suggestions for the future

To promote early intervention and prevention of psychiatric disorders in Korea, the following are essential : public relation, breaking, stigma among people, education of not only people but also physicians and restructuring health care delivery system.

Public relation

First of all, psychiatrists should have to improve their public relations. Psychiatrists should be trusted in their superiority and expertise as specialists for mental health problems by the people. They have to prove themselves to be really professionals for mental disorders through evidence from researches and satisfactory treatment results in referred patients. Psychiatrists' public relation with journalists, politicians and other community leaders are also important, as they can be partners with psychiatrists by establishing solidarity for joint advocacy for the importance of mental health, stigma and policy making.

People, especially those who have leadership and capability of policy making in the society, should understand that mental disorders are the most burdening disorders in the society now and in the future (Murray and Lopez 1996). Furthermore, they should know that early intervention and prevention are the most beneficial in cost-effectiveness for building the productive society. For these, evidences should be shown through researches.

Overcoming stigma

Stigma and prejudices against psychiatric disorders should be overcome. Stigma is one of the strongest obstacles which prevent patients from visiting for early intervention and proper treatment, especially in Korea. In paticular, prejudice other physicians have is one of the major targets of our anti-stigma campaign.

Education

Education should take place for improving the ability for early detection of mental health problems of non-psychiatric physicians. Education should be delivered also to other mental health professionals, such as traditional Chinese (herb) doctors, acupuncturists, and pharmacists and other related community leaders including school teachers and leaders religious organization who are close to patients. Family education, especially parent education, is most important, as they are the closest person who can detect early signs of mental health problems and are primary persons for caring patients.

Education of health professionals should include not only practical knowledge and skills for detecting and managing mental disorders but also understanding their limitation. They should know when to refer a patient to a psychiatrist. They should be familiar with other names of mental disorders called by ordinary people in a certain culture. These education should be given as continuous medical education and in regular interval.

Mental health policy

National health policy and health care delivery system are important in promoting early intervention and prevention in developing country like Korea and they should be restructured for these purposes in the future. This system should be well-balanced one between physicians' need and public needs. For this, mutual communication, understanding and cooperation between society and psychiatrists should be established. Of course, this cooperation should be based on ultimate welfare of patients.

Proper national guideline for early finding and referring should be made in Korea based on health concept and socio-cultural context in Korea. Guideline should be made based on consensus with non-psychiatrists ; how to find patients ; how to keep quality of care, what extent of responsibility ; when to make decisions for referring and to whom patients should be referred.

Community services

In long-term perspective, integrated community-based net-worked services seem to be one of the most efficient ways for early intervention and prevention. This service include education program, competence building, anticipatory guidance program, crisis intervention, hospitalization, case management, day care and social support systems. Researches should be accompanied for developing successful net-work for early intervention and prevention.

Roles of psychiatrists

For early intervention and prevention, psychiatrists should engage in advocacy, education, design implementation and services. Psychiatrists should study not only the way to overcome stigma, national mental health policy, educational programs and community services but also premorbid conditions, early signs, prodromal symptoms, risk factors and biological markers. All these study results should be informed to the public in easily understandable terms. Researches of psychiatrists for evidences will support policy makers and administers toward right direction.

Finally, as culture is different between countries, experiences of psychiatrists and results of studies in other countries should be communicated and shared to develop better strategies in the future.

References

1) Caplan, G. : Princioles of Preventive Psychiatry. Basic Books, New York, 1964.
2) Elpers, J. R. : Public psychiatry. In Sadick, B. J. and Sadock, V.A. (ed) : Comprehensive Textbook of Psychiatry. Lippincott Williams and Wilkins, Phialdelphia, pp. 3185-3199, 2000.
3) Kim, K. I. : Illness behavior and psychiatric practice in Korea. Mental Health Research, 17 ; 13, 1998.
4) Min, S. K., Kim, H. J., Oh, K. J. et al. : Model development of school mental health service. I. A school-based study on the emotional behavioral problems of elementary students. J. Korean Neuropsychiatric Assoc, 36 ; 812-825, 1997.
5) Min, S. K., Oh, K. J., Kim, H. J. et al. : Model development of school mental health service. II. Model development of school mental health service in Korean urban communities. J. Korean Neuropsychiatric Assoc, 368 ; 26-840, 1997.
6) Min, S. K., Kim, K. H. : Symptoms of hwabyung. J. Korean Neuropsychiatric Assoc, 37 ; 1138-1145, 1998.
7) Min, S. K. : A survey on help seeking behavior of patients with depression. Unpublished report, 2001.
8) Murray, G. I., Lopez, A. L. : The global burden of disease. Havard University Press, Boston, 1996.
9) Rhi, B. Y. : A preliminary study on the medical acculturation problems in Korea J. Korean Neuropsychiatric Assoc, 12 ; 97-109, 1973.

---

*Sung kil Min, M. D., Ph. D. : Yonsei University College of Medicine, Seoul Korea.

Early psychosis の早期発見と対応
The recognition and management of early psychosis

Patrick D. McGorry*

Summary

There is rapidly growing interest in early psychosis, where strategies for preventive intervention are becoming more realistic. There are essentially three preventive foci. The pre-psychotic phase is when most psychosocial impairment develops but the specifics of treatment remain difficult to research and apply. Secondly, while the extent of prepsychotic deterioration may mean that the total duration of untreated illness (DUI) may ultimately prove more critical, the duration of untreated psychosis (DUP) is a more realistic immediate target for early detection and intervention. Although DUP has not yet been conclusively demonstrated to be a malleable causal risk factor influencing outcome, early detection and engagement in treatment are well justified on clinical grounds, and are being systematically implemented in many countries. Once frank psychosis has become established, it makes no sense to withhold low dose antipsychotic treatment which has been shown to be increasingly safe and effective. Finally, first episode psychosis is comparatively more treatment responsive than multi-episode psychosis, and intensive phase-specific treatment appears to result in at least short term improvements in outcome and cost-effectiveness. It is probable that good adherence to low dose atypical antipsychotic medications and more intensive and skilled psychosocial treatment in this critical period of the illness (the first episode and the ensuing 2 - 5 years) will reduce the mortality, morbidity, costs of treatment, and ultimately the overall prevalence of psychotic disorders. Further research should test the strength of these propositions over the next few years. This may be expected to lead to an overwhelming case for more radical reform of mental health services.

Introduction

In recent years, psychiatry has witnessed a sustained surge of interest in early psychosis. After decades of unremitting pessimism, particularly in non-affective psychosis, a range of forces have combined to prise open the door sufficiently to allow preventive models to influence research and clinical care[1]. Because one of the obstacles to this shift is the Kraepelinian conceptual model itself[2], it is important to focus more broadly on early psychosis rather than schizophrenia alone. Psychosis is a more proximal and definable target, particularly since syndromal comorbidity and flux are common in the early phases of illness in young people, and delayed treatment is increasingly recognized in other serious mental illnesses, such as bipolar disorder[3]. There are three components of a preventive approach, namely pre-psychotic intervention, early detection and phase-specific intensive treatment during the critical period after diagnosis of first episode psychosis (FEP). These will be considered in chronological order.

Pre-psychotic intervention.

The logic for pre-psychotic intervention has a long pedigree, and recent descriptive and clinical research is providing increasing support for such subthreshold intervention[5,6]. While research interest has focused strongly on the duration of untreated psychosis (DUP) variable, the meticulous work of Häfner and colleagues[7,8] has shown that the more global concept of duration of untreated illness (DUI) may be even more critical for prevention and also help to short-circuit the debate (see below) as to whether DUP is confounded by a latent clinical severity factor. Although their research was retrospective in design, the Mannheim group[7,8] showed that deficits in social functioning were primarily established during the pre-psychotic phase. This confirms earlier work which showed that most people with subsequent schizophrenia are only very subtly, if at all, different from their peers and even less so from those who later develop an affective illness[10,11]. While an early vulnerability may exist in a proportion at least of cases, other environmental risk factors[12] and putative endogenous processes (the so-called "second hit")[13] clearly come into play during adolescence or later, though months or years prior to the emergence of the diagnostically defining features of psychotic disorder[7]. The level of social development achieved by the end of the prodromal phase, when the first psychotic symptom appears, determines the further social course of the disorder by setting a "ceiling". This effect has been termed "social stagnation" and complements the rather deterministic neurobiological concept of endogenous "deficit processes"[14]. While the pre-psychotic phase is critical, there is clearly scope for further biopsychosocial damage if DUP is also prolonged (see below).

It is possible to provide clinical access to the subgroup of young people who are at ultra high risk (UHR) of a first episode of psychosis, are already distressed and functioning poorly, and who are willing to accept professional help[5,6,18-20]. Yet even with excellent psychosocial care, 41% of operationally defined UHR patients make the transition to first episode psychosis within a 12-month follow-up period. One element of the research task is prediction, though it is important to be clear whether psychosis or schizophrenia is the predictive target - timing of schizophrenia diagnosis is probably affected by additional variables which may unnecessarily delay treatment[21]. Further conceptual complexity arises because frank psychosis is currently required at some stage for a diagnosis of schizophrenia. Within the schizophrenia concept, some have even proposed reintroducing non-psychotic forms of the disorder (Tsuang et al 2000), suggesting that psychosis is an epiphenomenon in schizophrenia. This is similar to the thinking of Huber and colleagues[22] and is a legitimate approach which ultimately could benefit many with disabling symptoms. However, several clinical and ethical issues need to be more fully addressed. At this stage, psychosis is a clearer target (and still more proximal than currently defined schizophrenia), at least for drug therapies, even though it occurs in a range of disorders. The new or atypical antipsychotic medications, while they may have broader spectrum effects than the older typical antipsychotic drugs, are still most potent in their effect upon positive psychotic symptoms. In other words they are still more antipsychotic than antischizophrenic.

Several clinical features, such as depression and various negative and positive symptoms, enhance the capacity to predict transition to psychosis in the ultra high risk group, even though a very diverse range of clinical features are present[19,20]. The work of the Bonn-Köln group has also shown that other specific clinical variables can possess substantial predictive power[22]. Contrary to our original hypothesis, hippocampal volume on MRI scan was normal at baseline in those UHR cases who later became psychotic, and significantly *larger* than in the non-psychotic cases, where it was *reduced* at baseline[20,24]. In a small subsample who have been rescanned after the transition to psychosis, significant amounts of volume loss have been demonstrated in the hippocampus and surrounding region[25].

A recent randomised controlled trial in this clinical population has shown a significant reduction in transition rate to psychosis for patients receiving specific treatment (ST) - very low dose atypical antipsychotic medication (risperidone) and cognitive therapy - in comparison to non-specific treatment (NST) - supportive psychotherapy and symptomatic treatment[26]. Clearly further research is required in this embryonic area and another study is in progress using olanzapine[27], though subject recruitment is difficult in the absence of a large scale first episode clinical focus[28]. In the meantime, psychosocial treatment -only with or without syndrome-based drug therapies treatments for distress and disability in young people seem eminently justifiable as components of youth-oriented health care, with early "rescue" once a certain threshold and persistence of positive symptoms is reached such that an ICD 10 or DSM IV diagnosis of clearcut psychotic disorder is reached[6,8].

Duration of untreated psychosis : Is it a causal risk factor and intervention point?

This focus is solely concerned with the timing rather than the quality of treatment. The currently accepted threshold for treatment with antipsychotic medication is at the first clear and sustained emergence of psychotic features. Despite this, for a substantial proportion of people, such treatment is delayed, often for very prolonged periods[29]. For others, especially in the developing world[30], treatment is never accessed. DUP, as a marker of delay in delivering effective specific treatment, is a potentially important variable in improving outcome in first episode schizophrenia, and more widely in first episode psychosis. Indeed, psychosis may be an easier and less conflicted target to detect than schizophrenia[2,21]. DUP is important because, unlike other prognostic variables such as genetic vulnerability, gender and age of onset, it is a potentially malleable variable which can become the focus of intervention strategies. While there are some studies which appear to cast doubt on the existence or persistence of the association (Craig et al 1999 ; Ho et al 2000 ; Barnes et al 2000), these studies, when looked at carefully, do not seriously challenge the correlational link. Furthermore, there is a strong literature supporting the association between DUP and both short and long term outcome[31]. This raises one obvious and central question. Is the association causal, that is, is delay (prolonged DUP) in treatment a risk factor for worse outcome? Or is the link due to a common underlying factor, namely a more severe form of illness which has a more insidious onset with more negative symptoms, more paranoid ideation, less salience and awareness of change and less willingness to seek and accept treatment?

Correlational research

Wyatt (1991)[32] and others have marshalled persuasive circumstantial evidence suggesting a link between delayed treatment and outcome. Loebel et al (1992)[33] showed that there was an independent association between DUP and time to and level of remission, though this association was not confirmed in later analysis[34,35]. There was no association evident between mode of onset or premorbid adjustment and DUP, a finding that has received support from other studies[9,36,37]. However, Verdoux et al (1998)[39] suggested that, because DUP was independently predicted by demographic and clinical variables, the association between DUP and poor prognosis was not likely to be causal. While there could be a latent severity factor intrinsic to the patient which gives rise to poor outcome and certain clinical features that contribute to delay in entry to treatment, eg negative symptoms, it could also be that these intrinsic clinical features produce poor outcome by delaying treatment (Figure 1). Even if we accept that the effect of DUP on outcome is likely to be confounded to some extent by other potential predictors of outcome, DUP remains a significant and important predictor after adjusting for the effects of these confounding variables[38]. Longer-term outcome is related to DUP as well, as shown by an elegant Irish study[10] in which the delay in treatment is most unlikely to have been affected by bias.

Experimental manipulation of DUP

The classic study of May et al (1976)[42] reanalysed by Wyatt (1991)[32] is the most compelling evidence in favour of a causal link. Essentially DUP, or more accurately, time to commencement of antipsychotic medication, was randomly varied in this comparison of psychological versus biological therapies. Delay in receiving antipsychotics led to significantly poorer short and medium term outcomes, interestingly even though treatment was not necessarily sustained by protocol. It is generally felt that to repeat such a study these days would pose ethical challenges, hence the pursuit of alternative designs.

An alternative, quasi-experimental design termed "adequate" has been proposed and implemented by McGlashan and colleagues[43]. This involves a two step process, first aiming to reduce the duration of DUP, and second estimating whether the outcome is correspondingly improved. The Scandinavian design involves an experimental sector where greatly enhanced detection systems have been systematically introduced and two control sectors where similar treatment was offered but detection was not improved[31,44]. The early results appear promising in having substantially reduced DUP in the experimental sector, however a number of unforeseen methodological problems have surfaced which may make interpretation complex. The enhanced detection intervention is powerful, so that, in addition to reducing DUP for those cases who would have been detected under usual conditions, previously untapped sources of cases are accessed. Certainly the treated incidence in the experimental sector has been substantially increased compared to the previous pilot study[45].

Firstly, brief self-limited psychoses, psychotic-like phenomena and non-clinically significant psychoses[46], which are more prevalent than previously realized[47], will be identified; secondly a long DUP subgroup similar to the untreated group described in Padmavathi et al (1998)[30] should also be detected. In our system in Melbourne, some of the first group have been channeled to the PACE clinic for potential prodromal patients[18], while the latter group have been clearly identified in a pilot study based on the Scandinavian design which actually showed more vigorous detection efforts resulted in a longer DUP[38]! It is likely that the Scandinavian study will clarify the issue because of the scope for DUP reduction in the local system and the power of the early detection intervention, provided the focus is confined to a subgroup of the sample. In any event it is not yet scientifically established whether delay is a genuine cause of poorer medium to long term outcome or merely an epiphenomenon. Other research designs can be contemplated and might be considered ethically justified, depending on the local level of untreated incidence and service quality.

Reality of delayed treatment

However, is it really necessary to reach the ultimate level of scientific evidence in order to advocate for early intervention? Some authors appear to think so (Ho et al 2000 ; Barnes et al 2000). On the other hand, McGlashan[31] regards delayed treatment as a major public health problem and regards it as "unequivocal that DUP, by itself, is reason enough for early intervention on a large and intensive scale." (p901). McGorry et al (1996)[50] and Lincoln et al (1998)[51] depict the range of negative psychosocial outcomes that result during the period of untreated psychosis. These include vocational failure, self-harm, offending behaviour, family distress, aggression, substance abuse and harm from others. Homelessness can occur in up to 15% of cases[52], and in two-thirds of these manifest before first treatment. From qualitative data, it seems obvious that the timing of entry to treatment is determined by a range of variables (Lincoln et al 1999). Some of these do seem to be related to clinical variables intrinsic to the patient and hence could be partially confounded in relation to prognosis. Others however, such as mental health literacy[53], accessibility and skill of health professionals, and even luck, are clearly extrinsic and potentially more independent and malleable[54]. Reducing DUP is almost certainly of clinical value, irrespective of whether there is in fact a limited window of opportunity (which may involve the prodrome, the period of untreated psychosis, *and* a period after entry into treatment) during which putative "deficit processes" are active or at their peak (31, 33, 55, McGlashan and Hoffman, 2000). This endogenous neurobiological notion can be extended to include the "critical period" idea[56], since adolescence and young adulthood involves a series of major developmental tasks, which if impeded or delayed through untreated illness, will be very difficult to subsequently master. Evidence in support of this broad concept of a limited window for secondary preventive intervention comes from a recent study by Carbone et al (1999)[29] which showed that for a range of values of DUP in first episode psychosis, one year outcome could be significantly enhanced by more intensive treatment only if the DUP was between one and 6 months. The logic of early detection has recently led to the establishment of a systematic national service response in the UK where 50 new early intervention teams for psychosis are being set up across the country.

In the developing world, the challenge is more commonly treatment delay of a permanent nature, i.e. widespread untreated prevalence. Tackling these public health problems has been inhibited by a paralysing ambivalence. This has arisen from the findings of the WHO studies which showed a better outcome for schizophrenia in developing countries where modern treatments are less freely available[57], and from the sense, reinforced by the meta-analytic study of Hegarty et al (1994)[41], that the outcome for schizophrenia in developed countries has not been improved by modern treatments. Recognising that sampling issues may partly explain the former finding[30], and failure to implement evidence-based practice the latter, may be important, especially given recent major advances in treatment.

Phase-specific intervention in first episode psychosis

Here the focus is on the quality of treatment, albeit during a putatively treatment-sensitive phase or "critical period". While perhaps less stimulating in a research sense, more intensive phase-specific treatment in first-episode psychosis and beyond is still the most feasible proposition for most clinicians and researchers interested in secondary prevention, since access to patients during this period is at least assured (Malla and Norman 2000). Several monographs have appeared on this subject recently[58-61].

Robinson et al (1999)[35] found that in first episode of schizophrenia or schizoaffective disorder there was a cumulative first relapse rate of 81.9% within the first 5 years after recovery. Discontinuation of drug therapy increased the risk of relapse by a factor of 5. Prolonged DUP did not predict increased risk of relapse in contrast to earlier work[62], however the New York sample was not a representative sample of first episode patients, had a much longer mean DUP and were treated during the 1980s with high doses of typical neuroleptic. These findings suggest that drug therapy should be continued for most if not all patients for longer than 12 months after recovery from a first psychotic episode. This is probably so for a substantial proportion, however it is important to discover who will not relapse and those who will not relapse for a long period. Furthermore, it is difficult to convince young people of the need for longer term medication after only one episode, especially if there has been a good remission, and it should be remembered that relapse prevention is not the sole consideration in treatment, but a means to an end. Other studies[63,64] have also stressed the persistence of symptoms and relapse-proneness of patients, however they also highlighted the limited capacity of any baseline variables to predict outcome, and emphasise the good functional outcome for about half of the patients at five year follow up. Power et al (1998)[66] reported on the initial treatment phase for an incident cohort of 231 patients entering the EPPIC program within a 12 month period. At 3 months after entry, 80% had responded to treatment and 63% had achieved remission. Conversely, a study of 12 month outcome from first episode affective psychosis revealed a much poorer than expected course of illness[65].

Home-based acute phase care is a specialised and highly appropriate component of the treatment of first episode psychosis[67], as are group-based recovery programs[68]. The novel antipsychotics are proving to be especially effective in early psychosis[69] and almost certainly superior in efficacy to and much better tolerated than the typical agents, though the latter have rarely if ever been used in appropriate doses[70,71]. Although North America seems strangely immune, the renaissance in (evidence-based) psychological therapies in psychosis is becoming productively focused upon early psychosis[72-76]. In general, the intensive treatment of young people at this phase of illness appears effective[77] and cost-effective[78] at least in the short-term. A secondary but important research question is whether it is possible to reduce the intensity of treatment for a proportion of patients over a longer time frame[56].

Finally, in developing countries where rates of untreated prevalence are high in many areas and mental health service budgets are low, what are the options for early intervention? Firstly, increasing the treated incidence is a key goal but this could focus preferentially on the early phases of illness ie the first 2 years or so post onset of symptoms, a potentially more treatment responsive period. Secondly, while in wealthy countries the advantages in tolerability, reduced side effects and marginally better efficacy, of the novel antipsychotics are affordable (though even here some countries have betrayed a puzzling ambivalence about this eg the UK), in countries where the mental health budgets are very meagre, it may be more cost-effective in the short term at least to spend the scarce mental health dollar on more professionals to deliver services and to increase the treated prevalence of psychosis in particular, than provide highest quality treatment to a select few. This will mean retaining conventional or typical antipsychotic medications for a little longer in such settings. In turn this means that they should be used much more resonsibly and safely than they have been used to date. Vastly lower doses must be employed (aiming for 2mg haloperidol equivalent per day for first episode cases, and 4mg per day for multiepisode cases) even in the acute phase. A small minority of cases will need higher doses but they should be required to demonstrate this using reasonable intervals of dosing eg 2 - 3 weeks. Acute phase behavioural problems and dysphoria should be managed with benzodiazepines in the first instance. This sort of regime will deliver most of the benefits of the atypicals except for the lower risk of tardive dyskinesia. Psychosocial management may also need to be quite different in different cultural settings.

Conclusion

The foundations for preventive interventions in early psychosis are firmly in place with an array of research endeavours and growing service reform and development in Europe, North America and Australasia. These are focusing on the pre-psychotic phase, the period of untreated psychosis and the early post-treatment period. In my opinion, there is sufficient, though perhaps not yet fully definitive evidence supporting these initiatives. It is vital that an evidence-based strategy continues to be pursued, however premature and excessive skepticism based on impatience or preconceived attitudes must be held in check to allow sufficient opportunity for this to fruitfully occur.

References

1) Mrazek, P., Haggerty, R. (eds) : Reducing risks for mental disorders : Frontiers for preventive intervention research. Washington, D.C., National Academy of Sciences, 1994.
2) McGorry, P. : A treatment-relevant classification of psychotic disorders. Australian and New Zealand Journal of Psychiatry, 29(4) ; 555-558, 1995.
3) Baldessarini, R., Tondo, L., Hennen, J. : Treatment delays in bipolar disorders. Americal Journal of Psychiatry, 156(5) ; 811, 1999.
4) Sullivan, H. : The onset of schizophrenia. American Journal of Psychiatry, 6 ; 105-134, 1927.
5) McGorry, P., Yung, A., Phillips, L. : "Closing in" : What features predict the onset of first episode psychosis within a high risk group? in The early stages of schizophrenia. Edited by Zipursky, R., Schutz, C., American Psychiatric Press, In press.
6) McGorry, P., Phillips, L., Yung, A. : Recognition and treatment of the pre-psychotic phase of psychotic disorders : Frontier or fantasy? in Early intervention in psychiatric disorders. Edited by Mednick, S., McGlashan, T., Libiger, J. et al. Netherlands, Kluwer, In press.
7) Häfner, H., Nowotny, B., Löffler, W. et al. : When and how does schizophrenia produce social deficits? European Archives of Psychiatry Clinical Neurosci, 246 ; 17-28, 1995.
8) Häfner, H., Löffler, W., Maurer, K. et al. : Depression, negative symptoms, social stagnation and social decline in the early course of schizophrenia. Acta Psychiatrica Scandinavica, 100 ; 105-118, 1999.
9) Barnes, T., Hutton, S., Chapman, M. et al. : West London first-episode study of schizophrenia : Clinical correlates of duration of untreated psychosis at first presentation to psychiatric services. Schizophrenia Research, 36(1-3) ; 12-13, 1999.
10) Jones, P., Rodgers, B., Murray, R. et al. : Child developmental risk factors for adult schizophrenia in the British 1946 birth cohort. The Lancet 1994, 344 ; 1398-1402.
11) Van, Os. J., Jones, P., Lewis, G. et al. : Developmental precursors of affective illness in a general population birth cohort. Archives of General Psychiatry, 54 ; 625-631, 1997.
12) Mahy, G., Mallett, R., Leff, J. et al. : First-contact incidence rate of schizophrenia on Barbados. British Journal of Psychiatry, 175 ; 28-33, 1999.
13) Rapoport, J., Giedd, J., Blumenthal, J. et al. : Progressive cortical change during adolescence in childhood-onset schizophrenia. Archives of General Psychiatry, 56 ; 649-654, 1999.
14) McGlashan, T. : Early detection and intervention of schizophrenia : rationale and research. British Journal of Psychiatry, 172 (Supplement 33) ; 3-6, 1998.
15) Amminger, G. P., Pape, S., Rock, D. et al. : Relationship between childhood behavioural disturbance and later schizophrenia in the New York High-Risk Project. American Journal of Psychiatry, 156(4) ; 525-530, 1999.
16) Lawrie, S., Whalley, H., Kestelman, J. et al. : Magnetic resonance imaging of brain in people at high risk of developing schizophrenia. The Lancet 1999, (353) ; 30-33, 1999.
17) Hodges, A., Byrne, M., Grant, E. et al. : People at risk of schizophrenia : Sample characteristics of the first 100 cases in the Edinburgh High-Risk Study. British Journal of Psychiatry, 174 ; 547-553, 1999.
18) Yung, A., McGorry, P., McFarlane, C. et al. : Monitoring and care of young people at incipient risk of psychosis. Schizophrenia Bulletin, 22 (2) ; 283-303, 1996.
19) Yung, A., Phillips, L., McGorry, P. et al. : Prediction of psychosis. The British Journal of Psychiatry, 172 (Supplement 33) ; 14-20, 1998.
20) McGorry, P. D., Phillips, L. J., Yung, A. R. et al. : The identification of predictors of psychosis in a high risk group. Schizophrenia Research, 36(1-3) ; 49-50, 1999.
21) Driessen, G., Gunther, N., Bak, M. et al. : Characteristics of early- and late-diagnosed schizophrenia : Implications for first-episode studies.

Schizophrenia Research, 33(1-2); 27-34, 1998.
22) Schultze-Lütter, F., Klosterkötter, J. : What tool should be used for generating predictive models? Schizophrenia Research, 36(1-3); 10, 1999.
23) Crump, N., McGorry, P., Yung, A. et al. : Developmental risk factors in the prediction of psychosis in at-risk young people. Submitted.
24) Phillips, L., Velakoulis, D., Pantelis, C. et al. : Non-reduction in hippocampal volume is associated with high risk of psychosis. Submitted Schizophrenia Research.
25) Pantelis, C., Velakoulis, D., Suckling, J. et al. : Progression of medial temporal lobe changes in psychosis : from high risk to chronic schizophrenia. Schizophrenia Research In press.
26) Phillips, L., McGorry, P., Yung, A. et al. : The development of preventive interventions for early psychosis : Early findings and directions for the future. Schizophrenia Research, 36(1-3); 331-332, 1999.
27) Cornblatt, B., Obuchowski, M., Ditkowsky, K. et al. : The Hillside RAPP clinic : A research/early intervention center for the schizophrenia prodrome. Schizophrenia Research, 36(1-3); 358-358, 1999.
28) Phillips, L., Yung, A., Hearn, N. et al. : Preventive mental health care : Accessing the target population. Australian and New Zealand Journal of Psychiatry In press.
29) Carbone, S., Harrigan, S., McGorry, P. et al. : Duration of untreated psychosis and 12-month outcome in first-episode psychosis : The impact of treatment approach. Acta Psychiatrica Scandinavica, 100; 96-104, 1999.
30) Padmavathi, R., Rajkumar, S., Srinivasan, T. : Schizophrenic patients who were never treated – a study in an Indian urban community. Psychological Medicine, 28(5); 1113-1117, 1998.
31) McGlashan, T. : Duration of untreated psychosis in first-episode schizophrenia : Marker or determinant of course? Biological Psychiatry, 46; 899-907, 1999.
32) Wyatt, R. : Neuroleptics and the natural course of schizophrenia. Schizophrenia Bulletin, 17; 325-351, 1991.
33) Loebel, A., Lieberman, J., Jose, M. et al. : Duration of psychosis and outcome in first-episode schizophrenia. American Journal of Psychiatry, 149(9); 1183-1188, 1992.
34) Robinson, D., Woerner, M., Alvir, J. et al. : Predictors of treatment response from a first-episode of schizophrenia or schizoaffective disorder. American Journal of Psychiatry, 156(4); 544-549, 1999.
35) Robinson, D., Woerner, M., Alvir, J. et al. : Predictors of relapse following response from a first-episode of schizophrenia or schizoaffective disorder. Archives of General Psychiatry, 56; 241-247, 1999.
36) Larsen, T., McGlashan, T., Johannessen, J. et al. : First-episode schizophrenia : II. Premorbid patterns by gender. Schizophrenia Bulletin, 22(2); 257-269, 1996.
37) Haas, G., Garratt, L., Sweeney, J. : Delay to antipsychotic medication in schizophrenia : impact on symptomatology and clinical course of illness. Journal of Psychiatric Research, 32; 151-159, 1998.
38) McGorry, P., Edwards, J., Harrigan, S. et al. : Duration of untreated psychosis in first-episode psychosis : Interpreting its influence. Schizophrenia Research, 36(1-3); 50, 1999.
39) Verdoux, H., Bergey, C., Assens, F. et al. : Prediction of duration of psychosis before first admission. European Psychiatry, 13; 346-352, 1998.
40) Scully, P., Coakley, G., Kinsella, A. et al. : Psychopathology, executive(frontal) and general cognitive impairment in relation to duration of initially untreated versus subsequently treated psychosis in chronic schizophrenia. Psychological Medicine, 27; 1303-1310, 1997.
41) Hegarty, J., Baldessarini, R., Tohen, M. et al. : One hundred years of schizophrenia : a meta-analysis of the outcome literature. American Journal of Psychiatry, 151; 1409-1416, 1994.
42) May, P., Tuma, A., Yale, C. et al. : Schizophrenia - a follow-up study of results of treatment, II : hospital stay over two to five years. Archives of General Psychiatry, 33; 481-486, 1976.
43) McGlashan, T. : Early detection and intervention with schizophrenia : Research. Schizophrenia Bulletin, 22(2); 327-345, 1996.
44) Johannessen, J., Larsen, T., Horneland, M. et al. : Strategies for reducing duration of untreated psychosis. Schizophrenia Research, 36(1-3); 342-343, 1999.
45) Larsen, T., Johannessen, J., Guldberg, C. et al. :

Early intervention programs in first-episode psychosis and reduction of duration of untreated psychosis (DUP). Schizophrenia Research, 36 (1-3) ; 345, 1999.
46) Van, Os. J., Ravelli, A., Bijl, R. : Evidence for a psychosis continuum in the general population. Schizophrenia Research, 36 (1-3) ; 57-58, 1999.
47) Verdoux, H., van, Os. J., Maurice-Tison, S. et al. : Is early adulthood a critical stage for psychosis proneness? A survey of delusional ideation in normal subjects. Schizophrenia Research, 29 ; 247-254, 1998.
48) Friis, S., Melle, I., Haahr, U. et al. : Threats to validity in outcome studies of early intervention in schizophrenia. Schizophrenia Research, 36 (1-3) ; 340, 1999.
49) Salzman, C. : Not all psychiatric research is bad. American Journal of Psychiatry, 156 ; 987-988, 1999.
50) McGorry, P., Edwards, J., Mihalopoulos, C. et al. : EPPIC : an evolving system of early detection and optimal management. Schizophrenia Bulletin, 22 ; 305-326, 1996.
51) Lincoln, C., Harrigan, S., McGorry, P. : Understanding the topogaphy of the early psychosis pathways. British Journal of Psychiatry, 172 (Supplement 33) ; 21-25, 1998.
52) Herman, D., Susser, E., Jandorf, L. et al. : Homelessness among individuals with psychotic disorders hospitalized for the first time : Findings from the Suffolk County Mental Health Project. American Journal of Psychiatry, 155 ; 109-113, 1998.
53) Jorm, A., Korten, A., Rodgers, B. et al. : Belief systems of the general public concerning the appropriate treatments for mental disorders. Soc-Psychiatry-Psychiatr-Epidemiol, 23 ; 1988-1998, 1997.
54) Lincoln, C., McGorry, P. : Pathways to care in early psychosis : clinical and consumer perspectives, in The recognition and management of early psychosis : A preventive approach. Edited by McGorry P, Jackson H. Cambridge, UK, Cambridge University Press, 1999.
55) Lieberman, J., Sheitman, B., Kinon, B. : Neurochemical sensitization in the pathophysiology of schizophrenia : deficits and dysfunction in neuronal regulation and plasticity. Neuropsychopharmacology, 17 ; 205-229, 1997.

56) Birchwood, M., Todd, P., Jackson, C. : Early intervention in psychosis : The critical period hypothesis. British Journal of Psychiatry, 172 (Supplement 33) ; 53-59, 1998.
57) Jablensky, A., Sartorius, N., Ernberg, G. et al. : Schizophrenia : manifestations, incidence and course in different cultures. A World Health Organization ten-country study. Psychol-Med-Monogr-Suppl, 20 ; 1-97, 1992.
58) McGorry, P., Edwards, J. (eds) : Early Psychosis Training Pack. Cheshire, UK., Gardiner-Caldwell Communications Ltd, 1997.
59) McGorry, P. E. : Preventive strategies in early psychosis : verging on reality. British Journal of Psychiatry, 172 (Supplement 33) ; 1-136, 1998.
60) Aitchinson, K., Meehan, K., Murrary, R. : First episode psychosis. London, Martin Dunitz Ltd, 1999.
61) McGorry, P., Jackson, H. (eds) : The recognition and management of early psychosis : A preventive approach. Cambridge, UK, Cambridge University Press, 1999.
62) Crow, T., Macmillan, J., Johnson, A. et al. : A randomized controlled trial of prophylactic neuroleptic treatment. British Journal of Psychiatry, 148 ; 120-127, 1986.
63) Vazquez-Barquero, J., Cuest, M., Castanedo, S. et al. : Cantabria first-episode schizophrenia study : three year follow-up. British Journal of Psychiatry, 174 ; 141-149, 1999.
64) Wiersma, D., Nienhuis, F., Slooff, C. et al. : Natural course of schizophrenic disorders : A 15-year followup of a Dutch incidence cohort. Schizophrenia Bulletin, 24 (1) ; 75-85, 1998.
65) Strakowski, S., Keck, P., McElroy, S. et al. : Twelve-month outcome after a first hospitalization for affective psychosis. Archives of General Psychiatry, 55 ; 49-55, 1998.
66) Power, P., Elkins, K., Adlard, S. et al. : Analysis of the initial treatment phase in first-episode psychosis. British Journal of Psychiatry, 172 (Supplement 33) ; 71-76, 1998.
67) Fitzgerald, P., Kulkarni, J. : Home-oriented management programme for people with early psychosis. British Journal of Psychiatry, 172 (Supplement 33) ; 39-44, 1998.
68) Albiston, D., Francey, S., Harrigan, S. : Group programmes for recovery from early psychosis. British Journal of Psychiatry, 172 (Supplement

33) ; 117-121, 1998.
69) Sanger, T., Lieberman, J., Tohen, M. et al. : Olanzapine versus haloperidol treatment in first-episode psychosis. American Journal of Psychiatry, 156 ; 79-87, 1999.
70) Remington, G., Kapur, S., Zipursky, R. : Pharmacotherapy of first-episode schizophrenia. British Journal of Psychiatry, 172(Supplement 33) ; 66-70, 1998.
71) Kapur, S., Zipursky, R., Remington, G. : Clinical and theoretical implication of 5-HT2 and D2 receptor occupancy of Clozapine, Risperidone, and Olanzapine in schizophrenia. Americal Journal of Psychiatry, 156 ; 286-293, 1999.
72) Haddock, G., Morrison, A., Hopkins, R. et al. : Individual cognitive-behavioural interventions in early psychosis. British Journal of Psychiatry, 172(Supplement 33) ; 101-106, 1998.
73) Jackson, H., McGorry, P., Edwards, J. et al. : Cognitively-oriented psychotherapy for early psychosis(COPE). The British Journal of Psychiatry, 172(Supplement 33) ; 93-100, 1998.
74) Edwards, J., Maude, D., McGorry, P. et al. : Treatment of enduring positive symptoms in first-episode psychosis : A randomised controlled trial of CBT and clozapine. Schizophrenia Research, 36(1-3) ; 278.
75) McGorry, P., Jackson, H., Edwards, J. et al. : Preventively-oriented psychological interventions in ealry psychosis, in Psychological Treatments for Schizophrenia. Oxford, England, Institute of Psychiatry, The University of Manchester, 1999.
76) Tarrier, N., Lewis, S. : SoCRATES - A CBT trial for the early stages of psychosis, in Psychological Treatments for Schizophrenia. Oxford, England, Institute of Psychiatry, The University of Manchester, 1999.
77) McGorry, P., Edwards, J. : The feasibility and effectiveness of early intervention in psychotic disorderrs : the Australian experience. International Journal of Clinical Psychopharmacology, 13(suppl 1) ; 47-52, 1998.
78) Mihalopoulos, C., McGorry, P., Carter, R. : Is phase-specific, community-oriented treatment of early psychosis an economically viable method of improving outcome. Acta Psychiatrica Scandinavica, 100 ; 47-55, 1999.

*Patrick D. McGorry : University of Melbourne Department of Psychiatry.

精神分裂病に対する早期マネジメントにおける最近の進歩

Expanding treatment objectives during the early course of schizophrenia

Barry D. Jones*

This meeting has focused on the idea of trying to find out whether an individual will develop schizophrenia, and if he/she is going to develop the disease, when to intervene, in order to prevent this dreaded disease from occurring. Those who work in this area of treating schizophrenia faces a dilemma because the course of the disease is not steady, and is often a deteriorating course. The belief though is that may be if we can intervene early enough, this deteriorating course can be stopped.

We take too long to treat our patients. An individual may develop the prodrome of schizophrenia when he/she becomes a teenager and then subsequently develop the first psychotic symptoms. We take too long to discover this, and depending on how long you have been ill prior to receiving treatment, the course of recovery is slowed while the percentage of patients that do recover is less. This is a tremendous challenge for us in medicine and in psychiatry to get to these patients with schizophrenia as early as we can.

That early intervention in this illness makes a difference is almost an established fact. What is unestablished is whether the type of intervention is important. Does it make a difference? There are many kinds of treatments for schizophrenia, but my focus will be to examine this issue from the perspective of the newer atypical antipsychotics. In other words its one thing to treat the patients early but are we going to use the older drugs on these patients? Or do we have an opportunity to avoid problems by using the newer drugs?

The development of newer antipsychotics over the last decade, has had the goal of trying to create a drug that has a similar pharmacological and clinical profile as Clozapine without the problems of Clozapine- in other words agranulocytosis. Risperidone, Quetiapine, and Olanzapine were developed with this goal in mind.

You can see that these drugs are very different from Haloperidol, which is very specific in blocking D2 receptors. The pharmacology of these drugs tends to be somewhat complex-especially as we move to drugs like Olanzapine and Clozapine, where many different receptors are targeted, as opposed to a selective activity such as Haloperidol's selectivity on Dopamine 2 receptors. Do this complex pharmacology make a difference for First-Episode patients?

Three studies and an abstract from the proceedings of this meeting are reviewed in this presentation. Data from our work with Olanzapine comparing it to higher doses of Haloperidol in first episode patients with schizophrenia will be shown, followed by a more recent study comparing Olanzapine to lower doses of Haloperidol in first-episode schizophrenia, and finally data from a third study which compares Olanzapine to Haloperidol and Risperidone in patients within the first 5 years of antipsychotic drug treatment. Each of these studies tells us about how the atypical antipsychotics are changing the treatment for schizophrenia in its early weeks and months, and even first few years when the treatment is obviously so important.

The first study was a comparison of Olanzapine and Haloperidol at doses that we might consider to be a little high for a first-episode patient. This study was not designed to look at first-episode schizo-

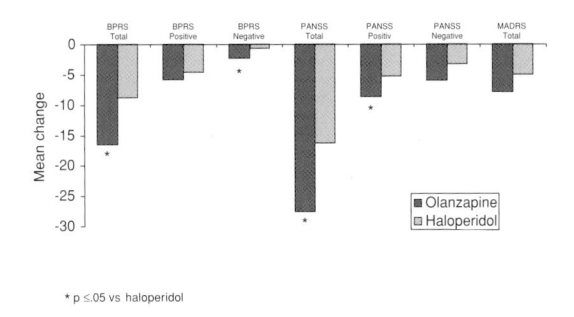

Figure 1 Efficacy scales : Mean change first episode patients - acute phase

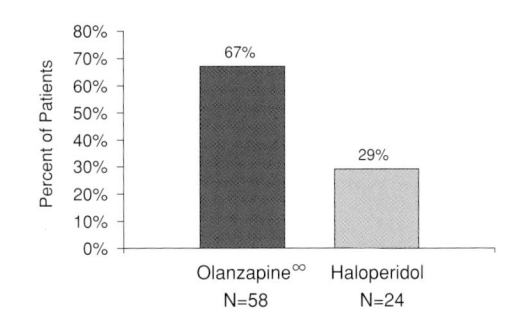

∞p = .003 vs haloperidol
[a] ≥40% improvement on BPRS Total (0-6) from baseline

Figure 2 Response rate[a] : First episode patients - acute Phase

phrenia. It was a double-blind randomized controlled study comparing Olanzapine to Haloperidol in close to 2,000 patients that looked at the diagnostic entities of schizophrenia, schizophreniform and schizoaffective disorder. Data shown are after 6 weeks of treatment. There were 2 treatment groups with doses at 5-20 mg of Olanzapine and 5-20 mg of Haloperidol-a reasonable dose of Haloperidol in a general population of patients with schizophrenia, but may-be not so in a First-Episode group who tend to be more sensitive to side-effects.

The first-episode sub-sample patients had to have no previous psychotic episodes when they entered in to this trial ; they had to have a length of current psychotic episode, less than or equal to 5 years and they had to be less than 45 years old. The subgroup was retrospectively picked out of a very large sample of patients. Patient characteristics were as follows : 59 Olanzapine-treated patients, 24 Haloperidol-treated patients ; more males-about two-thirds to one-third ; Age of Onset of the illness, 27 ; Length of Episode, 1 year on average ; slightly more than one-quarter in each group were Neuroleptic Naive.

The Olanzapine group tends to be treated with 5-10 mg with a subset getting larger doses. Haloperidol group tends to cluster around the 10 mg-dose, a small group receiving 20 mg. In terms of mean dose, Olanzapine is around 10-11mg, and Haloperidol is around 12-13 mg.

In terms of completion or discontinuation of the patients, more than two-thirds of the Olanzapine-treated patients are completing the 6-weeks of treatment, whereas only slightly more than one-third of the Haloperidol-treated patients are completing the 6-weeks. The reason for them not completing is either adverse events or lack of efficacy in the Haloperidol group. As a result, the clinical trial suggests that the atypicals, Olanzapine, offer a tremendous advantage in first-episode patients. Having said that, the dosing of Haloperidol is, again, somewhat aggressive for a First-Episode group. Efficacy results in terms of rating scale scores ; BBRS Total, BBRS Negative symptoms, PANSS Total, and PANSS Positive symptoms, all significantly improving on Olanzapine versus Haloperidol (Figure 1). And if we look at the efficacy from a different perspective, here we're looking at Olanzapine and response rates-greater than 40% improvement on the BPRS total at 6 weeks, about two-thirds of patients are achieving that milestone, less than a third on Haloperidol (Figure 2).

When we compare the two drugs in our First-Episode population versus our more chronic population in terms of this 40% improvement Olanzapine seems to really do well with the First-Episode group, even better than with the Multi-Episode group, which may simply reflect the fact that a

First-Episode population, has in general a better outcome when first treated with antipsychotics. But it doesn't seem to hold up when you look at Haloperidol within this study. And one of the reasons, that Olanzapine is doing so well in this particular study is that it is very well-tolerated. Parkinsonism is actually decreasing from baseline, and akathisia is decreasing from baseline, whereas with Haloperidol we're getting significant increases.

In the second study, "Olanzapine vs. Lower Dose Haloperidol," a study specifically designed to look at first-episode schizophrenia, and designed not just to look at short-term but also long-term efficacy and safety. Also the effects of these two different compounds were measured in terms of cognition and brain architecture using MRI and MRS. This study is one of the first to look potential brain anatomical changes in first-episode schizophrenia occurring with atypical antipsychotics versus the older drugs.

The study was a double-blind, randomized study that lasted 2 years. The length of this study is extraordinary compared to most clinical drug trials, but in first-episode it is important to study patients over an extended timeframe because we really are looking for longer-term effects. 262 patients were treated with Olanzapine in the same dosing range, as in the previous study-5 to 20 mg, but the Haloperidol dose could go down to 2 mg, a much more fair dose in a first-episode population.

The patient characteristics were younger than the last study that I showed you-more males, instead of two-thirds about four-fifths. The average dose of Olanzapine was 9 mg instead of 11 on average in the previous study. The Haloperidol group is treated with certainly half, if not a third of the dose that they received in the study that I showed you previously. So in this study, a reasonably fair comparison of these two drugs at doses that may be relevant clinically in the treatment of first-episode schizophrenia was carried out.

In terms of outcome, figures appear to support

	PANSS Total	PANSS Positive	PANSS Negative	MADRS Total	CGI - Severity
Olanzapine	-18.63	-7.30	-2.09	-2.97	-1.16
Haloperidol	-16.97	-7.17	-1.94	-1.02	-1.04

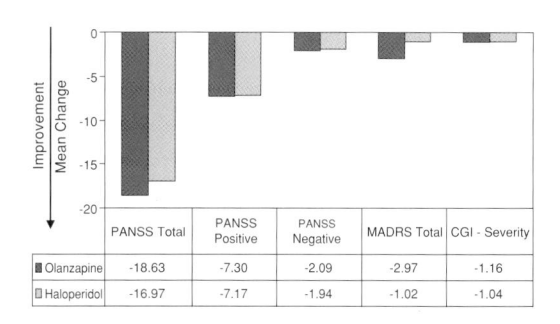

Figure 3　Efficacy scales : Mean change

Haloperidol much more so in this study. However Olanzapine is still doing better than Haloperidol on completion rates.

In terms of the efficacy data, Total PANSS, Positive PANSS, Negative PANSS, depression, and a clinical global impression of severity. Olanzapine is numerically superior, but it is not statistically significantly different on any one of these measures at 3 months compared to Haloperidol, when Haloperidol is dosed less aggressively (Figure 3).

On the other hand there is a statistically significant difference for the effects of Olanzapine and Haloperidol on neurocognition favoring Olanzapine. So even at 3 months, which is early, we are starting to see a neurocognitive effect that is differentiating the atypical drug Olanzapine from the conventional drug, Haloperidol.

This is not a surprising finding. As mentioned earlier, a comparative study of patients within the first 5 years of their disease was carried out looking at cognition comparing Olanzapine, Risperidone and Haloperidol. The study followed patients over 1 year. In the Haloperidol group, attention improves, but nothing else. The overall score is not significantly different from baseline. Risperidone does well on overall cognition and on two items, "Verbal" and "New Learning." The Olanzapine group, in this particular study, did extremely well on overall and a number of subitems on cognition. So these younger patients, treated with these atypical agents relative to the older drugs like Haloperidol, in fact, do improve their cognitive performance, and in some cases, quite dramatically.

Looking at the results of this study over time, on 52 weeks of Haloperidol treatment, you go from bad to worse. On 52 weeks of Risperidone and 52 weeks of Olanzapine, you go from bad to much better. And this improvement, although not back to the norm, is putting these people at an advantage to, possibly return to some form of normal life, because they are now able to use their cognitive abilities whereas before they were not.

We can thus say that there is at least some data to suggest that atypical antipsychotics are associated with improved cognition in first or early-episode schizophrenia. The next question is, "Is this improved cognition associated with brain anatomical changes?" This is important because it can be suggested that cognition improved because don't have as many side effects, such as extrapyramidal side effects. But if there's something also actually changing in their brain anatomically, then the association is more robust.

A study published in 1998 compared first-episode patients, chronic patients, and healthy controls.

The controls are fine, but the brains of the patients with first-episode schizophrenia and chronic schizophrenia show some signs of atrophy, specifically, in the frontal and the temporal lobe at baseline. They then followed these patients over a year, and found that on the left and the right side of the frontal cortex, the controls don't change much, and the chronic patients don't change much, although there's a little bit of a loss of frontal brain volume.

However the first-episode patients are changing much more dramatically, and also, it is only in the first-episode patients, that along with those changes, there's less improvement in negative symptoms, a decline in neurocognitive performance, and a treatment history of higher, conventional antipsychotic dose. This suggests that not only is there a neurocognitive decline but it's linked to brain anatomical changes with frontal volume decreasing, and temporal volume decreasing, and possibly associated with high doses of typical antipsychotics.

Going now back to the study of Olanzapine compared to lower dose Haloperidol in first episode schizophrenia. Let's look at MRI results in first-episode patients treated with either an atypical psychotic, in this case Olanzapine or Haloperidol. On Haloperidol on the right and the left side of the frontal cortex, gray matter decreases. With Olanzapine, there's no change. So once again, on the typical antipsychotics after 3 months in this study, there are neuroanatomical changes that are occurring that are not good, and would seem to represent frontal cortex atrophy and ventricular volume increase, which is not seen with atypical antipsychotic drug treatment. Furthermore as discussed previously this is associated with cognitive decline in the Haloperidol group. What does this all mean? Although the outcomes of using typical antipsychotics especially at conservative doses may be similar in terms of treating psychosis, the typical antipsychotics are allowing a neurodegenerative process in the brain associated with schizophrenia to progress. In contrast the atypicals especially Olanzapine seem to be able to arrest this process. That is why we need to get to our first episode patients as soon as possible. If we treat them early and with the newer drugs, perhaps we can stop the illness from progressing and keep schizophrenia in its more severe forms from emerging. At least that is the dream.

---

*Barry D. Jones, M. D. : McMaster University.

初回エピソード患者の治療における新しい非定型抗精神病薬の役割

The role of novel antipsychotics in the management of early/first episode psychosis

Tim Lambert*

Schizophrenia remains one of the most serious conditions to afflict mankind. It strikes persons in their prime and reduces both the quantity and quality of their lives. Treatments for the condition have improved but need to be optimized to improve long-term outcome. Additionally, many patients with this disease die younger than they should, and have abiding physical, psychological and social morbidities, despite treatment with antipsychotic medications. Hence appropriate treatments are crucial for Schizophrenia patients and particularly so for those experiencing their first episode of psychosis.

Before getting into the main topic, some predictors of poor outcome will be very briefly reviewed.

Gender is particularly relevant in first episodes. Males have earlier onsets with more severity (Iacono 1992) and outcome has been found to be worse (SSG, 1988). A window of between 17 and 24 years of age is described. All outcome dimensions, including suicide seem worse for males (Salokangas & Stengard 1990). Neurodevelopmental models favour the poorer outcome for males (Murray, O'Callaghan, et al., 1992). Females, on the other hand, appear to have a better pharmacological response (Szymanski, et al., 1995).

Symptom balance: The balance of positive vs. negative symptoms (NS) at the start of the illness suggests negative symptoms have a worse prognosis (SSG, 1988). When patients present with NS, they are usually primary (Peralta, Cuesta, et al., 2000). These symptoms may reflect changes in brain structures (supported by more recent MRI findings of frontal volume reductions). Negative symptoms are (collectively) a sign of ongoing changes in brain function, essentially for the worse and their presence clearly points to a reduced expectation of recovery.

Affectivity: Unlike the 'old days', mood symptoms are no longer considered as a good sign today, and there is suspicion that having a mood component early on may actually lead to a worse prognosis (Geddes, 1994).

Good *pre-morbid social functioning* and active *psycho-education* are also useful predictors of positive outcome. Among the predictors of poor outcome, the worst is arguably the duration of untreated psychosis (DUP), since if we fail to initiate antipsychotic treatment at an early stage, it may well lead to more severe symptoms and increased time to recovery. Both poor premorbid functioning and long DUP are significantly correlated with more negative symptoms and poorer global functioning at follow-up (Larsen, Moe et al. 2000). Hence, it is essential to try and measure negative symptoms and estimate the duration of untreated psychosis when we firstly admit a patient, and the DUP should be kept below 6 months (where possible).

Now we are going to look at the changes in the brain. The brain morphology changes reflect active toxic pathology - positive symptoms being a proposed marker of this process. For instance, when comparing an control brain with a chronic schizophrenic brain, the left is always smaller than the right in both control and the schizophrenic brain, although in the latter the volumes are significantly reduced. When we consider the brain volume of the first episode group in comparison to the chronic group we find that after a certain amount of time there is no difference between them. This suggests to us is that we have a limited time to intervene before the brain of first episode patients cannot be distinguished from that of chronic relapsing patients. Therefore we must intervene as quickly as possible to prevent the brain from experiencing the ongoing toxic event of psychosis. Put another way, the psychosis is a sign that something wrong is happening to the brain, and we should intervene as early as possible in order to prevent the brain from shrinking.

It is now accepted that the 2nd generation antipsychotics (the aconventionals) are popular treatment in such cases and are the first line treatment in many settings. Where the availability of these agents is reduced, *low-dose* conventionals can be prescribed as an alternative. However, for first episode patients, we need to be particularly cautious in the use of typical antipsychotics. In order to help explain the reason for this, we shall look at four areas of dopamine function in the brain

First, the pituitary infundibular area. In this circuit, dopamine is released from the hypothalamus and acts as a neurohormone that works as the prolactin releasing inhibiting factor. When dopamine binds to dopamine receptors on the lactotrophs, it results in the restraint of prolactin release. Therefore, since both atypical and typical agents block D2 receptors, prolactin can escape from the control of dopamine, and hyperprolactinaemia may result. The conventionals, as well as large doses of atypicals such as Risperidone (>6 mg) which is a tightly-bound drug with respect to D2 receptors, can cause hyperprolactinaemia. This can adversely effect sexual functioning, and may be of particular concern to younger, first episode patients.

Avoiding sexual side effects is particularly cru-

Table 1 Pituitary-infundibular system : Prolactinemic symptoms

	Risperidone (N=202)	Olanzapine (N=205)
Impotence	4 (2.0%)	1 (0.5%)
Ejaculation failure	3 (1.5%)	0 (0.0%)
Libido decreased	3 (1.5%)	1 (0.5%)
Anorgasmia	2 (1.0%)	0 (0.0%)
Breast pain male	2 (1.0%)	0 (0.0%)
Breast pain female	2 (1.0%)	1 (0.5%)
Sexual function abn.	2 (1.0%)	1 (0.5%)
Ejaculation disorder	1 (0.5%)	0 (0.0%)
Dysmenorrhoea	0 (0.0%)	2

Conley, 2001

Both Risperidone and Olanzapine have hyperprolactinemic effects, but OLZ is less than RIS, as predicted by D2 affinity

cial for compliance as side effects in general will often lead to rapid discontinuation of treatment in this group. The very loosely-bound dopamine antagonists Clozapine and Quetiapine, have little hyperprolactinaemia. Moderately binding drugs such as Olanzapine have hyperprolactinaemia only at the initial stages of treatment and in the main normalize with ongoing treatment. (Table 1). Even loosely bound drugs can have other potent adverse effects, and the long-term efficacy of some have yet been proven, Therefore, to conclude, we have quite a limited choice in the treatment for first episodes when we consider the need to avoid hyperprolactinaemia.

The second dopaminergic system to consider, is that of the meso-cortical dopamine projections (ventral tegmentum to pre-frontal cortex). This is an important system for us as these dopamine tracts have been imputed to subserve neurocognition, and thus mediate the ability to 'understand', to plan and judge for the future, to help us navigate through the complexities of daily living. Related to this circuit are the clinical syndromes of reduced motivation, language, emotion and affect, and other dimensions of function, which we label as 'nega-

Table 2 Mesocortical system : Negative neurocognitive symptoms

A typical neuroleptics improve negative symptoms where conventionals either do nothing or worsen them...

	Total Scores	Positive Symptoms	Negative Symptoms	EPS
Clozapine CLZ	CLZ>CPZ	CLZ>CPZ	CLZ>CPZ	CLZ<CPZ
Risperidone RIS	RIS>HPD	RIS>HPD	RIS>HPD	RIS<HPD
Olanzapine OLZ	OLZ>HPD	OLZ=HPD	OLZ>HPD	OLZ<HPD
Quetiapine QTP	QTP=HPD	QTP=HPD	QTP=HPD	QTP<HPD
Ziprasidone ZIP	ZIP=HPD	ZIP=HPD	?	ZIP<HPD

Adapted from Conley/Keith et al

tive symptoms'. These are thought to occur due to reduction of dopamine function. In first episodes of Schizophrenia, frontal lobe function is often already impaired by the time of first hospitalization or diagnosis. The 'hypofrontal' clinical picture, presumably one of hypodopaminergic function, is connected to both neuro-cognitive deficits and negative symptoms. Conventional antipsychotics may give worse outcomes with respect to negative and neurocognitive deficits since they block dopamine function in pre-frontal cortex, which is already presumed to be dysfunctional. The neuropharmacology of the atypicals is sufficiently different from conventionals with respect to enhancing pre-frontal dopaminergic function and it is for this reason that the atypical drugs, such as Clozapine, Risperidone and Olanzapine, are more efficacious in negative and neurocognitve symptom domains. (Table 2)

In distinguishing novel antipsychotics from older ones, the concept of improvement in frontal hypodopaminergic function is critical for understanding differential effects on social reintegration. For first episode patients, giving typical agents often decreases frontal functioning rather than enhances it, Needless to say, for effective community-based management atypicals are first line medications

Neurocognitive symptoms are improved very little with typical agents-in contrast to the atytpicals.

Improvements in NC function may predict return to work and better outcome in general.

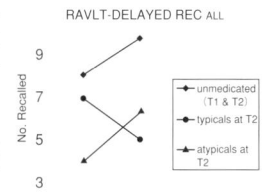

BASELINE 6 MONTHS
non-medicated vs typicals, p<0.05
atypicals, paired t(7) = −2.89, p<0.0

Pantels, Bewer et al.

Figure 1 Neurocognitive responses

when the gestalt of social competence is considered.

As mentioned neurocognitive deficit symptoms also should be considered at this point, since their improvement relates to better outcome. Some indicative data from the Melbourne Group are shown in Fig 1.(Figure 1). When patients are treated with atypicals, cognitve functions significantly improve, (a similar picture with unmedicated controls is also seen). In contrast cognitive functioning gets worse with conventionals. This suggests that conventionals are potentially 'poisoning' some of cognitive process. It is not difficult to conclude that high dose typical agents are likely to worsen frontal functioning, and thereby impair cognition and motivation - the worst possible effect one would desire in first episode patients.

Partly referable to the frontal systems, although presumably more extensively distributed than in just dopamine systems, is the disregulation of mood and affect in schizophrenia. Schizophrenia patients have increased cross-sectional rates of depression. It's reported that at least 20% of female schizophrenic meet the Hamilton Depression rating scale levels of marked depression at any time point. In our own services, we find that it would be commonplace to find 20% of the schizophrenia patients receiving SSRI antidepressants at any one time. The severity of depressive symptoms is correlated with positive symptoms but not with age, gender, or negative symptoms. This suggests that if we are successful in applying early intervention strategies to treat positive symptoms, we may see better outcomes with comorbid depressive symptoms. This is especially important considering lifetime prevalence of major depression in schizophrenia is 50% and that the suicide rate is 20 times the normal population. Depression may be even more prevalent in first-episodes as up to one third of patients can meet criteria for major depressive episode during their first episode break.

Depressive syndromes of schizophrenia appear to be responsive to the atypicals more so than to the conventionals (the conventionals are sometimes said to *induce* dysphoria, rather than relieve it). The thymoleptic or mood stabilizing properties of the newer agents, Olanzapine, Clozapine, and risperidone have been variously demonstrated. More recent data from a Risperidone verses Olanzapine RCT study that suggests that Risperidone also has very capable properties in amelioration of mood symptoms. This is particularly important for first episodes, as, in order to enhance compliance, we need to use the lowest possible doses of a single agent. As depressive phenomena are a major part of the presentation for many first episode patients, being able to give a medicine that has good effects on mood as well as negative and cognitive symptoms is obviously very useful. This is another reason for using atypical antipsychotics as a first line treatment.

The third dopamineric system we are concerned with are the motor tracts (the nigro-striatal tracts of the basal ganglia from substantia Nigra pars compacta to the caudate and putamen). Dopamine is essential for normal motoric responses. All conventionals are prone to cause neuroleptic-induced extrapyramidal symptoms (EPS) when given at doses required for antipsychotic effects. These occur in one form or another as a consequence of blocking dopamine-2 receptors in the basal ganglia. The first episode patient is much more sensitive to medication, and therefore EPS, and in some cases may develop dystonia on very low doses of typical agents. Studies have showed that first episode patients treated with even low doses of Haloperidol have much more EPS than those receiving standard or equivalent doses of novel antipsychotics. In general, atypical antipsychotics have less EPS than typical agents when used in monotherapy in the appropriate dose ranges - this was the source of the original appellation 'atypical'. Considering the fact that first episode patients are very sensitive to EPS, the best solution for drug naive patients is to start giving medication from a very low dose, possibly as low as a half dose of chronic patients. This will help to prevent the patients from developing dystonia as well as the other acute EPS such as akathisia and parkinsonism. Once patients experience dystonic (and other EPS) reactions they are loath to ever take medicine again. This is compounded by the low detection rates so that many patients experience these side effects without recourse to side-effect treatment and other EPS management. The importance and critical nature of dosing now comes into focus. The sensitivity of first episode patients makes them exquisitely susceptible to EPS if 'adult' doses are used. Antipsychotic effects (see below) are obtained with lower doses in both old and newer classes of medicine but conventionals still cause appreciable comparable EPS at lower doses. Atypicals are considered optimum in this situation as they have far reduced EPS and are equally (or better) equipped to reduce positive symptoms (Table 3).

The fourth dopaminergic schema to be presented is the meso-limbic system - projections from the midbrain VTA to the limbic nuclei. In affecting this system, we are able to consider the use of both old and new drugs. It is thought that positive symptoms are due to an overactivity of dopamine in the meso-limbic system, whereas negative symptoms are due to its effective underactivity (in meso-cortical systems). It is necessary to reduce dopamine function in the mesolimbic projections

Table 3 Nigro-striatal systems : Extrapyromidal symptoms

Atypical neuroleptics cause much reduced EPS and decreased longer term phenomena such as TD. EPS is a major cause of non-compliance in FEP...

	Total Scores	Positive Symptoms	Negative Symptoms	EPS
Clozapine CLZ	CLZ>CPZ	CLZ>CPZ	CLZ>CPZ	CLZ<CPZ
Risperidone RIS	RIS>HPD	RIS>HPD	RIS>HPD	RIS<HPD
Olanzapine OLZ	OLZ>HPD	OLZ=HPD	OLZ>HPD	OLZ<HPD
Quetiapine QTP	QTP=HPD	QTP=HPD	QTP=HPD	QTP<HPD
Ziprasidone ZIP	ZIP=HPD	ZIP=HPD	?	ZIP<HPD

Adapled from Conley/Keith et al

and enhance it in the projections to the frontal lobes. Only the novel antipsychotics are capable of fulfilling both actions in the one patient.

In contrasting the doses required for first-episodes, a number of early studies used doses of the medications which were higher than needed (Remoxipride vs. Thioridazine, 348 vs. 361 mg/day, Lambert et al 1995 ; Risperidone vs Haloperidol : 6.1 vs 5.6 mg/day, Emsley et al 1999). Emsley et al treated FE patients with haloperidol or Risperidone and found little difference in efficacy between the treatments. However, when doses were stratified into those <6 mg and those >6 mg per day, patients did as well on the lower doses with lower EPS. In addition, the tolerability of Risperidone was greater.(Emsley et al, 1999). McGorry et al(1977) presented early results of a very low dose strategy for first episodes. In this study, 2 mg RIS was commenced in non-affective FE patients : 60-70% responded in 4 weeks and non-responders, who had their doses increased to 4 mg/day then responded with good effect. In a number of studies examining low dose strategies with Risperidone, Kopala et al showed that RIS(2-4 mg) was more effective than higher doses (5-8mg) in terms of psychopathology and propensity to cause clinically significant EPS. A number o studies based on McEvoy's neuroleptic threshold concept also support that lower doses(usually not exceeding 4mg/day) of conventionals such as haloperidol are required for first episodes. Finally, Lieberman et al studied first episode patients in a RCT of haloperidol vs. olanzapine. The mean doses required were 9.1 mg for Olanzapine and 4.4 mg for haloperidol.Response rates were comparable but in terms of tolerability and quality of life, Olanzapine was superior(more completers and less EPS). Sanger and Lieberman(1999) conclude that novel antipsychotic agents such as olanzapine should be considered as a preferred option in first-episode psychosis, on the basis of both safety and efficacy advantages.

To summarize the issue of dosing strategies : first episode patients are proven to show a greater response to neuroleptic therapy than chronic patients due to neuroleptic sensitivity. Both older and newer drugs can show efficacy but if a medication such as haloperidol is used, 2 to 6 mg per day in monotherapy is optimal. Nevertheless, in Australia and many other countries, Haloperidol and other conventionals are not used for first episodes at all as their risk-benefit ratio is inferior to the aconventionals.

Conclusion

Novel antipsychotics(such as Olanzapine and Risperidone) should be first line treatments for psychosis due to improved effect on positive, negative, affective, and cognitive symptoms combined with low EPS and reduced side effect burden, especially hyperprolactinemia. Ultimately this leads to enhanced compliance through efficacy and tolerability. It is hoped that this will in turn reduce the period of DUP and lead to superior long-term outcomes for patients with first episode psychoses.

*Tim Lambert, M. D. : University of Melbourne.

予防的観点からみた ADHD 児の治療
―親訓練プログラムを通して―

Treatment of children with ADHD from the aspect of prevention : Parent Training Program

岩坂　英巳* 　飯田　順三** 　崎山　忍*** 　岸本　年史***

I. はじめに

ここ数年 ADHD に関して，医療・教育そして一般の方で関心が高まっているが，その理由として，①3～5％という頻度の多さ，②診断の難しさ，③総合的な治療計画の難しさ，④予後の多様さ，⑤昨今のマスコミ報道の影響で，学級崩壊や非行，少年事件と ADHD が結びつけられがちなことなどがあげられる。

特に診療場面で ADHD をもつ子どもの親や教師に説明すべきと思われることは，もともとは脳の機能障害であって，本人のわがままや親の養育の失敗ではないということと，経過の中であらわれる2次障害としての行為障害や Self-Esteem の低下などは，周囲の対応で変わるということである。

そこで，学校生活を困難にする ADHD 児への総合的な治療としては，全米での多施設共同の臨床的研究 MTA Study でも結論されているように，正確な診断ののちに，①薬物療法，②行動療法(親訓練，本人への SST)，③家族支援，そして④教育への介入・連携のコンビネーションを行うことである。そこで，本稿ではこの②と③にあたる，行動療法と家族支援を兼ねそなえた親訓練について奈良での試みを報告し，2次障害の予防という観点から若干の考察を行った。

II. 奈良県立医大親訓練の目的

奈良県立医大精神科では，Massachusetts 医療センター R. Barkley のプログラムと著者が98～99年留学中に参加したカリフォルニア大学ロサンゼルス校(UCLA)の Parent Training Program を参考にして，2000年2月より「奈良医大 ADHD 家族教室」を開始した。

親訓練の目的は，子どもの ADHD としての行動特徴を理解し，行動療法に基づく効果的な対応法を習得し，子どもの適応行動を増やすとともに，よりよい親子関係の獲得をめざすことである。また，親同士のサポート機能の育成も意識して行っている。

III. 親訓練の対象と内容

対象は，ADHD と診断された小学2～4年生児の親である。

方法は，1回1時間半のセッションを原則隔週で，1クール全10回を同一メンバー(1グループ5～6名)で行った。各回テーマを決めて学習，話し合い，練習を行い，さらにホームワークとして自宅でも練習し，グループ全体でステップバイステップで進んでいく。

内容は表1にあるように，①ADHD の医学的知識の講義とプログラムオリエンテーションを行い，ADHD は脳の機能障害であり，本人のわがままや親の育て方のせいではない，しかし周囲の対応によって経過がかわるので，その適切な対応法をこのプログラムで習得していく，という点を強調している。②子どもの行動を前後の状況からも観察する。表の右側〈　〉の内容はホームワークで，行動―対応―結果について観察記録をつけ，子どもの行動を客観的に観察する習慣をつけていく。③子どもの行動を良い行動，良くない行動，問題行動の3つに分ける練習を通して，良い注目の仕方をマスターしていき，④親子タイムでの「良いところさがし」で，子どもの行動のなかから，良い行動に注目してほめていく練習をくり返し行う。⑤前半5回のセッションでのメンバー

表1　プログラム全体の流れ

1) 講義「ADHDの医学的知識」と 　　プログラムのオリエンテーション	〈前評価〉
2) 子どもの行動の観察と理解 　　【ロールプレイ】	〈H.W.：行動—対応—結果〉
3) 子どもの行動へのよい注目のしかた	〈H.W.：行動の3つの類型分け〉
4) 親子タイムと良いところさがし	〈H.W.：親子タイムシート作り〉
5) 前半のふりかえり	〈H.W.：親子タイム〉
6) 子どもが従いやすい指示の出し方 　　【ロールプレイ】	〈H.W.：指示—反応—次にどうしたか〉
7) 上手なほめ方，無視の仕方 　　【ロールプレイ】	〈H.W.：行動—どうほめたか／ 　　行動—どう無視したか—その反応〉
8) トークンシステム	〈H.W.：トークンポイント表作り〉
9) タイムアウトと後半のまとめ 　　【ロールプレイ】	〈H.W.：警告—反応—次にどうしたか／ 　　トークンポイント表〉
10) 全体のまとめ 　　【ビデオフィードバック】 　　【家族の自信度再記入】	〈後評価お願いとブースターセッション〉
11) 修了パーティ（親も子どもも参加）	

のがんばりの結果，親子のやりとりがスムーズになり，良い注目をすることが上手になっていることをフィードバックするとともに，親子タイムの継続を指示する。

後半5回は，子どもの行動に対しての具体的な対応法をロールプレイもまじえて練習していく。⑥ADHDの不注意，持続できないなどの特徴をふまえて，より従いやすい指示の出し方の練習，⑦〜⑨3つに分けた行動に対しての，上手なほめかた，無視の仕方，そしてトークンとタイムアウトの仕方について練習を順次行っていく。最終の，⑩メンバーへのポジティブフィードバックとしてのセッション前半と後半でのビデオ比較や訓練前後での評価尺度の変化を皆で確認しあい，今後の親子のやりとりへの自信と習得した対応法の継続を確認する。また，⑪修了パーティとして，子どもにも参加してもらい，親へは修了証書の授与，子どもへは親子タイムやトークン表でのがんばりを賞して，メダルの授与などを行い，メンバー間の親睦を深め，半年間にわたるプログラムを終了した。

次に，プログラムのいくつかの重要なポイントを説明する。まず，行動の3つの類型分けとは，子どもの行動を親からみて①好ましい行動，すなわち増やしたい行動，②好ましくない，すなわち減らしたい行動，そして③破壊的で他人を傷つける可能性があり，すぐ止めるべき行動に分ける。そして，①好ましい行動に対しては，すぐ，具体的にほめる，②好ましくない行動には無視，すなわち余計な注目をしないことで子どもに今の行動が良くないことを気づかせ，良い行動に変わればすぐほめる，③問題行動には，まず警告を発し，本人に従うチャンスと責任を負わせ，それでも従わなかった時はタイムアウト，罰を与える。ここで重要なのは，このようにして一貫性をもって対応することで，子どもに正しい行動を気づかせ，身につけさせていくということである。

次に親子タイムとは，子どもにとって特別な時間で，①親は干渉せずに子どもとかかわり，②子どもは，自分の好きな遊びをする，ただしTVゲームなどはだめで，対人関係の必要な遊びをする。③親は子どものやっていることをよく観察して，実況するように声を出したり，いいなと思うことをどんどんほめていく。

このような親子タイムを行うことで，親は子どもの良い行動への注意の向け方が上達し，すぐ具体的にほめる習慣がつく。子どもは叱られずに，良い注目をうけることが多くなり，その結果，親

表2　対象者の背景と訓練効果

学年	性別	亜型	併存障害	薬物	行動調査票	子どもの気分尺度	親の自信度	親のGHQ
小2	M	混合型	ODD，LD	リタリン	54→42↑	39→28↑	68→88↑	33→16↑
小4	M	混合型	ODD，MR，夜尿	リタリン	7→16↓	27→22↑	40→48↑	14→22↓
小4	M	混合型	LD，CD	リタリン セレネース	57→56	39→28↑	41→54↑	48→42↑
小4	F	不注意優勢型	MR，恐怖症	リタリン	29→36↓	19→27↓	39→74↑	14→36↓
小4	F	混合型	境界知能，チック	リタリン	36→22↑	0→0	40→80↑	14→12
小2	M	混合型	ODD，LD	リタリン	44→24↑	31→24↑	73→73	48→22↑
小2	M	混合型	ODD，LD，不安障害	リタリン	10→10	39→42	65→77↑	10→43↓
小3	M	混合型	ODD，OCD，恐怖症	リタリン	30→35↓	29→29	65→70↑	26→12↑
小3	M	不注意優勢型	境界知能，夜尿	リタリン	17→18	32→24↑	58→79↑	29→33
小3	M	混合型	LD，癲癇性脳波異常	テグレトール	35→11↑	32→24↑	72→68	30→15↑
小3	M	多動衝動優勢	ODD	リタリン	36→16↑	25→25	79→83	13→24↓

学年は訓練開始時学年
ODD：反抗挑戦性障害　CD：行為障害　LD：学習障害　OCD：強迫性障害　MR：精神発達遅滞
評価尺度　改善：↑　悪化：↓　不変：矢印なし

子のやりとりがスムーズになり，子どものSelf-Esteemの高まりも期待される。

Ⅳ．親訓練の効果

訓練前の評価尺度としては，子どもの評価として，DSM-Ⅳに準拠した山崎らによるADHD-RS親用・教師用，行動の全般評価のCBCL(Achenbach)，子どもの気分やSelf-Esteemの目安となるDepression Self-rating Scale for Children(Birleson)，そしてSM社会生活能力検査，親の評価は，心身健康度GHQ60と子どものADHDの受容や行動への対応の自信を評価する上林らによる家族の自信度評価票，そしてTK式親子関係テストを行った。訓練後には，ADHD-RS，DSRSC，GHQ，家族の自信度評価票を再評価し，効果判定を行った。

訓練参加者の子どもの背景と訓練前後の評価尺度の変化を表2に示した。表の上5名が第1期，下6名が第2期で，年齢は小学2年から4年で，男児9名，女児2名であった。併存障害は，LD5名，ODD(反抗挑戦性障害)6名，不安障害圏3名などであった。薬物は全員が服用しており，10名がリタリン，行為障害を伴う1名がセレネース，1名がテグレトールであった。

訓練効果をみてみる。各評価尺度で，改善は↑，悪化は↓，不変は無矢印で示した。

行動そのものは，評価期間中にリタリンを開始した1期の小4女児と，2期小3男児で行動が改善しているのを除けば，小2で2名，小3で1名と年少児で行動改善がみられており，年少児ほど行動改善がみられやすかった。子どもの気分尺度は，1名のみ悪化で，他は不変か改善。親の自信度は，1期の全員，2期も不変3名はいずれも訓練前から自信度が高かったため変化なしとなっているだけで，訓練後には全員高い自信度を持てるようになっていた。また，行動そのものの改善・悪化によって，子どもの気分や親の心身健康度が影響をうけやすい傾向がみられた。

訓練効果の理解を深めるために，典型例をひとつ提示する。

〈症例〉

小学2年男児で，主訴は落ち着きがない，宿題ができない，指示に従えない。ODDとLDを合併するADHD混合型。ADHDの家族負因あり。訓練前後で評価尺度の変化した項目を具体的にあげると，行動面では，順序立ての困難，忘れやすい，妨害，かんしゃく，指示に従えない，達成できないなどADHD-RSの多くの項目で改善。子どもの気分面でも，DSRSCの項目で，何をしても楽しい，いじめられても「やめて」といえる，やろうと思ったことがうまくできる，家族と話すのが好きだなどがよくなっていた。これらより，自分に「やればできる」という達成感，自信がでてきて，気分が明るくなり，親子関係も良くなってきていることが示唆された。親の自信度も，本人の成長を焦らずに見守る，不適応行動に対処する，本人のADHDへの自分の不安をへらすなど多くの項目で自信が持てるようになっていた。親のGHQも改善しており，特に身体的疲労度が改善していた。本ケースは，反抗的だった子どもが親子タイムをとても楽しみにし，母親も親子タイムを通してほめる習慣がついた，本人といて楽しいと感じられるようになったと語り，苦手だった宿題も指示に従ってできるようになった。

V．考察とまとめ

高橋らによると，アメリカではSelf-Esteemに焦点をあてた一般学童の精神保健1次予防活動のモデルがオレゴン州などで行われている。それは，「不適切なSelf-Esteemが，学習上の問題，無断欠席，破壊的行動や自殺，薬物依存などにつながる恐れがある」「Self-Esteemを高め，学童期の行動特徴を変化させることは，将来の精神障害や適応障害の発症予防や再発予防に効果的である」というデータに基づいている。つまり，ADHDの2次障害のひとつである行為障害などの予防には，Self-Esteemを高め，学童期の行動特徴を変化させていくことが重要である。

また，学校精神保健の立場から，Self-Esteemを変容させていくためには，学級での個別配慮，コミュニケーション技能を育成するプログラムの活用，ハイリスク児への早期発見・早期介入，家族のプログラム参加の促進などが重要であるとされている。CHADD（全米のADHD自助組織）でも，親訓練の最も大切な効果は，行動変容だけでなく，親子のSelf-Esteemの改善である，と会報に述べられている。

今回の奈良医大親訓練にて，子どもの行動特徴は年少児ほど改善しやすいこと，子どものSelf-Esteemが達成感や親子のスムーズなやりとりによって改善すること，親の子どもへの対応の自信回復がみられることなどがわかった。以上から，このような親訓練的プログラムを学童期早期から行うことは，ADHD児の2次障害の予防に有効である可能性が示唆された。

---

*奈良県心身障害者リハビリセンター
　Hidemi Iwasaka : Nara Prefectural Rehabilitation Center.

**奈良県立医大看護短期大学部
　Junzo Iida : Colledge of Nursing, Nara Medical University.

***奈良県立医大精神医学教室
　Shinobu Sakiyama, Toshifumi Kishimoto : Department of Psychiatry, Nara Medical University.

学校の精神保健とその問題の予防：注意欠陥多動障害(ADHD)
ADHD in terms of prevention

原田　謙*

A disciplinary facility for children is one of the facilities in which the author works as a part-time psychiatrist. This facility is unique in that three married couples of teachers work as parents looking after several children to correct their antisocial behavior. The author has been involved in care in this facility for 4 years. Most children who enter this facility will be diagnosed as having conduct disorder(CD) according to DSM-IV[1]. Many of the children are very restless and careless, and are regarded as having attention-deficit/hyperactivity disorder(ADHD).

In this article, ADHD and ADHD-related disorders were reviewed from the viewpoint of prevention based on the investigation of the children in a disciplinary facility.

Subjects

The subjects were 33 children, consisting of 28 boys and 5 girls, aged 12-16 years, who were in Facility A between April 1999 and March 2001. The mean age was 13.6 years at interview. The purpose of the investigation was orally explained to the subjects at interview, and the consent was obtained in writing from their parents or guardians.

Methods

The female teachers as the mother were interviewed using the semi-structured interview method, which was produced by National Center of Neurology and Psychiatry based on the structured interview of Berkley et al[2]. The author also interviewed all children and diagnosed their conditions according to DSM-IV, and if children were diagnosed as having ADHD, oppositional defiant disorder(ODD) or CD, the times of the occurrence of the disorders were investigated by asking questions of their parents or guardians using a questionnaire. The ages at the occurrence of the disorders were statistically examined using the Kruskal-Wallis method. Comparisons of groups were performed using the Bonferroni/Dunn method. Psychosocial problems were examined using the records of examination performed at admission and by interviewing the male teachers as the father.

Results

Of the 33 children, 26 consisting of 21 boys and 5 girls were diagnosed as having CD. Table 1 shows the comorbid behavioral and developmental disorders in the CD children. According to DSM-IV, subjects who are diagnosed as having CD are not diagnosed as having ODD, but in this study, overlap of both CD and ODD was allowed for better understanding of the characteristics.

Of the 26 CD children, 17 were diagnosed as having ADHD(65%), and 18 were diagnosed as having ODD(69%). Eight children were diagnosed as having mental retardation(MR) with an IQ less than 70(31%), and 2(8%) were diagnosed as having pervasive developmental disorder (PDD).

Figure 1 shows the psychosocial problems in the CD children, of which divorce between the actual parents was noted for 18 children(69%), followed by abuse in 12(46%) and mothers with mental disorders such as schizophrenia and mental retardation in 5(19.2%).

Table 1 The comorbid behavioral and developmental disorders in the CD children.

No	sex	age	ADHD	ODD	MR	PDD
1	F	13	○	○	○	
2	M	13	○	○	○	
3	M	15	○	○	○	
4	F	13	○	○		
5	F	15	○	○		
6	M	12	○	○		
7	M	12	○	○		
8	M	12	○	○		
9	M	14	○	○		
10	M	14	○	○		
11	M	15	○	○		
12	M	15	○	○		
13	M	11	○		○	
14	M	12	○		○	
15	M	14	○		○	
16	F	14	○			
17	F	15	○			
18	M	13		○	○	
19	M	12		○		
20	M	13		○		
21	M	14		○		
22	M	15		○		
23	M	15		○		○
24	M	13				○
25	M	15			○	
26	M	14				

Note ; ADHD ; Attention-Deficit/Hyperactivity Disorder, ODD ; Oppositional Defiant Disorder, CD ; Conduct Disorder, MR ; Mental Retardation, PDD ; Pervasive Developmental Disorder.

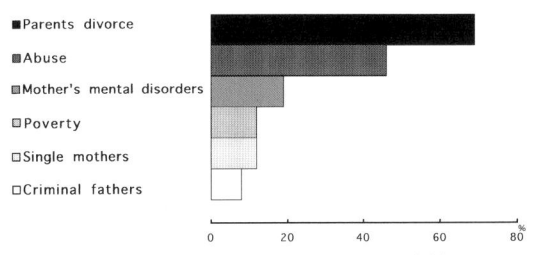

Figure 1 Psychosocial problems in the CD children

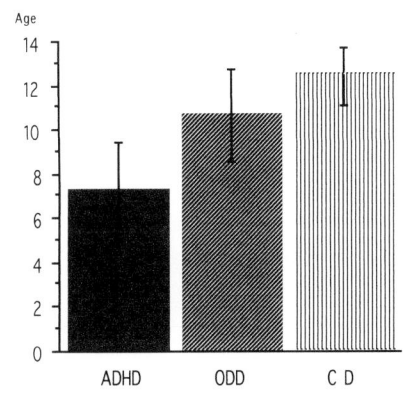

Figure 2 The age at the occurrence of ADHD, ODD and CD in 22 children with adolescent-onset type of CD.

Figure 2 shows the ages at the occurrence of ADHD, ODD and CD in 22 children with adolescent-onset type of CD. The mean age at the occurrence was 7.3 years in ADHD, 10.7 years in ODD, and 12.4 years in CD. There were significant differences in the age at the occurrence between ADHD and ODD and between ODD and CD (P< 0.01).

Discussion

It is controversial whether biological or psychosocial factors are more important as the risk factors of CD[15,19]. Gender[16], genetic factors[3,4], difficult temperament[14] are regarded as biological, and factors such as, socioeconomic disadvantage, marital discord and/or poor family functioning, poor parenting, child abuse and neglect, familial substance abuse and psychiatric illness and negative peer relationships and role model are regarded as psychosocial[7,11]. CD, which is considered to be a heterogeneous disorder, is caused by one of the above factors or their combination[6]. Recently, the complication of CD with ADHD has been drawing attention[9,13,17].

Epidemiological studies[5,18,20] indicated that ADHD was complicated with CD at a rate of 18~23%. In 55~85% of children who had been diagnosed as having CD, complication with ADHD was reported, indicating that preexisting ADHD markedly affects the occurrence of CD.

How is ADHD complicated with CD? The key to understanding the process is in the concept of ODD (Table 2). ODD is a pattern of negativistic, hostile, and defiant behavior. A criterion is considered met only if the behavior occurs more frequently than is typically observed in individuals of comparable age and developmental level[1].

ODD is regarded as the developmentally preceding stage or prodrome of CD. Epidemiological

Table 2 Diagnostic criteria for oppositional defiant disorder by DSM-IV

A. A pattern of negativistic, hostile, and defiant behavior lasting at least 6 months, during which four (or more) of the following are present:
(1) often loses temper
(2) often argues with adults
(3) often actively defies or refuses to comply with adults requests or rules
(4) often deliberately annoys people
(5) often blames others for his or her mistakes or misbehavior
(6) is often touchy or easily annoyed by others
(7) is often angry and resentful
(8) is often spiteful or vindictive
B, C, D are omitted.
Note : Consider a criterion met only if the behavior occurs more frequently than is typically observed in individuals of comparable age and developmental level.

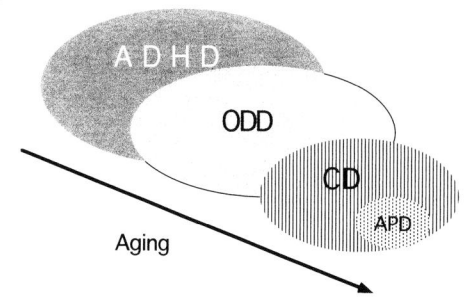

Figure 3 DBD movement

The author considers that the transition in the behavior disorders with aging can be called "DBD movement". Note ; ADHD ; Attention-Deficit／Hyperactivity Disorder, ODD ; Oppositional Defiant disorder, CD ; Conduct Disorder, APD ; Antisocial Personality disorder.

studies[5,18,20] indicated that ADHD was complicated with ODD at a rate of 30~45%, and 25% of children who were diagnosed as having ODD were diagnosed as having CD by re-examination performed 3~4 years later[10].

During the period of growth, about 40% of ADHD schoolchildren, who are very aggressive, satisfy the diagnostic criteria of ODD, and about 30% of ODD show CD symptoms with development of mental and physical ability around adolescence. Furthermore, 40% of CD juveniles become diagnosed as having antisocial personality disorder, and more often commit brutal crimes[22].

In DSM-IV, ADHD, ODD and CD are considered to be related with each other, and categorized into attention-deficit and disruptive behavior disorder (DBD). The author considers that the transition in the behavior disorders can be called "DBD movement" (Figure 3).

The results obtained in this study serves as evidence of DBD movement. Of the 26 CD children, 12 were diagnosed as having ADHD and ODD. The age at the occurrence of ADHD was the lowest, followed by ODD and CD. These findings indicated that about half the children reached CD in the course of DBD movement.

Various methods such as psychodynamic psychotherapy, psychopharmacological treatment, group therapy, behavior therapy and family therapy including parenting skills training have been used for the treatment of CD children. However, none of them is considered effective on its own in treating adolescent patients with severe CD[21].

According to Loeber[12], since the treatment of CD is less effective because it is difficult to correct troublesome behaviors due to the fixation of personality with growth, it is important to treat the disorder in the "reversible" ODD stages. In other words, ODD is a critical point to stop the development of DBD movement, and early diagnosis of ODD in ADHD children and intensive treatment would prevent CD or suppress CD symptoms.

To verify this hypothesis, it is necessary to examine the prognosis in treatment and non-treatment groups of children with both ADHD and ODD, randomly divided. However, this kind of study is unrealistic, because appropriate comparisons are difficult, and because there are ethical problems in deliberately leaving some of the children untreated.

Since ADHD and ODD children and their surrounding adults are very concerned about the symptoms, it is necessary to treat the disorder appropriately. The author considers it important to reduce the number of children in whom ADHD and ODD advances to CD by early treatment, even if a little.

Lastly, since ADHD is also a risk factor of anxiety and mood disorders in children[8], which is not discussed in this paper due to space limitations, appropriate treatment of ADHD can also prevent these mental disorders.

References

1) American Psychiatric Association : Diagnostic and statistical manual of mental disorders. Forth ed., American Psychiatric Association, Washington, D.C., 1994.
2) Barkley, R. A. and Murphy, K. R. : A clinical workbook Attention-deficit hyperactivity disorder 2ed. The Guilford Press, New York, 1998.
3) Eaves, L., Silberg, J., Hewitt, J., Rutter, M. : Analyzing twin resemblance in multisystem data : genetic applications of a latent class model for symptoms of conduct disorder in juvenile boys. Behav. Genet., 23 ; 423, 1993.
4) Faraone, S., Biederman, J., Chen, W., Milberger, S. : Genetic heterogeneity in attention-deficit hyperactivity disorder (ADHD) : gender, psychiatric comorbidity, and maternal ADHD. J. Abnorm Psychol., 104 ; 334-345, 1995.
5) Faraone, S. V., Biederman, J., Keenan, K. et al. : Separation of DSM-III attention deficit disorder and conduct disorder : evidence from a family-genetic study of American child psychiatric patients. Psychol. Med., 21 ; 109-21, 1991.
6) Forness, S., Kavale, K., King, B., Kasari, C. : Simple versus complex conduct disorders : identification and phenomenology. Behav. Disord., 19 ; 306-312, 1994.
7) Frick, P., Lahey, B., Loeber, R., Stouthamer-Loeber, M. : Familial risk factors to oppositional defiant disorder and conduct disorder : parental psychopathology and maternal parenting. J. Consult Clin. Psychol., 60 ; 49-55, 1992.
8) Geller, B. and Luby, J. : Child and adolescent bipolar disorder : A review of the past 10 years. J. Am. Acad. Child Adolesc. Psychiatry, 36(9) ; 1168-1176, 1997.
9) Hechtman, L., Weiss, G. : Controlled prospective fifteen year follow-up of hyperactives as young adults : non-medical drug and alcohol use and anti-social behavior. Can. J. Psychiatry, 31 ; 557-567, 1996.
10) Lahey, B. B., Loeber, R., Stouthamer-Loeber, M. et al. : Comparison of DSM-III and DSM-III-R diagnoses for prepubertal children : changes in prevalence and validity. J. Am. Acad. Child Adolesc. Psychiatry, 29 ; 620-626, 1990.
11) Lahey, B., Piacentini, J., McBurnett, K., Stone, P. : Psychopathology in the parents of children with conduct disorder and hyperactivity. J. Am. Acad. Child Adolesc. Psychiatry, 27 ; 163-170, 1988.
12) Loeber, R., Lahey, B. B., Thomas, C. : Diagnostic conundrum of oppositional defiant disorder and conduct disorder. J. Abnor. Psychol., 100 ; 379-390, 1991.
13) Maziade, M. : Should adverse temperament matter to the clinician? In ; Temperament in Childhood, Kohnstamm, G., Bates, J., Rothbart, M., eds. Chichester, England : Wiley, p.421-435, 1989.
14) Maziade, M., Caron, C., Cote et al. : Psychiatric status of adolescents who had extreme temperaments at age 7. Am. J. Psychiatry, 147 ; 1531-1536, 1990.
15) Offord, D. : Conduct disorder : risk factors and prevention. In : Prevention of Mental Disorders. Alcohol and Other Drug Use in Children and Adolescents, OSAP Prevention Monograph 2, Shaffer. D., Philips, I., Enzer, N., eds. Rockville, M. D. : United States Department of Health and Humans Services, p.273-297, 1990.
16) Offord, D. : Prevention of behavioral and emotional disorders in children. J. Child Psychol. Psychiatry, 28 ; 9-19, 1987.
17) Offord, D., Boyle, M., Racine, Y., Fleming, J., Cadman, D. : Outcome, prognosis, and risk in a longitudinal follow-up study. J. Am. Acad. Child Adolesc. Psychiatry, 31 ; 916-923, 1992.
18) Pelham, W. E., Gnagy, E. M., Greenslade, K. E. et al. : Teacher ratings of DSM-III-R symptoms for the disruptive behavior disorders. J. Am. Acad. Child Adolesc. Psychiatry, 31 ; 210-218, 1992.
19) Plomin, R. : The Emanual Miller Memorial lecture 1993 : genetic research and identification of environmental influences. J. Child Psychol, Psychiatry, 35 ; 817-834, 1994.
20) Spitzer, R. L., Davies, M., Barkley, R. A. : The DSM-III-R field trial of disruptive behavior disorders. J. Am. Acad. Child Adolesc. Psychiatry,

29 ; 690-697, 1990.
21) Steiner, H. et al. : Practice parameters for the assessment and treatment of children and adolescents with conduct disorder. J. Am. Acad. Child Adolesc. Psychiatry, 36(10 Supplement) ; 122S-139S, 1997.
22) Zoccolillo, M., Pickles, A., Quinton, D., Rutter, M. : The outcome of childhood conduct disorder : implications for defining adult personality disorder and conduct disorder. Psychol. Med., 22 ; 971-986, 1992.

---

*信州大学医学部精神医学教室
Yuzuru Harada : Department of Psychiatry, Shinshu University School of Medicine.

不登校の下位分類と対応

The subclasses of school refusal for management

笠原　麻里[*]

I. 不登校の異種性

「学校恐怖症」「登校拒否」と変遷してきた概念は，今日「不登校」として，疾病概念としてではなく，さまざまな異種性の病態を含む現象名として扱われている。つまり，「不登校」は一病態ではなく，その子どもにとっての心理発達のステップをのりこえるための表現や，環境の変化に適応できなくなっているサイン，また，ある病態の一側面の表現型であると捉えることができる。

II. 国府台病院の統計

当国立精神・神経センター国府台病院児童精神科を受診した不登校の子ども達について，1995年および2000年の統計を示す（表1）。

また，これらの不登校をあらわす子ども達の，初診時の主たる問題について，診断別患者数を示す（図1）。内訳は図のようにさまざまな病態が含まれている。

III. 不登校の下位分類

このように多岐に渡る要素をはらむ不登校という現象に対応するために，齊藤の提唱する登校拒否の四型の下位分類（1989）を示す（表2）。

IV. 症例検討

以上の不登校の下位分類に照らして，具体的な対応について検討する。

1. 過剰適応型不登校

症例　麻奈）初診時中1女子。父は開業医，母は主婦。麻奈は生来健康で，成績もよく，小学校から一貫教育の名門校に通っていた。診察室ではニコニコと笑顔を見せ，しっかりした話し方をし

表1　国立精神・神経センター国府台病院児童精神科外来を受診した不登校

・1995年
　外来新患数　　　　322名
　不登校をともなう者　193名（全体の59.9%）
　　　　　　　　　　男子108名，女子86名
　　　　　　　　　　平均年齢12.6±2.5歳

・2000年
　外来新患数　　　　576名
　不登校をともなう者　225名（全体の44.0%）
　　　　　　　　　　男子121名，女子104名
　　　　　　　　　　平均年齢12.2±2.5歳

た。麻奈は面接の中で「学校へ行くのは嫌いじゃない」といい，登校すると友人との交流もあり，部活動までこなして夕方遅く帰宅したが，朝になると頭痛や気持ち悪さを訴え，週に2〜3回欠席していた。この時過剰不安障害と診断された。中2になるとほとんど登校できなくなったが，中3時，欠席が多いと進学できないことから，登校を再開した。しかし，気分は抑うつ的だった。麻奈は登校できないと苛立つ一方で，「学校に行こうと思うけれど，出かけているうちに家がなくなっているような気がする。」と不安を訴えた。麻奈は徐々に両親の不仲に触れ始め，自宅では殆ど話しをしない両親の思いを伝達する役割を麻奈自身が担っていることが明らかになった。高校には一応進学したが，全く登校せず退学，美術系の専門学校へ通う夢をようやく父に話すことができ，アルバイトで入学金をためている。

症例麻奈の考察）成績もよく，しっかり者の長女として，家庭内の調整役を担いつづけていた麻奈が，不登校という形ではじめて挫折した時，麻奈自身，その背伸びしてきた自己像をすぐに修正することはできなかった。「平気」を装う麻奈の背後には両親の離婚の危機という耐えがたい不安

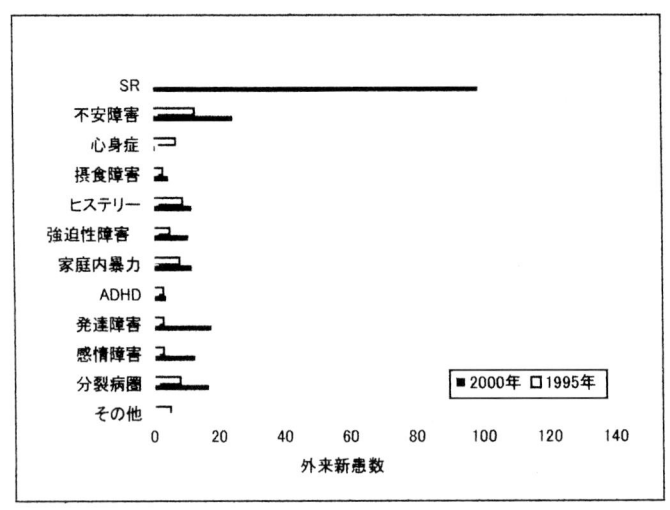

図1　国府台病院児童精神科を受診した不登校児の内訳

があることを治療者と共有していく過程の中で，麻奈は身の丈の自己像を手に入れていったものと考えられる。

2．受動型不登校

症例　タケシ）初診時小5男子。両親健在，父は自営業。明らかな発達の遅れはなく，初語1歳2カ月だったが，その後おしゃべりを余りしない子で，ことばが遅れているのではないかと母は心配していたという。幼稚園は，年中時まで母子分離困難で，年長時のみ通園した。園では友達の輪の中に入りニコニコしているような子だった。小学校入学後，成績は中位で，いつも数人の仲間とゲームなどして遊んでいた。小4の時，忘れ物をしたことを担任に叱られてから，不登校気味。朝起きられず，支度も遅いため，母は嫌がるタケシを無理に着替えさせて，何度か学校へ引っ張って行き，父も強く叱責した。しかし，タケシは次第にどんなに起こされても布団から出ることができなくなり，小5になって受診した。診察室のタケシは，口元は笑おうとしているが，視線はおどおどし，元気のない様子で，2，3返事をした後は，殆ど話しをしなかった。対照的に同席の母親はよく話し，タケシのことはすべて代弁するかのようであった。治療者の母親ガイダンスで，ある程度見守ることが大切と伝えられると，母は当初納得のいかない様子だったが，徐々に受け入れ，

表2　不登校の下位分類(齊藤，1989)

過剰適応型	：内面の依存欲求を完全に隠し，仲間関係に過剰適応的。背伸びし，超自我不安が強い。
受動型	：元来消極的。前思春期の仲間集団の勢いや，学校の厳しさに圧倒される。
衝動統制未熟型	：衝動統制が未熟であることにより，仲間関係に不適応を生じる。
分類不能型	：多彩な神経症症状や問題行動がみられ，対人関係は著しく不安定である。

小6の頃には登校刺激が減り，タケシは自宅での生活を楽しみ始めていた。しかし，中学入学に際して母は，「登校刺激はない方がいいので」と制服も作らず，教師からの電話も断ってしまった。タケシは遊びに来ている弟の友人と交流したり，夏休みには好きな釣りをしに自転車一人旅に出たりと，自発性を見せていたが，教科書を開くことは一度もなく，中学へは決して行こうとせず，時に弟に激しい暴言をぶつけていた。中学3年になった時，母は「タケシが行きたいというまで，待ちます」と進路選択にも硬い態度であったため，治療者はタケシに自発性が出てきていること，義務教育後の進路選択は真の意味で自由であるべきことを母に伝え，タケシとこれからのことを話し合う時期であると告げた。タケシは中学最後の1年間で「高校進学」を決め，これまでの学習の進度と通学の可能性を自ら判断し，公立の通信制高校へ入学，現在高2で，趣味の合った友人と釣り

にいったりしている。

症例タケシの考察）元来消極的なタケシに対し，母は過度に支配しすぎてきた。不登校というタケシの行動にも，当初は強引に登校させることで，後には「登校刺激を与えない」という名目の，いわばdouble bind的な支配をしていることに，母自身は気づいていなかった。タケシの不登校は，特に中学年代になってから，passive-aggressiveな意味合いが強くなっていたと考える。中3からは，母子別席で面接を行うことで，治療者はタケシ自身に対しては補助自我的に，母親には子どもの思うままの行動を見守ることができる距離を保つアドバイザーとして接することができたものと考えている。

3．高機能広汎性発達障害の不適応

症例　ショウ）初診時小5男子。幼少時期から超然とした雰囲気があり，話し言葉の発達は遅れた。実父からの暴力を受けていたという。両親の離婚を機に，小4時転居。転校先の学校で，些細なことで思い通りにならないと椅子を振り上げ，教室を飛び出すようになった。「教室は怖い」と言いだし，不登校になったため，受診した。ショウは表情の変化が乏しく，話し言葉に抑揚の欠ける子どもだが，全般的知能の遅れを認めなかった。病院内学級の利用を決め，通級したが，当初はお弁当箱を取り出したらフタがずれていたなど些細なことで激しいパニックを頻発。院内学級の教諭や母親がじっくりとこれに対応し，現実的な理解をその都度冷静に呈示し続けたところ，徐々に情緒的に落ち着きをみせていった。

症例ショウの考察）衝動統制未熟型の不登校を呈した高機能PDDのケースである。自己のあり様と周囲との不釣合いについて，児なりに自覚的になり，これまでには生じなかった情緒的混乱を起こすようになったものと思われる。

症例　由利）初診時中1女子。元来マイペースで変わった子だと母が述べている。身体発育，言語発達に遅れはない。小学校時代，友人を自らは求めず，仲間が盛り上がっても「バカみたい」と，いつもさめていた。文化祭ではおどけ役を演じ，「こういう時は，派手にやるものよ」と淡々という。もともと着る物にはうるさかったが，中学入学に際し制服を嫌い「こんなセンスのないものは着れない。でも制服を着ないと学校には入れない。だから中学へは行かない」と宣言して不登校になった。

症例由利の考察）親しみをもった対人関係を結ばず，集団から孤立する傾向にある子どもである。本人の考え方には柔軟性が乏しく，独自の判断で行動してしまう傾向があり，学校側への協力を要請するなど，環境面の調整を図りつつ，社会性の発達を支えることが必要である。

V．不登校の子どもの心に関する考察

これまで述べてきたように，不登校それ自体が，子どもの心のさまざまな変化をあらわす危険信号としての側面を持つため，単に不登校をさせないようにとだけ働きかけることは本質的ではないと思われる。

さらに，不登校という状態において，不安・抑うつの高まり，家族内葛藤の高まり，自己同一性の模索などが生じる。これは，家庭内暴力，強迫症状，転換症状，身体化障害，さらなる不安・抑うつを呈する場合もある。このような状況は子ども自身のみならず，周囲をも悩ませるという点も考慮しなければならない。

このように，複雑な表現型としての不登校という現象から，その子どもの変化を的確に読み取り，その後の心理発達を支え社会性を育むように，その子どもに合った水先案内をすべきであろう。不登校というサインに早期介入することは，その子どもの社会性の発達を支えるため，あるいは疾病の兆しに対応するうえで重要であると思われる。

---

*国立精神・神経センター国府台病院児童精神科
Mari Kasahara : Department of child and adolescent psychiatry, National center of Neurology and Psychiatry, Kohnodai hospital.

不登校の早期介入

Early intervention in school refusal

山崎　透*

I. はじめに

不登校は，我が国の学校精神保健における重要な課題の一つであり，児童精神科臨床においても援助や治療の主な対象の一つでもある。文部省の報告によれば，不登校児童の数は年々増加傾向にあり，平成11年度に不登校を理由に年間30日以上欠席した小中学生は約13万人にのぼり，これは，全生徒数の1.1％にあたる。したがって今後，不登校の予防や早期介入の視点に立った取り組みが重要になると思われる。本報告では，まず，演者が考える，不登校という現象の捉え方やその予防や早期介入の方法について述べる。次に，不登校児童の多くがその直前や初期に訴える，腹痛や頭痛といった身体化症状に関する臨床研究について報告し，不登校の予防や早期介入の視点から考察してみたい。

II.「子どもと学校環境の関係性の障害」としての不登校

著者は，不登校現象を「子どもと学校環境の関係性の障害」の視点から捉えることにしている。それは，以下のような理由による。学校恐怖症に代表される個人原因論や，その対局にある学校原因論といった，不登校を一つの要因から捉える方法では，不登校の多様な現象を理解することは困難であるばかりでなく，周囲がいわば「犯人探し」に終始して，肝心の子どもの援助がおろそかになってしまうという事態を招く場合もある。その点，不登校を，学校環境の持っている特性と，子どもの特性のいわばミスマッチの結果起こる現象である，と捉えるこの視点は，犯人探しをするのではなく，学校と，家庭環境を含んだ子ども両者の特性を冷静に見つめていく姿勢を促進するのに役立つと思われる。それは同時に，その子や家族にどのような援助が適切なのか，一方の当事者である学校はどのように環境を改善していくべきなのかといった手がかりを提供してくれることになる。

III. 不登校の予防／早期介入

不登校の予防や早期介入としては，以下の3つの方法が考えられる。

1）不登校の学校要因について改善していく。

ラターらは，ロンドンの12の中学校において生徒の出席率に影響を及ぼす学校要因について調査研究を行い，学習面の重視，授業における教師の行動，教師の相談しやすさ，生徒の主体的参加態度，教職員の士気の高さと協調性，などが出席率と有意な関係がある，としている。また，レイノルズは，学校規模が小さい，規則が守られる，生徒自治が行われている，学校と保護者の緊密度が高いといった傾向が強いほど出席率が高い，と報告している。さらに，フォーゲルマンは，教員異動率が高いほど欠席率が高いと報告している。このような学校要因を改善していくことは，不登校のみならず，学校精神保健の様々な問題の予防に有効と思われるので，今後教育界がハード・ソフトの両面から学校環境を整備していくことが望まれる。

2）不登校になる前に，子どもの心理的危機を示すサインを捉え適切に対応する。

不登校の発現はしばしば突然のように見えるが，実際には登校をめぐる葛藤は不登校の始まるずっと前から高まっている。こうした葛藤の高まった状態でなお学校にとどまっている子どもは，その内面の危機を様々な形で表現している。その代表的なものが腹痛や頭痛などの心身症的な身体

症状である。その他，予期不安，無気力や抑うつ感，イライラ感，不潔恐怖や洗浄強迫など，様々なサインが認められる場合がある。こうした子どもの発するサインを教師や親がきちんと受け止め，子どもに何が起こっているのかを理解し適切な対応をしていくことで，不登校の発現を未然に防げるケースも少なからずあると考えられる。

3）不登校の初期に適切な介入をしてその長期化を防ぐ。

ただしここでいう介入とは，子どもに何か働きかけることを指すわけではない。ケースによっては，まず，安心して学校を休める環境を整えることが必要な場合があり，こうした環境の調整も介入に含まれる。しかし，初期の不適切な対応のために不登校が長期化し，心理的発達の停滞や青年期に至る長期の引きこもりなどの問題が生じることも事実である。したがって不登校の初期に，教師や親，時には相談機関も含めた援助者たちが，その子どもの状態や学校の状況を冷静に分析し，子どもの心理的成長をサポートするような適切な対応をしていくことが，長期の引きこもりなどの問題の予防に寄与するものと考えられる。

Ⅳ．不登校と身体化症状に関する臨床研究

1）不登校の随伴症状に関する研究

対象は不登校を主訴に，演者が以前勤務していた，国立精神・神経センター国府台病院児童精神科を受診した小中学生165名ある。不登校に伴う随伴症状を調査したところ，頭痛や腹痛といった身体症状が最も多く，120名（73%）であった。

2）一般中学生を対象にした身体化症状と不安抑うつ感に関する調査研究

一般中学生769名を対象に，頭痛や腹痛といった各身体症状について，調査時期からさかのぼって3カ月間持続し，1週間に一度以上の頻度で出現しているかどうかをチェックしてもらったところ，約78%の中学生が何らかの身体症状を訴えていて，平均では一人当たり2.1個の身体症状を訴えていた。また，男子より女子が，1・2年生より3年生の方が有意に多く訴えていた。また，一人当たりが訴えた身体症状数と，CDI（小児用抑うつ尺度）およびSTAIC（小児用状態―特性不安検査）の関係をみると，いずれとも正の相関関係を示していた。以上のことから，一般中学生においても，身体症状は不安や抑うつ感といった心理的状態と密接な関係があることが示唆された。

3）不登校と身体化症状に関する追跡調査

対象：対象は，不登校を理由に国立精神・神経センター国府台病院児童精神科を受診した小中学生のうち，器質的異常の認められない身体症状を不登校の理由の一つとして訴え，身体症状の経過を追跡し得た177名である。

方法：まず，初回面接でDSM-Ⅲ-R診断基準を用いた診断を行い，それをもとに不安型，抑うつ型，身体表現型の3型に分類した。類型別の度数は不安型が103名，抑うつ型が16名，身体表現型が58名であった。加えて初診時点では，小児科などの他科受診状況，身体症状に対する親の態度，各身体症状の出現時期，精神症状（分離不安，過剰不安，パニック，解離，抑うつ，強迫）の有無などに関する調査を行い，作成した個人票に記載した。そして，初診以後，各身体症状の経過を追跡し，身体症状が完全に消失したか，時に訴えても社会生活には影響を及ぼさなくなった時期を「消失時期」と同定し，各々の持続期間を月単位で算出した。そして一症例ごとに何らかの身体症状を訴えていた期間を「身体症状の全持続期間」として月単位で算出しました。さらに身体症状数と不登校の期間についても算出した。なお，平均追跡期間は2年1カ月であった。

結果および考察：対象全体でどのような身体症状が出現していたかをみると，腹痛が53.1%と最も多く，以下頭痛，嘔気，発熱，倦怠感，の順に多く出現していた。身体化症状の出現時期では，不登校開始前一カ月以内に身体症状が出現した者が全体の54%を占めていた。不登校発現3カ月以内までを含めると，全体の71%を占めており，身体化症状が，不登校の前駆症状や初期症状として重要であることを示唆している。身体化症状の持続期間は平均11.7カ月であり，1カ月以内に消失している者が6%，1〜3カ月が24%，3〜6カ月が19%，などとなっており，2年以上身体症状が持続している者は19.2%であった。これは，従

来言われてきたような，身体化症状は周囲に危機的状況を知らせるメッセージの役割を終えると速やかに消失してしまうという症例ばかりではなく，身体症状を長期間に渡って訴え続け治療が展開しない症例も少なからず存在していることを示している。

各調査項目について類型間で分布に有意差を認めたのは，初診前の身体症状消失率，親の態度，身体症状の全持続期間の3項目であった。初診前の消失率は，不安型が33.0％と最も高く，身体表現型が8.6％と最も低いという結果であった。身体化症状に対する親の態度は，不安型と抑うつ型では「否定的に捉え登校を指示していた」が最も多く，身体表現型では「身体疾患と捉え，身体治療に専念していた」が最も多いという結果であった。また，身体症状の全持続期間では，不安型が最も短期間で中央値4.0カ月，身体表現型が11.5カ月と最も長期間持続していた。また，調査期間中に不登校が改善した45名の類型間で比較検討を行った（類型別度数は不安型25名，身体表現型19名，抑うつ型1名のため抑うつ型は関東から除外した）ところ，身体表現型は不安が他に比べて，身体化症状の全持続期間，不登校期間とも有意に長いという結果であった。精神病理学的な類型別の特徴は以下のようにまとめることができる。不安型は，1）身体化症状が短期間に改善しやすい，2）治療前に症状が消失してしまう頻度が高い，3）身体表現型と比べて短期間で再登校に至る傾向がある，といった特徴が明らかとなった。抑うつ型は，1）治療前の消失率と全持続期間は不安型と身体表現型の中間に位置しているといった特徴が認められた。身体表現型は，1）身体化症状が遷延しやすい，2）治療前に症状が改善する頻度が少ない，3）不登校も不安型に比べて長期化する傾向があるといった特徴がみとめられた。これまで不登校に伴う身体化症状は，不登校初期の葛藤の表現や一過性の症状として捉えられ，治療の中で重要視されることは少なかった。しかし，身体表現型に代表されるような，身体症状をどう取り扱うかが治療の重要なテーマとなる症例も，不登校児童の中に少なからず存在していることをこれらの結果は示していると考えられる。

次に，身体化症状が不登校の経過とどのような関係にあるのかをみるために，不登校期間が同定可能な再登校群45名について，不登校の期間と身体症状の全持続期間の相関関係を検討したところ，両者の間には統計学的に有意な正の相関が認められた。これは，前駆症状や初期症状として出現した身体化症状を訴えている期間の長さが不登校全体の経過に影響を及ぼす可能性があることを示していると考えられる。言い換えれば，適切な対応によって身体化を訴えている時期を短縮することが不登校の長期化を防ぐことにもつながる可能性を示唆している。

次に，身体化症状の経過がどのような要因によって影響を受けているかを分析するために，身体症状の全持続期間を目的変数，各症状の有無を含む27項目を説明変数として重回帰分析を行った（R^2乗値＝0.531）。説明に有効な変数を整理すると，身体化症状の遷延には，1）個体側の要因，2）子どもを支える家族側の要因，3）身体化症状を取り扱う医療側の要因が関わっている，とまとめることができる。個体側の要因としては，年齢による言語化能力の未熟さ，精神病理学的な感情表出の困難さ，あるいは強迫的な身体へのこだわりといったことが遷延化の要因となりうることを示唆している。また，家族側の要因としては，身体症状を詐病や怠けだと否定的に捉えて登校を強制したり，身体症状がよくなれば登校できるだろうと考えて身体の治療に専念するといった，子どもが身体症状にしがみつかざるをえない家族の対応が遷延化の一因になっていることを示唆している。なお，もう一つの環境側の要因として，教師を始めとした学校側の対応が考えられるが，客観的な評価が困難なため今回は調査することができなかった。医療側の要因として，先行研究では，身体診療科が身体疾患と考えて精査を続けること，過剰な保証をあたえること，初期の段階で関わる治療者の身体化に対する認識不足などを，身体化症状の遷延化の要因としてあげている。今回の調査では詳細に検討することはできなかったが，少なくとも精神科と身体診療科の身体化に関するコンセンサスの形成や治療の連携の必

要性を示唆していると考えられる。

V．まとめ

1）不登校は「子どもと学校環境の関係性の障害」として捉えると理解しやすく，援助や治療の手がかりも得られやすい。

2）不登校の予防／早期介入には以下の3つの方法がある。

①不登校の学校要因を改善する。

②不登校になる前に，子どもの心理的危機を示すサインを捉え適切に対応する。

③不登校の初期に適切な介入をしてその長期化を防ぐ。

3）不登校と身体化症状に関する臨床研究から以下のことが示唆された。

①身体化症状は子どもの心理的危機を示すサインや不登校の初期症状として重要な意味を持っている。

②身体化症状の遷延化と不登校の長期化は密接な関係がある。

③身体化症状に適切な対応をすることは，不登校の発現や長期化を防ぐ有効な手だてとなりうる。

---

*静岡県立こころの医療センター

Toru Yamazaki : Shizuoka Prefectural Mental Care and Rehabilitation Center.

家庭の精神保健とその問題の予防
―「社会的ひきこもり」をめぐって―

Mental health of family and the prevention of its problems
Hikikomori or a type of social withdrawal prevalent in Japanese adolescents

白石　弘巳*

Introduction

As one of the issues concerning the mental health within a family, *hikikomori* or the problems of children who shut themselves in their rooms for long period of time even after reaching their adolescence began to be actively discussed by media in the late 90s. Social withdrawal can be observed not only in Japan, but also in other countries. But it has become a big social problem in Japan so as to attract attention and curiosity from abroad.

Hikikomori is a problem of a family as a whole as well as of an individual. The family members try to help the individual solve the problem, but it is not easy. It is known that it sometimes brings about serious domestic violence. In this paper, the author will discuss the problem of *hikikomori* from the standpoint of its prevention with some comments about its statistics, nature, and background.

Definition

Hikikomori is not a nosological entity, but a syndrome. Saito (1998) defines *hikikomori* as follows : "a withdrawal which becomes apparent by a person's late 20s ; which continues longer than 6 months ; and the cause of which is hard to be attributed to other mental diseases." The withdrawal caused by schizophrenia and other mental diseases, which makes the subject unable to take a social part in daily lives, is a great problem as well. But what is to be noted now is the withdrawal behavior lacking psychotic symptoms. There is a possibility that this *hikikomori* is a partial symptom of various mental disorders, such as social phobia, panic disorder, obsessive-compulsive disorder, avoidant personality disorder and schizoid personality disorder. There is also a possibility that it is a prodromal syndrome of schizophrenia. We cannot say that any of the specific diseases previously mentioned is prevailing. The core of the question seems to be that, no matter what the underlined disease is, psychological and social factors contribute to it and act as instigator to the withdrawal phenomenon. So irrespective of the background diagnosis, we should make much of the psycosocial factors in therapeutic approach. In this sense, it is clinically significant to summarize them into "nonpsychotic *hikikomori*."

Facts about *hikikomori*

The number of those who withdraw are presumed to be approximately in the "several hundred thousands" (Saito, 1998). This comes from the fact that the junior high school students who don't go to school or high school students who quit their schools are respectively more than 100,000. A magazine said that there was "a tragedy of 1,000,000 withdrawing people." (Bungei Shunju, August '99) If that were true, it would equal the number of schizophrenic patients in Japan. But the precise number is still unknown, as the large scaled research has not been practiced yet. It is necessary to grasp the precise number of *hikikomori* in order to take countermeasures for the problem.

According to the questionnaire done by an association of the parents of socially withdrawing children (Saitama Shinbun, January 19, 2001) the average age of the withdrawing individuals is at 22 years and 9 months old ; the most frequent onset is at 17 years old ; 17% of them has withdrawn for more than 10 years and about 80% has caused some domestic violence including that of words. Saito (1998) also pointed out that overwhelming majority of the subjects are male ; 68.8% of the trigger to their withdrawal were their stopping to go to school ; the length of time from the occurrence of the problem till the visit to treatment facilities was long ; the class of the families are often higher than middle and the extraordinary conditions such as divorce or husbands' living apart from their families for jobs, were rather few.

Recently the increasing number of the subjects are said to have begun communicating through the Internet or meeting regularly with each other. But these people, whose degree of *hikikomori* is comparatively less severe, are also too sensitive to human relations to take part in the society sufficiently. Even when they begin some part time job, some of them stop that and withdraw again.

Hikikomori and family

Generally when a member of a family has some psychiatric disease or behavioral problems, his or her family have to take, whether they want or not, one or more of the following roles : (a) cause, (b) victim, (c) the obstructing factor for the solution, (d) the supporter for the solution.

The trigger for *hikikomori*, most frequently pointed out, is the stress experienced out of the family. The older the age of onset, the less domestic events are referred to as direct causes. As *hikikomori* is prolonged, it unavoidably assumes to be a domestic problem. Many families are eager to solve the problem though actually, they can't function as the suitable supporter for the solution. They often become the obstructing factor for the solution. For example, when the family members' coping pattern is a "directing type", they try hard to take the subject out of the house. If this stimulation of taking out is inappropriate, the subject will have more stress, which will lead to a vicious circle.

When their coping patterns are "taking care type", the family will fulfill the subject's whims and desires all too eagerly. But that will decrease the subject's ability to confront his anxiety, which leads to another vicious circle. In view of the resemblance to the research of the emotional expression in schizophrenia, the family of "directing type" is apt to believe that the subject could and should live a not-withdrawing life and take a critical attitude to him. On the contrary, the family of "taking care type" has a problem of being emotionally involved. Both coping patterns latently have risks to lead to domestic violence if the tension within the family grows. The "letting alone type", the third coping pattern, is compared to the low EE in schizophrenia research, but it rarely produces the positive support for a solution.

When *hikikomori* is prolonged, among the above-mentioned four roles of the family members, the "victim" occupies a large part. They often suffer from violence, health problems of those who take care of the subject, the discord between the husband and the wife and social inadaptability of the members other than the subject. There is also a possibility that it leads to the dispersion of the family, murder of the children and a whole family suicide, though they are few.

The social and cultural problems as the background of *hikikomori*

Saito pointed out that many of *hikikomori* cases occurred in middle class families or higher. The fact that those who have been the center of the Japanese economic prosperity so far produced many cases of *hikikomori* would disclose the essential problems concerning the Japanese post war society itself. After the World War II, Japan succeeded in the industrialization and commercialization, made a high economic growth. The occupational population of the primary industry, which had occupied almost 50% of all by 1950s, fell to 7% in 1990. In this process, the population concentrated in big cities while that of the rural areas became sparse. The family structure also altered. The aging of the society is proceeding at a surprising speed. No wonder the family function changed, too. Working women increased, and they became economically more independent. The total specific rate of birth was the third lowest in the world in 1996. Japanese families have become richer, but the members are busy working on their own businesses and have less time to be relaxed at home. The function of members' mutual support decreases. In particular in urban areas, the association with relatives and commitments to the local activities have become less. They now need the help of outsiders for bringing up their children.

Sato (1986) images a healthy family as follows: (a) they are on a good term (the husband and the wife, in particular), (b) all the members can say anything to each other, (c) they share a significant time, (d) it has an atmosphere of mutual support, (e) it is open to the outer world. How many Japanese families fit these images?

Japanese children have been expected to get high education no matter what their wills are and much money has been invested for their education. It sounds very paradoxical that, according to a recent survey, that only 16% of Japanese high school students answers "I positively agree" to study focusing on the preparation for the entrance examination, while 53% of American students do so. Japanese students showed far less interest in getting high status in the society or contributing to the society than American students. These data show the introvert view of life opposed to that of their parents' ways of living.

Therapeutic approaches to *hikikomori*

In origin, *hikikomori* has a positive meaning as a refuge from the stress in social activities before they are prepared for that. The principle of the treatment to specific cases is to keep the positive significance of *hikikomori* as well as to reduce its negative influence. In the case of *hikikomori*, the family members are apt to receive services for problem-solving before the subject, but we want to emphasize the importance of direct approach to the subject, independent from the programs for the family members. It is essential to construct a relation with the subject and to try to keep that. It is important for the supporters to maintain a stance to listen to the subject and to help the subject's self-determination. They should not easily judge the effect of intervention only by seeing if they can go out or not. From the author's experience, those who could come to the outpatient office by themselves recovered little by little as time went on. Of course with those who could not come, therapists should try to make a good relationship, if necessary, by visiting their homes many times or communicating with them through phone calls and letters. It may be necessary to improve their skills for that. It is regrettable that many subjects, who need the therapists' visits, are left for long without getting those chances.

According to Rund (1990), patients recovered from schizophrenia say the triggers for recovery were: (a) recovery of a feeling of trust in their own faith and ability, (b) the warm support by their family, (c) the encounter with a good therapist, (d) the encounter with the peer clients with mental disorder. These factors will have the same therapeutic effect in *hikikomori*, which is not caused by mental disorder. It is necessary for the family members to stand the ambiguous condition and to gain energy to live with the subject. The author proposed that the desirable conditions for the recovery of the families were (a) having the knowledge of the disease to find it not easy to cure and, at the same time, to have hope, (b) contacting with the subject with both warmth and strictness, (c) feeling thankful for the medical facilities but being able to request orders to them easily, (d) making much of their own lives as well as contacting with the subject, (e) supporting the subjects from their back, ready to come to the front if necessary to deal with the society. The purpose of psychoeducation is to empower family members to accomplish the tasks, which are easy to mention but difficult to perform. For this, there should be not only stereotyped supply of information but also the exchange between experienced family members and eager professionals.

In the process of these interventions, if necessary, medical treatments, communication techniques and problem solving method are introduced. It is important to assist self-help groups and to recommend the clients to attend them. It is also worth trying to make use of voluntary activities groups. Taking advantage of these groups can be expected to lead to the third prevention.

When it is necessary to intervene in the crisis such as violence, the most important matter to be considered is to assess what effect can be expected from their involuntary admission to the mental hospital. It must be avoided to the utmost to send them to the hospital in order to keep them out. The best way should be to try to settle the situation by the intervention of a third person. If there is no alternative, the person who is at the risk of being the victim of violence should take an emergency refuge out of the house. If violence happens, they should call the police and strictly treat the case.

In the condition where the number of the withdrawing people is still unknown, the comprehensive program for *hikikomori* response is hard to make. But at least, if they come to the mental health and welfare centers or medical facilities for consultation, we should make more practice and research to be able to effectively intervene.

The primary prevention of *hikikomori*

As the primary prevention of *hikikomori*, we may well considerate to practice screening the children of high risk at elementary schools and junior high schools. But the principle of community health is to promote the possibility of self-discovery and self help activities by the supply of information. After that, it becomes important to ensure the system where people can consult at ease. If we dare use the term prevention, we should understand that *hikikomori* is just one of domestic problems and prepare some places where, even if there were no apparent problems, a husband and a wife can consult or have group sessions. The author thinks that the principle of the modern family problem is that of married couples.

Furthermore, *hikikomori* is a warning to the modern Japanese society. Considering this view, it is essential that we take interest and take active part in making a social system that will enable families to live healthy lives.

References

1) Rund, B. R. : Fully recovered schizophrenics : A retrospective study of some premorbid and treatment factors. Psychiatry, 53 ; 127-139, 1990.
2) Sato, E. : Kateinai komyunikeishon (Intrafamilial communication). Keiso Syobo, Tokyo, 1986. (in Japanese)
3) Saito, T. : Shakaiteki hikikomori (Social withdrawal). PHP Kenkyusho, Tokyo, 1998. (in Japanese)

---

*東京都精神医学総合研究所
Hiromi Shiraishi, M.D., Ph.D : Tokyo Institute of Psychiatry.

職場の精神保健とその問題の予防

Preventive aspects of occupational mental health

倉林るみい*

I. Introduction

Occupational medicine used to put emphasis on taking care of patients with occupational disease. Occupational medicine today emphasizes prevention more than therapy, and so does occupational mental health. Furthermore, the aim of occupational mental health today is not only to prevent illness, but also to promote employees' mental health. In that sense, occupational mental health aims to treat all employees, from healthy ones to those who fall ill.

This article shows the current situation and agenda of occupational mental health. Some measures for stress management for employees are also introduced.

II. Mental health from the standpoint of a research topic in occupational medicine

Nowadays, occupational mental health is considered an important area in occupational medicine. Figure 1[1] shows the best ten among 58 research topics based on short- and long-term priority considering occupational health needs, degree of importance and urgency, and usefulness of research results. Fifty experts in various areas of occupational health discussed and selected these topics for the conference on occupational health research strategies in the 21st century, held in 1998 with the support of the former Ministry of Labour[2]. The Ministry was merged with the former Ministry of Health and Welfare to become the Ministry of Health, Labour and Welfare in 2001. In Figure 1,

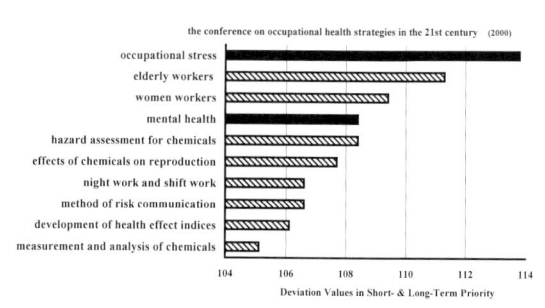

Figure 1 Top Ten Priority Topics for Occupational Health Researches during 2001 to 2010

mental health ranks fourth among the 58 research topics. Job stress, which overlaps a good deal with mental health, comes at the top of the list. Considering the fact that there are only a few mental health experts among the fifty selectors, you can see how much mental health is spotlighted as an important topic in the workplace in Japan in this century.

III. Mental health from the standpoint of health management in companies in Japan

According to national surveys on the state of employees' health[3] conducted every five years, more than 60% of Japanese employees had strong anxiety, worry and stress concerning their job and working life in 1997. The rate has been increasing considerably (Figure 2).

The Japanese workplace itself is changing. The lifetime employment system and the seniority system, which have been considered traditional in Japan, are being phased out. Instead of these systems, the ability-oriented system was introduced. In addition to that, technological innovations and

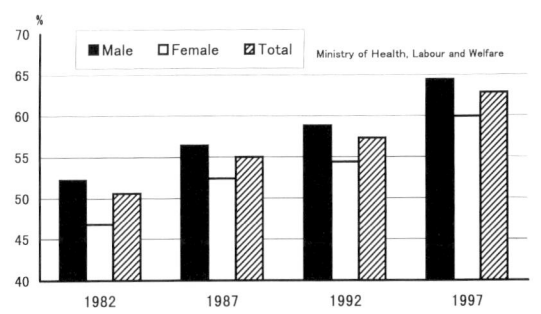

Figure 2 Percentage of Japanese employees with strong anxiety, worry and stress related to their work

Figure 3 Suicide rate in Japan

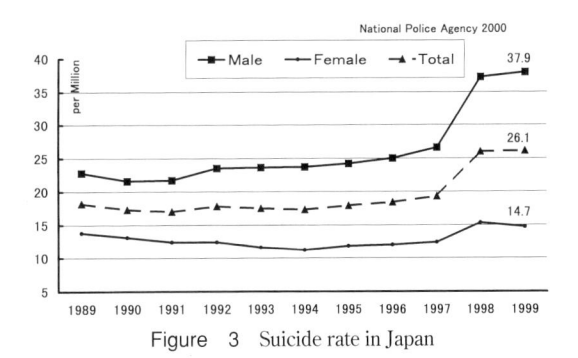

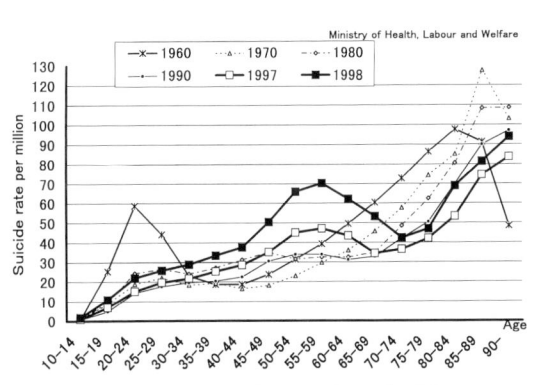

Figure 4 Suicide rate in Japan (male)

diversification of employment styles also cause many new problems. And the business recession in the past eight to ten years has been causing re-structuring and down-sizing, which can be stressful for many employees.

Because of this situation, not only experts in occupational health, but also employers of Japanese companies now take an increasing interest in mental health.

Japanese employers used to regard mental health management as one of the welfare services for their employees, but now there are two new factors which make Japanese employers pay much more attention to mental health management. One is cost-benefit. Some studies calculated the cost of medical treatment and labor loss caused by occupational stress in employees, and they pointed out that good stress management could save cost. The other factor is risk management. For several years, some cases of suicide by employees were recognized as work-related accidents due to overwork. In some cases, employers had to pay a lot of compensation as a result of losing court cases.

IV. Karo-jisatsu : suicide from overwork

In 1998, the suicide rate[4] had remarkably increased in Japan, and since 1998, more than thirty thousand people have committed suicide every year. The increasing suicide rate is shown in Figure 3. Figure 4[5] shows the transition in the male suicide rate in Japan in the past forty years. In 1960, the rate for young adults was very high. In 1997 and in 1998, however, the rates for men in their forties, fifties and sixties were high. Compared with 1997, it is obvious that the rate for middle-aged men in 1998 had increased. In 1998, suicide by men in their fifties had increased by 54% compared with the previous year. As for women, no peak in the middle-aged group was noticed (Figure 5)[5]. This middle-age peak was observed only in men.

In the workplace in Japan now,"karo-jisatsu," a type of suicide, receives much attention."Karo" means overwork and "jisatsu" means suicide. Karo-jisatsu is suicide by those in a depressive state due to overwork.

The suicide of 24-year-old employee of a big advertising company in 1996 is a typical example. During 17 months, there was no day on which he did not work. Complaining of sleep disturbance and fatigue, finally he committed suicide by hang-

Table 1 Karo-jisatsu cases approved for workers' compensation (all cases are male) as of March 1999

Case	Year	Victim's Age and Job	State of Work	Having Seen Psychiatrist (+)
1	1979	31y engineer	overtime work and promotion	(+)
2	1984	25y office worker	overtime work for one month	(−)
3	1985	30y press factory worker	overtime work and promotion	(−)
4	1988	28y engineer	overtime work	(−)
5	1991	41y leading hand in iron foundry	overtime work and promotion	(±)
6	1991	24y employee of advertising co.	overtime work	(−)
7	1995	24y sauce factory worker	overtime work	(±)
8	1997	26y computer programmer	overtime work	(−)
9	1998	37y construction co. site leading hand	overtime work	(−)
10	1999	53y scout of professional baseball team	difficult work	(−)

ing. Worker's compensation was granted in his case. It used to be very difficult to have suicide recognized as a labour accidents, because it was regarded as the result of employees having chosen to kill themselves of their own free will. Now the way of judging these cases is changing. In 1999, the Ministry of Labour made the guideline for approval of labour accidents on mental disorders[6].

Table 1 shows the list of karo-jisatsu cases where workmen's compensation was approved as of March 1999. All cases are men. The sixth case was already been shown. Of the cases listed in this table, the fact that only one saw a psychiatrist is regrettable. A plus-minus (±) mark means that the victim had seen a doctor but not psychiatrist.

A national policy for preventing suicide, especially karo-jisatsu, and promoting employees' mental health are urgently needed.

V. Practice of occupational mental health as to preventive aspects

The Ministry of Labour, taking the above situations into consideration, issued the guidelines for mental health promotion for employees in 2000[1,7]. According to these guidelines, four types of mental health care are recommended for the workplace.

1. Self-care : Employees themselves think about what kind of stress they suffer and how to get rid of it.
2. Care by managers : Team leaders and superi-

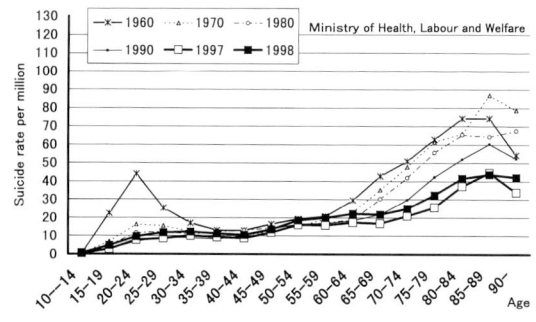

Figure 5 Suicide rate in Japan (female)

ors should improve the working environment, and if necessary, advise each employee how to promote his/her mental health.
3. Care by professional health care staff in a company : Industrial physicians, health supervisors, public health nurses and mental health staffers should assess and improve the working environment in cooperation with supervisors, and acquire a greater understanding of the mental health issues among employees. They should refer employees needing psychiatric treatment to clinics and hospitals and support them in their rehabilitation.
4. Care by service resources outside of a company : It is recommended that employers make use of occupational mental health facilities outside of their company, for example, regional industrial health centers and prefectural industrial health promotion centers.

These staffers are recommended to be mutually

engaged in these four type of the activities. For example, to promote "self-care" and "care by managers" activities, it is very important for the professional health care staff to have training programs for employees and managers.

EAP(Employee Assistance Program) is a good means for promoting mental health of employees. Small companies which cannot afford to have their own professional mental health care staffers can make use of EAP with at reasonable cost.

References

1) Kurabayashi, L. : Work stress : current situations, agendas, and stress management. Seishin Igaku (Clinical Psychiatry), 142 ; 1016-1022, 2000 (in Japanese)
2) Ministry of Labour : Healthy work life in 21st century Japan. National occupational health research strategies, The conference on occupational health research strategies in 21st century, 2001
3) Ministry of Labour : Survey on state of employee's health. 1982, 1987, 1992, 1997 (in Japanese)
4) National Police Agency : Statistics of suicide in 2000, 2001 (in Japanese)
5) Ministry of Health and Welfare : Statistics of suicide in 1998, 1999 (in Japanese)
6) Ministry of Labour : Guideline for approval of labour accidents on mental disorders. 1999 (in Japanese)
7) Ministry of Labour : Conference report on mental health care for employees : mental health promotion in workplace. 2000 (in Japanese)

---

*独立行政法人産業医学総合研究所
Lumie Kurabayashi, M. D. : Division of work stress control, National Institute of Industrial Health.

アルコール・薬物乱用の予防：内科と精神科の連携によるアルコール依存症早期治療と早期回復を目指して

Strategy for early intervention and recovery of patients with alcohol dependence : psychiatric liaison with physicians

渡辺　省三[*1]　高瀬幸次郎[*2]　広藤　秀雄[*3]　木村　光政[*4]　西村　晃[*5]　奥田　喜朗[*6]
藤本　昌雄[*7]　小島　裕治[*8]　井上　淳[*9]　遠藤太久郎[*10]　猪野　亜朗[*10]

The number of alcoholic patients referred to psychiatric specialists is small and most of them are often serious in a late stage of the illness, suggesting physicians' awareness is necessary for patients to receive psychiatric treatment of alcohol dependence at an early stage. To push on with psychiatric liaison with physicians as a strategy for early intervention and recovery of patients with alcohol dependence, we organized the Mie Association for the Study of Alcohol-related Diseases (MASAD) consisted of doctors, nurses, public nurses, and medical social workers. The meeting was held every 6 months at district general hospitals and about one hundred participants shared the information to support patients with alcohol-related physical, psychological and social problems. Activities of the MASAD brought up a marked increase in referral of alcoholic patients to psychiatric specialists, but the outcome of half the referred patients was still unsatisfactory. This evidence indicates that psychiatric liaison with physicians should be done at an earlier stage of the illness to realize a goal of the treatment of alcohol dependence.

Introduction

The amount of alcohol consumption and the number of patients with alcohol-related organ disorders are increasing in Japan. In general hospitals, physicians treat primarily physical diseases to save the patients' lives, but in many cases they fail to give proper advice on the underlying cause of alcohol misuse. Many physicians are likely to be pessimistic about curing alcohol dependence because alcoholic patients often resume drinking and show poor prognosis for life due to relapses of the illness. Probably for this reason, the number of patients referred to psychiatric specialists is very small and most of them are often too late to recover from the illness. This evidence suggests that physician's awareness is necessary for patients to receive good advice and/or psychiatric treatment of alcohol dependence at an early stage. To carry out a strategy for early intervention and recovery of patients with alcohol dependence, we organized the Mie Association for the Study of Alcohol-related Diseases (MASAD) in 1996. In this paper, we describe the circumstances of the MASAD and its activities achieved until now.

Background of organizing the MASAD

In 1972, four young psychiatric doctors started special medical care of patients with alcohol dependence at Mie Prefectural Takajaya Hospital (presently named the Mental Care Center, Prefecture of Mie) and volunteers of patients formed the meeting for supporting abstinence. They constructed an abstinence-house to which an apartment house for single patients and an outpatient clinic were set up as an annex.

Cooperation with district health centers and public health nurses was started along the right lines in 1988, and the number of patients who received the advice about their alcoholic problems was gradually increased. Two years later, the Mie Network Association for Aid to Patients with Alcoholic Problems was organized by volunteers from fields of medical service, social welfare, administrative organ, school, legal profession, and labor union in Mie Prefecture. The network members listened to special guests' lectures on the current therapy of alcoholism, and exchanged the information on alcohol-related problems of their patients. The network association prepared a pamphlet of "*For you having more than 100 units of γ GTP !*" for screening alcohol misuse at the industrial physical examination. In the process, some network members brought up an important problem ; if they refer suspected patients of alcoholic diseases to general hospitals, physicians only treat organ disorders without intervention to underlying alcohol dependence of the patients.

In fact, Ino, *et al*. revealed that 85% of patients with alcohol dependence had been admitted to general hospitals due to alcohol-related diseases, and after that the patients had not receive any psychiatric treatment for 7.4 years until they had visited the Mental Care Center. In addition, at their initial visit to the general hospital, withdrawal symptoms and abnormal drinking behavior had been detected in 77% and 96%, respectively, of the patients[1]. This finding indicates that physicians have to recognize underlying alcoholic dependence of patients at an early stage of the illness, and to provide them psychiatric liaison therapy for the recovery. On the other hand, patients' denial or lack in awareness of drinking problems often hindered completing the treatment and many physicians had not a useful way to develop psychiatric liaison by adjusting problems between patients and their families. Physicians had also little opportunity to know the outcome of patients referred to specialists, and sometimes they tended to be pessimistic or skeptical about psychiatric liaison therapy due to the treatment failed cases. Under these delicate situations, the MASAD was organized on February in 1996 to develop a cooperation among doctors, nurses, public health nurses, and medical social workers for supporting the recovery of patients with alcohol dependence at an early stage.

Outline of the MASAD

The MASAD is conducted by 35 managers constituted of 28 doctors, 5 nurses, and 2 medical social workers from whole area of Mie Prefecture and its activities are backed up by the prefectural and district medical associations and by the prefectural societies of nurses and medical social workers. The MASAD meeting is held every 6 months at the conference room of a district general hospital at which a manager in charge of the meeting is working. A director of the hospital gives an opening remark about alcohol-related problems at each MASAD meeting and it is a good message for the hospital staffs and participants to know that the hospital will take a positive attitude toward the alcoholic problems.

A subject for discussion in the meeting is decided by representatives of the MASAD managers : (i)At the case conference, two main themes of the cases difficult to care and the treatment of serious withdrawal symptoms were the subject of discussion and thirty-seven cases were presented and discussed until now. (ii)Patients recovered from the illness and their families talked about their experience of alcoholic problems (4 cases) and it was impressive to the attendants. (iii)Studies carried out by the MASAD were reported and discussed ; 1,484 staffs of general hospitals were surveyed the sense to medical problems of alcoholic patients using questionnaires in July, 1998, and the result was reported elsewhere[2]. A study on the outcome of alcoholic patients received psychiatric liaison therapy is now in preparation for publication. (iv)Three special lectures on physical, psychiatric, social, and family problems of alcoholic patients were given to attendants of the meeting.

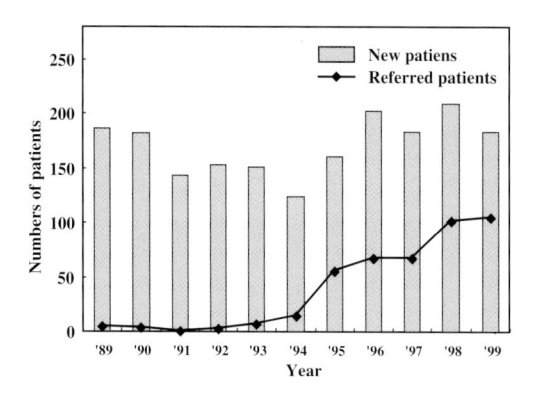

Figure 1 Changes of Numbers of Referred Patients to the Mental Care Center

Table 1 Outcome of 326 Referred Patients to the Mental Care Center

	Numbers of Patients
In the hospital	18 (5.5%)
Outpatient clinic (stable)	108 (33.1%)
Outpatient clinic (unstable)	13 (4.0%)
Interruption of the care	56 (17.2%)
Missing	104 (31.9%)
Died	15 (4.6%)
Chang the doctor	12 (3.7%)

The MASAD meeting was held at eight hospitals in five cities for five years and about 100 (ranging from 77 to 146) persons attended the meeting every time. At the time of the survey in 1998, 64% of medical staffs answered that they wanted to attend the MASAD meeting if it would be held at their hospitals. In addition, more than 70% of persons who had ever attended the MASAD meeting made an answer that the meeting was useful for them to care alcoholic patients[2]. This result encouraged the MASAD members and accelerated the MASAD activities.

Fruits of the MASAD activities achieved until now

At the MASAD meeting, about 100 participants shared the information to support patients with alcohol-related physical, psychological and social problems every time, and thereby the close cooperation of the MASAD members for the treatment of alcoholic patients was promoted. Physicians came to recognize their responsibility for underlying alcohol dependence of patients, and referral of patients to specialists and psychiatric liaison with physicians markedly increased in number (Figure 1).

The MASAD members of nurses, public nurses and medical social workers interchanged the information about nursing care of patients with alcohol dependence twice a year and this activity stimulated doctors' awareness of alcoholic problems.

In 1999, the MASAD prepared an own pamphlet of "Is your drinking habit OK ? " for early intervention, which included self-records for daily drinking and flowcharts for checking alcoholic organ disorders, drinking habits, CAGE and ICD-10 questionnaires, and guide-lines for doctors. Two thousand copies of this pamphlet have been sold (@200 yen) and those are available to both patients and doctors.

One of the district general hospitals held the MASAD meeting on February in 1997, and that was the opportunity for starting a regular meeting to talk about alcohol and health in the hospital. This meeting was held every 4 months for alcoholic patients and the families, at which the attendants listened to a doctor's lecture on alcohol-related diseases and talked with hospital staffs of doctors, nurses, and medical social workers, and with a psychiatrist as a guest adviser.

These MASAD activities are likely to grow physicians' awareness of underlying alcohol misuse of patients, and to promote psychiatric liaison with physicians. As shown in Figure 1, the number of patients referred to specialists of the Mental Care Center in Mie Prefecture began to increase in a preparatory period for organizing the MASAD, and markedly increased thereafter. Especially, the percentage of referred patients in all new patients visited the Mental Care Center has accounted for 50 per cent or more every year after 1998.

Future problem of the MASAD activity for early intervention to alcoholic patients

Although referral of patients to psychiatric specialists has been certainly increasing, their outcome is still unsatisfactory : A survey of the outcome of 326 referred patients to the Mental Care Center was carried out on March in 2000, which revealed that about half the patients interrupted to receive the care of psychiatric specialists, and were missing or died (Table 1). This result gave us a future problem that psychiatric liaison with physicians for the recovery of patients with alcohol dependence should be done at an earlier stage of the illness. Therefore, the MASAD is planning to start the two-days course to learn skills for early intervention in alcohol dependence on this July and about 80 persons including doctors, nurses, public health nurses, and medical social workers are making an application for participating in the course so far.

Thus, though there are many medical and social hurdles to be cleared, we would do patiently continue our trial of psychiatric liaison with physicians as a strategy for realizing a goal of the treatment of alcohol dependence.

References

1) Ino, A., Endo, T., and Nishiyama, M. : Cooperation between general doctors and specialists for the treatment of alcoholism. Jpn. Med. J., 3768 ; 28-32, 1996 (in Japanese).

2) Endo, T., Ino, A., Takase, K., Watanabe, S., Suzuki, H., and Kataoka, C. : Actual state of psychiatric liaison with physicians for the treatment of alcohol-related diseases. Jpn. Med. J., 3901 ; 37-42, 1999 (in Japanese).

---

[1]三重大学保健管理センター
Shozo Watanabe (physician) : Health Administration Center, Mie University.

[2]三重大学医学部
Kojirou Takase (physician) : Mie University School of Medicine.

[3]市立四日市病院
Hideo Hirofuji (physician) : Yokkaichi City Hospital.

[4]四日市社会保険病院
Mitsumasa Kimura (physician) : Yokkaichi Social Insurance Hospital.

[5]鈴鹿中央総合病院
Akira Nishimura (physician) : Suzuka Central General Hospital.

[6]済生会松坂総合病院
Yoshiro Okuda (physician) : Saiseikai Matsuzaka General Hospital.

[7]伊勢市立病院
Masao Fujimoto (physician) : Ise City Hospital.

[8]山田赤十字病院
Yuji Kojima (physician) : Yamada Red Cross Hospital.

[9]伊勢慶応病院
Jun Inoue (physician) : Ise Keio Hospital.

[10]三重県立こころの医療センター
Takuro Endo (physician) and Aro Ino (psychiatrist) : Mental Care Center, Mie Prefecture.

アルコール・薬物乱用の予防：BDIM (Before-Discharge Intervention Method) によるアルコール依存症の否認への気付効果について

Therapeutic effects of Before-Discharge Intervention Method (BDIM) for alcoholics

猪野　亜朗* 　　林田　基**

Introduction

It is extremely important in the early phase of alcohol dependence treatment for the patient to recognize his／her own denial (Anderson, D. J., 1981) of alcohol-related problems. Conventional treatment methods such as psychological educational classes, self-help groups, and naikan therapy (a form of Japanese introspective psychotherapy) sessions are often ineffective in overcoming his／her denial. To help alcoholics achieve a more meaningful level of awareness of their alcohol dependence and remain in long-range treatment, Aro Ino has developed the Before-Discharge Intervention Method "BDIM" (Aro Ino, Motoi Hayasida, 2000), a modified version of the intervention method by Johnson (Johnson, V. E., 1980, 1986).

We conducted a clinical trial of the BDIM and wish to report its outcome results here.

Subjects

The study reference population consisted of alcoholics hospitalized at Mental Care Center, Prefecture of Mie for alcohol dependence syndrome and their family members.

The study patients were those 153 patients who, after their initial medical examination, were admitted to the hospital and discharged during the 2 year period beginning January 1, 1996, and ending December 31, 1997, and were capable of attending the hospital's follow-up clinic.

Procedures

The patients were assigned to either group I or II, depending on which day of the week they reported to the hospital for admission. Each group of patients had one physician in charge. Both physicians had 27 years of experience in clinical psychiatry, including a course they took on alcohol dependence syndrome treatment at the National Institute on Alcoholism- Kurihama National Hospital. Patients attended educational classes on alcohol-related matters in an open atmosphere and specialized alcohol dependence syndrome ward. There were no substantive differences in treatment provided between groups I and II with the exception that the BDIM was employed only with group I patients and their families.

Administration of BDIM

Excluded from administration of the BDIM but included for the outcome evaluation were 12 patients whose families were not able to participate in the BDIM for various reasons, 9 patients who were depressed, schizophrenic or violent, 4 patients with cognitive and／or memory deficits, 5 patients who prematurely dropped out of inpatient treatment, and 1 patient who refused to participate in the BDIM.

Outcome evaluation

The intervention outcome evaluation was conducted on the behaviors of all group I and II partients during a total of 4 months, that is, for two

Table 1 Characteristics of Study Patients

	W/spouse		W/nonspouse		Alone		Total	
Treatment groups	I	II	I	II	I	II	I	II
Number of inpatients	47	56	8	15	20	7	75	78
Number of females	3	4	1	3	1	2	5	9
Mean ages (years) at admission	55	52.2	47.1	47.5	48.6	47.7	52.5	50.9
Standard deviations of age at admission	10.3	10.3	17.4	12.7	10.7	11	11.9	11.1

calendar months before and for two calendar months after 2 years after discharge.

Behavioral outcome variables included ① the patient's and ② family members' attendance at hospital outpatient follow-up sessions and/or local self-help group (Danshukai) meetings and ③ the patient's abstinence.

In this study, a single attendance by a patient and/or family member during the 4 months evaluation period moved the subject into the "attendance yes" category.

Structured Before-Discharge Intervention Method (BDIM)

1) A patient and his/her family members comprehended and agreed to receive the BDIM.

2) Those patients who were depressed, shizophrenic and violent were excluded from administration of the BDIM.

3) The BDIM was employed between 3 and 10 days before discharge.

4) To help family members write their messages (letter), the physician met with them to explain the purpose of the BDIM and provided them with the instructional manual.

5) To write an effective message to the alcoholic, each participant was advised to mention in his/her message the following items:

1. The reason for deciding to participate in the intervention.
2. Some positive things that the participant could recall about the patient before his/her drinking problems developed.
3. Three to five present and three to five past episodes of the patient's problem drinking.
4. That he/she understood that the patient's problem drinking was attributable to the disease of alcohol dependence syndrome.
5. That he/she hoped that the patient would return to his/her former self, that is, without drinking problems.
6. That he/she hoped that the patient would meet the challenge to remain abstinent.
7. That he/she would remain committed to help the patient achieve abstinence.

6) The intervention was attended by the patient, family members and physician.

7) Each family member delivered his/her message to the patient one by one.

8) The patient was instructed to respond to the message with a comment or a statement about his/her emotional reaction.

9) After the intervention was over, the original written messages were given to the patient and copies were filed in the hospital patient chart.

10) The physician sometimes asked the patient that he/she would reply to family members by letter.

Results

Table 1 and 2 show the results of treatment.

Discussion

When the BDIM was added to the therapeutic program for alcohol dependence syndrome, those patients living with their spouse or significant other

Table 2 BDIM, Outcome, and Living Arrangements

	W／spouse		
	Group I	Group II	Total
A．Number of subjects(Number of BDIM ： %)	47(37：79%)	56(0：0%)	103(37：36%)
B．Patients' attendance at hospital follow-up sessions and／or self-help group meetings	21(45%)	15(27%) p＜0.1	36(35%)
C．Family members' attendance at hospital follow-up sessions and／or self-help group meetings	14(30%)	7(13%) p＜0.05	21(20%)
D．Patients' and family members' attendance at hospital follow-up sessions and／or self-help group meetings	14(30%)	7(13%) p＜0.05	21(20%)
E．Abstinence of the patients who and family members attended follow-up sessions and／or self-help group meetings	11(23%)	5(9%) p＜0.05	16(16%)
F．Abstinence of the patients who attended follow-up sessions and／or self-help group meetings	17(36%)	11(20%) p＜0.1	28(27%)

in group I did significantly better than their counterpart in group II in five behavioral treatment outcome variables. We contend that the BDIM is useful to motivate these patients to perform these behaviors which, in turn, will improve the prognosis of alcohol dependence syndrome. We grant, however, that the current study was not conducted in a random patient assignment design and, therefore, needs to be interpreted with some caution. Further research is appropriate.

Conclusion

The administration of BDIM to a group of patients living with their spouse or significant other is significantly effective in producing the following positive behavioral variables.

1) Patients' attendance at hospital follow-up sessions and／or self-help group meetings

2) Family members' attendance at hospital follow-up sessions and／or self-help group meetings

3) Patients' and family members' attendance at hospital follow-up sessions and／or self-help group meetings

4) Abstinence of the patients who and whose family members attended hospital follow-up sessions and／or self-help group meetings

5) Abstinence of the patients who attended hospital follow-up sessions and／or self-help group meetings

References

1) Anderson, D. J.：Professional Education 9, The Psychopathology of Denial. Hazelden, Minnesota, pp33-34, 1981.
2) Ino, A., Hayasida, M.：Before-Discharge Intervention Method in the Treatment of Alcohol Dependence. Alcohol Clin. Exp. Res., 24 (3)；pp373-376, 2000.
3) Johnson, V. E.：I'll Quit tomorrow：A Practical Guide to Alcoholism Treatment. Harper & Row, San Francisco, 1980.
4) Johnson, V. E.：Intervention：How To Help Someone Who Doesn't Want Help. Johnson Institute, Minneapolis, Minnesota, 1986.

＊三重県立こころの医療センター
Aro Ino：Mental Care Center, Prefecture of Mie.
＊＊横浜舞岡病院
Motoi Hayashida：Yokohama Maioka Psychiatric Hospital.

Table 2 BDIM, Outcome, and Living Arrangements

	W／nonspouse			Alone			Total		
	Group I	Group II	Total	Group I	Group II	Total	Group I	Group II	Total
A.	8(4:50%)	15(0:0%)	23(4:17%)	20(3:15%)	7(0:0%)	27(3:11%)	75(44:59%)	78(0:0%)	153(44:29%)
B.	1(13%)	5(33%) n.s.	6(26%)	4(20%)	1(18%) n.s.	5(19%)	26(35%)	21(27%) n.s.	47(31%)
C.	0(0%)	0(0%) n.s.	0(0%)	1(5%)	0(0%) n.s.	1(4%)	15(20%)	7(9%) $p<0.1$	22(14%)
D.	0(0%)	0(0%) n.s.	0(0%)	1(5%)	0(0%) n.s.	1(4%)	15(20%)	7(9%) $p<0.1$	22(14%)
E.	0(0%)	0(0%) n.s.	0(0%)	1(5%)	0(0%) n.s.	1(4%)	12(16%)	5(6%) $p<0.1$	17(11%)
F.	0(0%)	2(13%) n.s.	2(9%)	2(10%)	1(12%) n.s.	3(11%)	19(25%)	14(18%) n.s.	33(22%)

痴呆の早期発見・治療・予防
―初期アルツハイマー病の追跡研究から―

Preventive aspects of dementia : early intervention, treatment and prevention in dementia

宇野　正威*

はじめに

　アルツハイマー病(Alzheimer's Disease : AD)は、記憶障害に始まって、漸次認知機能が全体的に低下し、その多くは重症痴呆に至る痴呆性疾患である。ADに対する初めての薬剤として認可されたドネペジルは痴呆症状をある程度改善する作用はあるが、その進行を抑制する効力を持たない。そのため、痴呆の予防のためには、ADをできるだけ早期に発見し、多少とも効果の示唆されている薬剤と、生活指導・リハビリテーション活動で対処する必要がある。

I. アルツハイマー病の早期診断

　アルツハイマー病の進行は、健忘期(初期)、混乱期(中期)と痴呆期(末期)の3段階に分けられる。健忘期は顕著な記憶障害を呈するが、その他の知的機能はほぼ正常範囲であり、日常生活もある程度の援助があれば可能である。混乱期にはいると、理解力・思考力も漸次低下するため、日常生活上混乱を来すことが多くなる。早期診断は、健忘期の段階で診断することであり、その際、健常高齢者がしばしば訴える良性老人性もの忘れとの鑑別が重要である。そのためには、記憶を中心とする神経心理学的検査によりADに特有の近時記憶障害を、および画像検査により海馬領域の萎縮と局所脳血流量低下を明らかにすることが必要である。

1. 初期ADの記憶とその他の認知機能

　「もの忘れ」を愁訴として来院する患者の中に、自覚的に想起障害を訴える群と、家族が記銘障害に気付く群がある。前者は人名の度忘れなどを中心とし、全体的な知的低下はない。その多くは、良性もの忘れに相当する。一方、後者の特徴は、日常的に交わされる会話をすぐに忘れる、という家族の訴えである。多くは、時間見当識障害を伴い、また複雑な作業は拙劣になっている。Hughesらは、日常生活における広い範囲の知的機能を含んだ評価表 Clinical Dementia Rating (CDR)を開発し、初期痴呆を総合的に把握しようとした。CDRは記憶だけでなく、見当識、判断と問題解決、社会参加、家庭生活と趣味、セルフケアーの6項目からなる。各項目ごと0、0.5、1、2、3に5段階評価し、それを総合して、痴呆の重症度を5段階、すなわち　0：痴呆なし、0.5：痴呆疑い、1：軽度、2：中等度、3：重度に分類する。CDR 0.5ないしCDR 1が初期ADに相当する。

2. 近時記憶障害と遅延再生障害

　記憶障害には、記憶した情報を意識にのぼらせることが困難な想起障害と、新しい情報の取込みが侵される記銘障害がある。ADでは早期から後者の記憶障害、とくに"誰がいつどこで何をした"というニュース情報の取込みが顕著に障害されている。記憶は、一回的体験の'想い出'(エピソード記憶)と、繰り返し学習による'知識'(意味記憶)に分けられる。ADはとくにエピソード記憶の著しい障害を特徴とするので、その診断のためには、エピソード記憶のパラダイムである論理的記憶(物語再生)と単語リスト記銘の検査が中心となる。武蔵病院では、1)物語再生：15語句から成る物語の直後再生と30分後の遅延再生、2)10単語記銘検査：10個の日常語を用い、5回の反復学習、30分後再生、カテゴリー・Cueによ

る再生，再認の検査を中心に行っている。これらの検査の中で，初期ADの特徴は，物語再生と単語記銘の遅延再生の障害で，健常者との鑑別にももっとも有効である。

3．MRIとSPECT

AD脳の神経病理学的研究によると，病変は早期から海馬傍回と海馬に出現し，しだいに大脳皮質全体に広がる。これに対応して，MRI上早期から海馬と海馬傍回の萎縮と側脳室下角の拡大が観察される。

一方，SPECT上，早期には側頭葉内側部に，しだいに側頭葉外側部と頭頂葉後部の局所脳血流量の低下が見られるようになる。最近，非常に早期のADにおける局所脳血流の研究が詳しく調べられるようになり，帯状回後部の脳血流低下が目立つことが特徴的とされている。しかし，局所脳血流低下部位はADの発症年齢と関係があり，若年発症では帯状回と頭頂葉内側部，高齢発症では前頭葉において早期から局所脳血流量が低下する。

II．初期ADの位置付けと症状の進行

1．初期ADの基準

われわれの症例群については，次の基準を満たしているとき'初期AD'とした。すなわち，①日常生活上，最近の出来事についての記銘が極めて劣っている，②記憶検査のうち，物語再生検査と10単語記銘検査の両方で，遅延再生の成績が際だって低下している，③MRIかSPECTによって，側頭葉内側部の構造的変化あるいは機能低下が示唆される，の条件を満たす場合をADの可能性が高いとした。そうして，記憶と見当識以外の知的機能がほぼ保たれ，日常家庭生活レベルの低下も僅かであり，MMSE 24点以上，HDS-R 21点以上の場合を初期ADとした。

武蔵病院の症例を，CDRと対応させると，大部分はCDR 0.5に，一部はCDR 1に相当した。CDRの6項目のそれぞれの得点を比較してみると，おおよそ次のようなパターンを示している。①記憶：0，0.5，1，2，3の5段階評価のうち，多くは1，一部2，②見当識：0.5あるいは1，③判断力と問題解決：0あるいは0.5，④社会適応：0あるいは0.5，⑤家庭状況および趣味・関心：0あるいは0.5，⑥パーソナルケア：0である。そうして，総得点は1.5～4.0の間に分布した。なお，記憶の項目が0.5の場合には，ADは考えがたく，正常範囲ないしは別の痴呆性疾患を考える。

記憶障害のみの著しい症例をどのように位置付けるかについては議論がある。ADと診断し得るかの問題であり，Pertersonらは，ADに先立つ病態像として，Mild Cognitive Impairment（MCI）という概念を提唱した。その診断基準は，①自覚的な記憶愁訴と家族によるその確認，②その年齢としては異常な記憶力低下，③記憶以外は正常の認知機能，④運転や家計などの日常生活活動を行う能力は保たれていること，⑤痴呆はない，である。MCIと診断された患者を追跡すると，1年にその12％が，4年で約半数がADを発症するので，PetersonはMCIは正常老化と痴呆の過渡期であるという。Petersonらが研究対象とした症例の中でMCIと診断された群はCDR 0.5に属し，CDR総得点は平均1.5であった。われわれの初期ADの大部分はCDR 0.5，総得点では1.5～4.0点の間に分布しているので，MCIは全体としてわれわれの初期ADよりさらに早期を捉えているようである。

2．症状の進行

健忘期は数年間持続し，混乱期に入ると比較的急速に進行する。われわれの初期AD群では，3年以内は症状の進行は著しくはなかった。MMSEの得点で見ると，多くは年間変化率が1ないし2点の低下であった。健忘期に数年留まった後，次のような認知機能の低下が出現する。第一は，道具を使用した行為系列の障害が目立って来ることである。とくに女性の場合には，もともと料理の好きな人であっても，その手際が遅くなり，炊事そのものを避けるようになる。これは，実行機能の障害という観点から見ると前頭葉機能の低下であり，道具を使用した行為系列の障害という観点から見れば頭頂葉機能の障害という性質をもつ。第二は，会話の少なくなることである。一対一で

話せば，言語理解に著しい障害があるとは思えないが，一家団らんの場などでの言葉数が少なくなる。普通の会話では，個々の単語の意味を理解するだけでなく，文脈を通じての理解が必要であるが，後者の機能が落ちてきているため，グループの中での会話について行くことが困難になる。この状態がさらに進行すると，一対一で分かりやすく話しても理解できないようになる。

III. 早期治療

アルツハイマー病の早期診断の目的は，記憶をはじめとして知的機能全体の低下を少しでも抑制することである。しかし，われわれが使用できる薬剤であるドネペジルは痴呆症状を少し改善するが，疾患の進行を抑制することはできない。そこで，他の薬剤の効果も検討しながら，症状の進行を少しでも抑制し得るような生活指導・リハビリテーション活動が必要となる。

1. 薬物療法

アルツハイマー病の認知機能低下に対する治療薬として日本で最初に認可されたのはドネペジルである。この薬剤は軽度から中等度の患者に対して，認知機能面（記憶，見当識）と意欲・自発性の面での効果がある。MMSEでは，約2点の増加であり，患者の知的レベルを約1年前に戻すことに相当する。しかし，疾患の進行を抑制することはできぬため，その後症状は漸次進行する。

痴呆症状を直接改善することはないが，その進行を少しは抑制するのではないかと期待されているのは，ビタミンEとセレギリンである。両薬剤は，プラセボと比較すると機能の低下速度が減退し，ナーシングホームへの入所までの期間が長くなる。この研究では，ビタミンEの大量療法（2000IU/日）が使用されているが，日本ではその量を適用することはできない。またセレギリンはパーキンソン病に対する薬剤としてのみ日本では認可されている。

治療薬として，症例数は少ないが，治験の進められているのは，エストロゲン，および非ステロイド系抗炎症剤である。アメリカの国立老化研究所がボルチモアで行っている縦断研究によると，いずれの薬剤も長期に服用している場合，AD発症の危険率が服用していない場合と比較して約半分に低下するというが，エストロゲンはすでに発症しているADに対しては治療効果は否定的である。

2. 非薬物的介入

非薬物的アプローチとして，われわれが行っている生活指導とリハビリ活動の試みを紹介する。生活指導の考え方は，健忘期から混乱期に移行する際の症状の進行を少しでも抑えるためには，どのような生活の仕方が必要かということである。その第一は，創造的な手作業，すなわち道具と手を使いながら，何かを作り出すような行為系列を，日常生活の中に，楽しみとして位置付けることである。陶芸，プラモデルなどの趣味でもよし，また日常的に炊事を行っている場合はできるだけ続けるよう指導する。第二は，多くの人との会話の場をできるだけ頻回に持つことである。配偶者の存在は，それだけでも効果が大きいが，デイケアなどを通じて多くの人と交わり，より多くの言語コミュニケーションをもつことが大切であろう。

リハビリテーション活動としては，リアリティ・オリエンテーション，回想法，音楽療法などが知られているが，われわれは芸術造形研究所の協力を得ながらアートセラピーを試みている。これはアメリカのエドワーズによって開発された絵画教授法などに由来する方法を用いており，パステル画，陶芸，工作，オブジェなどさまざまな創作活動を指導している。予備的な結果ではあるが，WAIS-Rで検討したところ，一部の下位項目で成績の上昇も見られた。

おわりに

現在行われている薬物治療・非薬物的介入は，ある程度の効果をもつ。しかし，記憶障害に関しては，3年の経過でみると，やはり進行しており，多くはその後全体的な知的機能も漸次低下して行く。当然のことながら，疾患の進行を抑制する薬物の開発が必要である。アルツハイマー病は，脳にアミロイドβタンパクの蓄積する疾患

であり，そのβタンパクの生成を阻害する，蓄積を抑制する，分解を促進するメカニズムについて基礎的な研究が急速に進んでいる。ADの発症の予防あるいは進行を抑制する薬剤開発の可能性もみえてきており，アメリカではワクチン療法の臨床試験が開始されている。アルツハイマー病の病態機序に基づく本格的な薬剤が一日も早く臨床の場に現れることが期待される。

文　献

1) Homma, A., Takeda, M. et al. : Clinical efficacy and safety of donepezil on cognitive and global function in patients with Alzheimer's disease. Dement. Geriatr. Cogn. Disord., 11 ; 299-616, 2000.
2) Hughes, C. P., Berg, L. et al. : A new clinical scale for the staging of dementia. Br. J. Psychiatry, 140 ; 566-572, 1982.
3) Iwata, N., Saido, T. et al. : Metabolic regulation of brain Aβ by neprilysin. Science, 292 ; 1550-1552, 2001.
4) National Institute on Aging : Progress report on Alzheimer's disease, 2000.
5) Petersen, R. C., Smith, G. E. et al. : Mild cognitive impairment ; clinical characterization and outcome. Arch. Neurol., 56 ; 303-308, 1999.
6) Sano, M., Ernesto, C. et al. : A controlled trial of Selegiline, Alpha-tocopherol, or both as treatment for Alzheimer's disease. N. Engl. J. Med., 336 ; 1216-22, 1997.
7) 宇野正威：アルツハイマー型痴呆の早期診断と早期治療. 小椋力, 倉知正佳編：臨床精神医学講座 S3巻　精神障害の予防. 中山書店，東京，p.57-64, 2000.
8) 宇野正威, 朝田隆ほか：もの忘れ外来―武蔵病院におけるアルツハイマー病早期診断―. 老年精神医学雑誌, 11 ; 1195-1202, 2001.

---

*国立精神・神経センター武蔵病院（現：吉岡リハビリテーションクリニック）

Masatake Uno : National Center of Neurology and Psychiatry（Present address : Yoshioka Rehabilitation Clinic）

精神分裂病の性・年齢別分布
Age and gender distribution of schizophrenic patients

菊池　美紀* 　木下　裕久* 　道辻俊一郎* 　宇都宮　浩* 　中根　允文*

I. はじめに

　精神分裂病の疫学で共通してみられる所見として，女性の平均発病年齢が高いことである。また発症が早い場合は慢性化（男性）し，発症が遅い場合の転帰は良好（女性）という，2種の症状モデル仮説があることはよく知られている。

　当教室は1979～1980年に「重度精神障害の転帰決定要因に関する WHO 共同研究（WHO Collaborative Study on Determinants of Outcome of Severe Mental Disorders）に参加し，この中で上記仮説が正しいかどうかの検討をこれまで行ってきたが，今回は女性の発症年齢が男性よりも遅いか否かに関してデータ解析を行ったので報告する。加えて他施設のデータも紹介し，若干の考察も加えてみた。

II. 研究方法

1. 重度精神障害の転帰決定要因に関する WHO 共同研究

　本研究は1970年代後半に，社会的，文化的にそれぞれ異なる10カ国12施設で同時に開始され，その後2年間の追跡調査が行われた。参加施設は，Aarhus（Denmark），Agra & Chandigarh（India），Cali（Colombia），Dublin（Ireland），Honolulu & Rochester（USA），Ibadan（Nigeria），Moscow（USSR），Nagasaki（Japan），Nottingham（UK），Prague（Czechoslovakia）で，全施設合わせて最初のスクリーニングで1535名が選ばれ，うち1379名に関して追跡がなされた。

2. 対象
1) 初診時年齢が15歳以上55歳未満
2) 受診前の1年内に6カ月以上長崎市内に居住していること

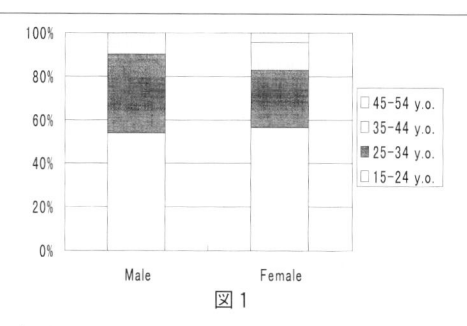

図1

3) 今回は初回の精神科受診であること
4) 過去1年間に審査基準を満たす精神症状や行動異常が認められること

なお器質性脳障害，アルコールまたは薬物依存による中枢神経系障害，重度精神遅滞が除外された。

3. 方法

　長崎市内に在住で新たに精神疾患に罹患した者がどの精神科施設に受診するかの予備調査が行われ，長崎市内および近郊の30の病院，医院，保健所などが特定され，これらの施設に研究の協力をお願いし，case finding network とした。そして1979～1980年の2年間，毎日，初診の精神障害者の受診の有無を尋ね，本調査の対象に採用される可能性のある症例に対して研究員がその施設を訪問し，該当例であれば患者および家族に同意を得て聞き取り調査を行っていった。

4. 初回接触時の評価項目
1) PPHS（Psychiatric and Personal History Schedule）（WHO, 1978）
2) DPS（Diagnostic and Prognostic Schedule）（WHO, 1978）
3) PSE-9（Present State Examination 9 th edition）（Wing et al., 1974）
4) Life Event Schedule（WHO, 1978）
5) KAS（Katz Adjustment Schedule）（Katz et

表1　性別発症年齢分布

AGE SEX	15-24 (%)	25-34 (%)	35-44 (%)	45-54 (%)	Total (%)
Male	33 (54.1)	22 (36.1)	6 (9.8)	0 (0)	61 (100)
Female	26 (56.1)	12 (26.1)	6 (13.0)	2 (4.3)	46 (100)
Total	59 (55.1)	34 (31.8)	12 (11.2)	2 (1.9)	107 (100)

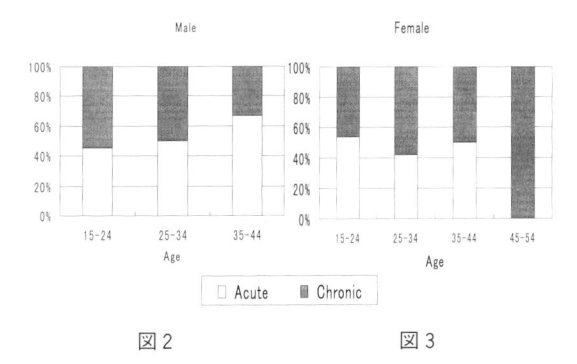

表2　発症様式（男性）

AGE (Male)	15-24 (%)	25-34 (%)	35-44 (%)	Total (%)
Acute	15 (50.0)	11 (36.7)	4 (13.3)	30 (100)
Chronic	18 (58.1)	11 (35.5)	2 (6.5)	31 (100)
Total	33 (54.1)	22 (36.1)	6 (9.8)	61 (100)

表3　発症様式（女性）

AGE (Female)	15-24 (%)	25-34 (%)	35-44 (%)	45-54 (%)	Total (%)
Acute	14 (63.6)	5 (22.7)	3 (13.6)	0 (0)	22 (100)
Chronic	12 (50.0)	7 (29.2)	3 (12.5)	2 (8.3)	24 (100)
Total	26 (56.5)	12 (26.1)	6 (13.0)	2 (4.3)	46 (100)

図2　　　　　図3

al., 1963)

III. 結　果

　対象となったのは男性61名，女性46名（計107名）で，初回接触時の平均年齢は男性24.8±7.5歳，女性27.0±8.9歳（計25.8±8.2歳）で，女性の方が平均年齢が高かった。この初回接触時年齢を発症年齢と考えて，性別発症年齢分布を示した（表1，図1）。年齢構成別の割合で男女の有意差は認めないものの，女性の方が高年齢層に占める割合が高く，45歳以上の晩発例もあった。
　次に発症様式に関しては，1カ月以内に発症した急性発症およびそれ以上の期間を経て発症した慢性発症に男女の有意差はなく，年齢別でも有意差は認めなかった。しかし男性の方が若年層に慢性発症が多い傾向が見られた（表2，図2，表3，図3）。
　一方共同研究を行った他の11施設に関しても女性の方が平均発病年齢が高いというデータが示されているが，唯一Pragueで女性の方が若年発症の傾向があると報告されている。

IV. 考察とまとめ

　今回の調査で，女性の発病年齢が男性よりも高い傾向は認められた。これまで精神分裂病の初発年齢の男女差に関しては様々な施設で調査がなされており，女性の晩発を報告している最近のデータとしては，Angermeyer & Kuhn(1988), Goldstein et al.(1990), Gureje(1991), Ohaeri(1992), Hafner et al.(1993), Faraone(1994), Gorwood et al.(1995), Szymanski et al.(1995)などが挙げられる。
　一方女性の早発を報告したデータも数少ないがあり，1992年にHambrechtらが行った調査では，イスラム圏で女性の早発が報告されている。また1993年にBeiserらが行った調査では，ICD-9による診断では初発年齢に性差はないとあったが，DSM-IIIを用いると女性の方に早期の症状発現が見られると報告している。
　このように診断基準がもたらすバイアスをはじめ，性差への様々な影響因子，さらには標本サイズなどを検討しながら，発病年齢の性差に関する仮説を今後も検証していく必要があると考える。

---

*長崎大学医学部精神神経科学教室
Miki Kikuchi, Hirohisa Kinoshita, Shunichiro Michitsuji, Hiroshi Utsunomiya, Yoshibumi Nakane : Department of Neuropsychiatry, Nagasaki University, School of Medicine.

精神分裂病発症とライフイベント
Relationship of life events to onset of schizophrenia

木下　裕久*　　宇都宮　浩*　　菊池　美紀*　　今村　芳博*
中根　秀之*　　石崎　裕香*　　中根　允文*

I. はじめに

当教室が1979年から80年にかけて行った『重度精神障害の転帰決定要因に関するWHO共同研究』の対象となった107例の初発分裂病患者のうち，評価可能であった80例に対し，発症前3カ月間に体験した日常生活上の出来事についてWHOのLife Event Scheduleを用い調査した。この一部はすでに，当教室の石澤らによって発表されたが，今回新たに，年代別の視点と家族問題の視点から分析を行った。

II. 結　果

対象者80例は，男性44名，女性36名で平均年齢は24.8才であった。このうち発症前3カ月に何らかのライフイベントを体験した人は，表1のように男性44名中35名(79.5％)，女性36名中28名(77.8％)，全体では80名中63名(78.8％)であった。また80名中50名が1カ月以内の急性発症，30名が緩徐に発症した慢性発症であった。表2は，ライフイベントの有無と発症様式との関係であるが，全体でイベントがある群に急性発症が多く，特に男性でイベントが有る35名中28名(80％)が急性発症であり，統計学的に有意であった。次にライフイベントを以下の8種類に分類し，他の要素との関連を調べた。8つとは，①職業・学業，②健康，③恋愛及び結婚，④経済，⑤転居・移動，⑥人間関係，⑦その他，⑧家族である。図1，表3では，性別とライフイベントの種類を検討した。仕事・学業は統計的には性差は出ず，女性で結婚及び恋愛問題に関するイベントが多く，また家族に関するイベントが多いことが統計学的に有意であった。表4では，発症形式とライフイベントの種類の差を男女別に検討した。男性では，人間関係のイベントが慢性発症例に多く，統計的に

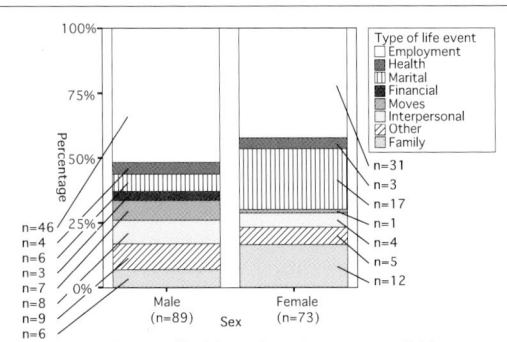

図1　性別とライフイベントの種類

有意だった。また女性では，家族のイベントが慢性発症で多かった。また，全体では慢性発症で，健康のイベントが統計的に有意に多く，家族のイベントが多い傾向があった。

表5は，各年代別のライフイベントの種類である。10代では，仕事・学業が多く，20代では，恋愛・結婚が多く，40代以降では経済的イベントが多いことがいずれも統計的に有意であった。また30代では家族のイベントが多い傾向があった。

III. 考　察

今回の結果だけでは，ライフイベントが分裂病発症の直接原因となりうるかどうかの判断はできないが，ライフイベントの有無が分裂病の発症形式に関連があり，性別，年代別で，イベントの種類に特徴がみられたことは，ライフイベントが，分裂病発症に関して，生物学的脆弱性に加えて何らかの引き金的役割を果たす可能性を示唆している。今後，再発時や追跡調査時の結果を分析し，ライフイベントが，病勢や転帰にどのように影響するのか検討していきたい。

*長崎大学医学部精神神経科学教室
　Hirohisa Kinoshita, Hiroshi Utsunomiya, Miki Kikuchi, Yoshihiro Imamura, Hideyuki Nakane, Yuka Ishizaki, Yoshibumi Nakane : Department of Neuropsychiatry, Nagasaki University School of Medicine.

表1 年代別分布とライフイベントの有無

Event positive [N]／Total [N] (%)

Sex	Age				
	15–19	20–19	30–39	40–54	Total
Male	14/18 (77.8%)	14/17 (82.4%)	5/7 (71.4%)	2/2 (100.0%)	35/44 (79.5%)
Female	9/9 (100.0%)	12/17 (70.6%)	5/6 (83.3%)	2/4 (50.0%)	28/36 (77.8%)
Total	23/27 (85.2%)	26/34 (76.5%)	10/13 (76.9%)	4/6 (66.7%)	63/80 (78.8%)

表2 ライフイベントの有無と発症様式

Sex	Type of Onset	Life event					
		−		+		Total	
Male	Acute	2	22.2%	28	80.0%	30	68.2%
	Chronic	7	77.8%	7	20.0%	14	31.8%
	Total	9	100.0%	35	100.0%	44	100.0%
Female	Acute	2	25.0%	18	64.3%	20	55.6%
	Chronic	6	75.0%	10	35.7%	16	44.4%
	Total	8	100.0%	28	100.0%	36	100.0%
Total	Acute	4	23.5%	46	73.0%	50	62.5%
	Chronic	13	76.5%	17	27.0%	30	37.5%
	Total	17	100.0%	63	100.0%	80	100.0%

表3 性別とライフイベントの種類

Type of life event	Sex					
	Male		Female		Total	
Employment	46	(51.7%)	31	(42.5%)	77	(47.5%)
Health	4	(4.5%)	3	(4.1%)	7	(4.6%)
Marital	6	(6.7%)	17**	(23.3%)	23	(14.2%)
Financial	3	(3.4%)	0		3	(1.9%)
Moves	7+	(7.9%)	1	(1.4%)	8	(4.9%)
Interpersonal	8	(9.0%)	4	(5.5%)	12	(7.4%)
Other	9	(10.1%)	5	(6.8%)	14	(8.6%)
Family	6	(6.7%)	12*	(16.4%)	18	(11.1%)
Total	89	(100.0%)	73	(100.0%)	162	(100.0%)

**P<0.005　*P<0.05　+P=0.058 (evaluated by Fisher's exact test)

表4 発症様式とライフイベントの種類

Type of Onset	Type of life event	Sex					
		Male		Female		Total	
Acute	Employment	40	(54.1%)	24	(45.3%)	64	(50.4%)
	Health	2	(2.7%)	1	(1.9%)	3*	(2.4%)
	Marital	6	(8.1%)	14	(26.4%)	20	(15.7%)
	Financial	3	(4.1%)	0	(0%)	3	(2.4%)
	Moves	6	(8.1%)	1	(1.9%)	7	(5.5%)
	Interpersonal	4*	(5.4%)	3	(5.7%)	7	(5.5%)
	Other	7	(9.5%)	5	(9.4%)	12	(9.4%)
	Family	6	(8.1%)	5**	(9.4%)	11+	(8.7%)
	合計	74	(100.0%)	53	(100.0%)	127	(100.0%)
Chronic	Employment	6	(40.0%)	7	(35.0%)	13	(37.1%)
	Health	2	(13.3%)	2	(10.0%)	4*	(11.4%)
	Marital	0		3	(15.0%)	3	(8.6%)
	Financial	0		0	(0%)	0	(0%)
	Moves	1	(6.7%)	0	(0%)	1	(2.9%)
	Interpersonal	4*	(26.7%)	1	(5.0%)	5	(14.3%)
	Other	2	(13.3%)	0	(0%)	2	(5.7%)
	Family	0	(0%)	7**	(35.0%)	7+	(20.0%)
	合計	15	(100.0%)	20	(100.0%)	35	(100.0%)

**P<0.025　*P<0.05　+P=0.062 (evaluated by Fisher's exact test)

表5 年代別のライフイベントの種類

Type of life event	Age					
	15–19	20–29	30–39	40–54	Total	
Employment	32* (61.5%)	33 (47.1%)	11 (39.3%)	1 (8.3%)	77	(47.5%)
Health	3 (5.8%)	0	2 (7.1%)	2 (16.7%)	7	(4.3%)
Marital	0	15* (21.4%)	5 (17.9%)	3 (25.0%)	23	(14.2%)
Financial	0	0	1 (3.6%)	2* (16.7%)	3	(1.9%)
Moves	4 (7.7%)	3 (4.3%)	1 (3.6%)	0	8	(4.9%)
Interpersonal	5 (9.6%)	4 (5.7%)	1 (3.6%)	2 (16.7%)	12	(7.4%)
Other	5 (9.6%)	8 (11.4%)	1 (3.6%)	0	14	(8.6%)
Family	3 (5.8%)	7 (10.0%)	6+ (21.4%)	2 (16.7%)	18	(11.1%)
Total	52 (100.0%)	70 (100.0%)	28 (100.0%)	12 (100.0%)	162	(100.0%)

*P<0.025　+P=0.064 (evaluated by Fisher's exact test)

初発分裂病の発症前特徴

Characteristics of symptoms before the onset of schizophrenia

石崎　裕香*　　今村　芳博*　　宇都宮　浩*
木下　裕久*　　道辻俊一郎**　　中根　允文*

　精神分裂病における発症前特徴と，分裂病罹病後の症状，社会適応能力などの分裂病の長期経過との間に関連性があると諸研究により指摘されているが，我々のデータにおいて発症前特徴が罹病後の症状や経過の指標となりうるか検討する。

　研究方法は前述と同様，1979～80年にかけて行った『重度精神障害の転帰決定要因に関するWHO共同研究』の一環として調査した107例の初発分裂病患者を対象とし，特に思春期の発症前行動特徴に注目した。

　我々の調査で用いた質問項目を「行為障害様特徴」と「分裂病様特徴」の2つのカテゴリーに分け，これらの質問で明らかにあるとするものが1つでもあればその発症前特徴があるとした。

1．発症様式と発症前特徴

　図1にみられるように，急性発症群において分裂病様特徴がある症例が有意に多かった。

　慢性発症群については分裂病様特徴がある症例が有意に多いとも，また，行為障害様特徴がある症例が急性発症群よりも有意に多いとも言えなかった。発症前特徴と発症様式との関係は有意ではなかった。

2．初診時診断と発症前特徴

　図2にみられるように，初診時のICD-9診断が破瓜型の症例群において分裂病様特徴を示した症例は有意に多い結果となった($p=0.023$)。妄想型において分裂病様特徴がある症例が有意に多いとは言えなかった。初診時診断と発症前特徴との関係は有意ではなかった。

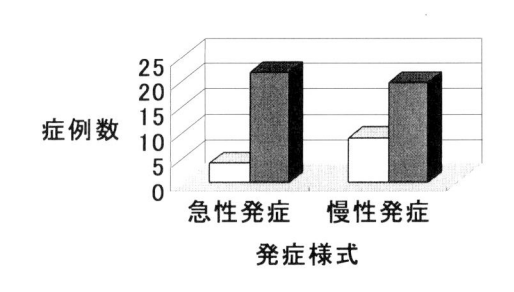

図1　発症様式と発症前特徴

3．社会適応能力と発症前特徴

　15年目転帰調査におけるDASの簡略版の全体評価を用い社会適応能力の指標とした。

　「非常に良好な適応状態」「良好な適応状態」「適応状態は良い方」という評価を受けた3つの群を『適応良好』群とし，「不十分な適応状態」「極めて貧弱な適応状態」「深刻な適応状態」という評価を受けた3つの群を『適応不良』群とした。結果は表1に示す。

　図3に示すとおり15年目転帰調査で適応良好群において分裂病様特徴を示した症例は有意に多い結果となった($p=0.034$)。適応不良群においては，分裂病様特徴がある症例が有意に多いとはいえなかった。また，行為障害様特徴を持つものが，適応不良群に多いというわけでもなかった。社会適応能力と発症前特徴との関係は有意ではなかった。

まとめ

　思春期の発病前特徴について，急性発症群において分裂病様特徴がある症例が有意に多かったが，発症様式と発症前特徴との関係は有意でなか

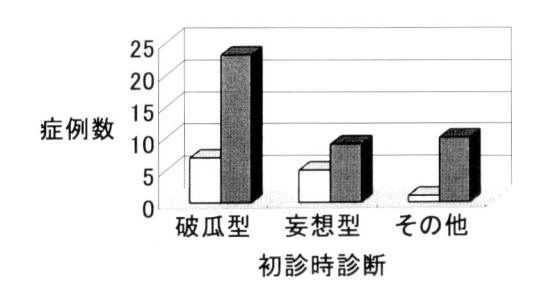

図2 初診時診断と発症前特徴

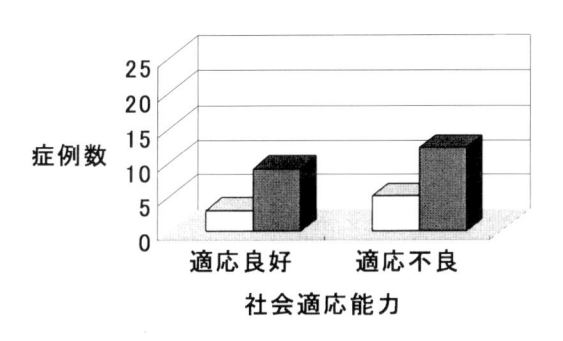

図3 社会適応能力と発症前特徴

表1 社会適応能力（WHO/DASの簡略版）

適応状態	n	（%）	良・不良
非常に良好な適応状態	6	（11.3）	
良好な適応状態	8	（15.1）	41.5%
適応状態は良い方	8	（15.1）	
不十分な適応状態	18	（34.0）	
極めて貧弱な適応状態	11	（20.8）	58.5%
深刻な適応状態	2	（3.8）	
計	53		

った。

また、初診時診断が、破瓜型群に分裂病様特徴を示した症例が有意に多かったが、初診時診断と発病前特徴との関係は有意でなかった。

15年目転帰調査で適応良好群において分裂病様特徴を示した症例は有意に多い結果となった。適応不良群においては分裂病様特徴がある症例が多いとは言えなかった。社会適応能力と発症前特徴との関係は有意ではなかった。

考　察

分裂病様特徴をもつ症例が発症様式においては急性発症群、初診時診断においては破瓜型群において有意にみられ、かつ15年目転帰においては適応良好群に有意にみられた。これらの結果はいくつかのハイリスク研究で指摘されているように、いわゆる分裂病様症状というものが分裂病の特定の亜型に特異的な所見でないものの、発病後の分裂病症状を示唆する可能性があるといえる。

発症前特徴と社会適応能力との関係は有意ではなく、様々な調査にて、発症前特徴が経過予測因子となる可能性が指摘されているが、今回の調査からは、明らかな経過予測因子は指摘できなかったが、今後はさらに詳細なる病前行動特徴と経過との関連を解析し、検討したい。

*長崎大学医学部精神神経科学教室
Yuka Ishizaki, Yoshihiro Imamura, Hiroshi Utsunomiya, Hirohisa Kinoshita, Yoshibumi Nakane : Department of Neuropsychiatry, Nagasaki University School of Medicine.

**長崎市立市民病院心療内科・精神科
Syunichirou Michituji : Department of Psychosomatic Medicine and Neuropsychiatry, Nagasaki City Municipal Hospital.

日本における初発分裂病の精神病未治療期間(DUP)について
DUP(Duration of Untreated Psychosis) of first episode schizophrenia in Japan

水野　雅文* 　　山澤　涼子* 　　三浦　勇太* 　　渡邊衡一郎*
山下　千代* 　　村上　雅昭* 　　鹿島　晴雄*

近年,精神分裂病の発病予防や早期発見・早期介入の重要性が議論されている[4]。長期化・重症化の防止には,発症後の速やかな介入が必要と考えられ,欧米を中心として精神病の未治療期間 Duration of Untreated Psychosis(以下 DUP)についての検討がなされている[2]。DUP の短縮は急性期症状の軽減と長期予後の改善にきわめて重要であることが指摘されているだけでなく,今後精神科臨床研究における対象者の基礎的データとして重視される可能性が極めて高い。しかしながら,本邦ではこれまで DUP に関する検討はなされていない。本研究では都内2施設において,初発の精神分裂病ケースの DUP を調べた。

I. 対　象

対象は,平成11年4月1日から平成12年3月31日までの間に,都内2施設にて生涯初めての精神科受診をし,この時点で精神病状態がみとめられ精神分裂病と診断された者52名とした。

今回調査を行った施設は,大学病院と精神科指定病院である。前者をA,後者をBとし,対象者はAが34名,Bが18名であった。性別は,男性19名,女性33名。Aでは男性13名,女性21名,Bでは男性6名,女性12名であった。平均年齢は37.4±15.6歳。Aでは36.4歳,Bでは39.2歳で,施設間に有意差は認めなかった。

Beiserら[1]や Sartorius ら[5]の論文においては,対象者を15歳から54歳の間に限定しており,今回の研究でもこれらに倣う形で15歳から54歳に対象を絞ると対象者数は41名で,Aは28名,Bは13名であった。性別は,男性17名,女性24名。Aでは,男性14名,女性14名,Bでは男性3名,女性10名であった。平均年齢は30.0±8.1歳で,Aは30.0歳,Bでは30.3歳で,両施設間に有意差は認められなかった。

II. 方　法

DUP は,今回の調査においては,精神分裂病と診断された者において,精神病状態の発現から,生涯初めての向精神薬処方開始までの期間,と定義した。診断は ICD-10を用いた。

また,精神病状態とは,シュナイダーの一級症状のうち少なくとも1つ,もしくは ICD-10の精神分裂病診断ガイドラインにおける(a)から(d)の症状のうち少なくとも1つを,自他覚的にみとめることを指すこととした。いずれもいわゆる陽性症状を指しており,陰性症状や,社会的機能の低下は含まない。

調査方法としては,前述の対象者のカルテ調査を行い,DUP を調べるとともに,同居者の有無,初診時の社会参加の有無,受診経路,併発症の有無を調査し,DUP との関連について検討した。社会参加とは,会社や学校に通うなど,何らかの社会活動に参加していることをさす。

III. 結　果

1. 全対象者の DUP

全対象者の DUP を調べたところ,その平均値は17.6±26.9カ月であった。

施設間で比較すると,Aでは13.1カ月,Bでは26.1カ月で,施設間において有意差が認められた。また,中央値は5カ月で,Aでは3カ月,Bでは10.5カ月であった。

2. 15歳から54歳の DUP

対象を15歳から54歳とした場合の DUP の平均

は，11.1±18.7カ月であった。この数値は，Beiserら[1]やLoebelら[3]による海外の先行研究の結果とほぼ一致している。施設間で比較すると，Aでは10.3カ月，Bでは12.7カ月であり，2施設間に有意差は認められなかった。また，中央値は3.5カ月で，Aでは2.5カ月，Bでは6カ月であった。

3．同居者・社会参加による差異

同居者の有無によってDUPに違いがあるかどうかを調べたが，同居者がいる場合は12.0カ月，いない場合は9.1カ月で，有意差は認めなかった。また，社会参加の有無では，社会参加している場合のDUPは8.5カ月，していない場合は13.3カ月で，社会参加をしているほうがDUPは短いことが示唆された。

4．受診経路

受診経路としては，直接来院した人が29人と，全体の70%を占めた。その他の受診経路は，大学病院と単科病院で大きく異なり，大学病院は，企業の診療所が2人，他科からの紹介が3人であったのに対して，単科病院では措置が2人，保健所が3人であった。大学病院にはクリニックからの紹介が，単科病院には他の総合病院からの紹介が各々1件ずつあった。

また，薬物依存，アルコール依存を含めた精神疾患の併発は見られなかった。

IV．考　察

海外の調査に倣って対象を15歳から54歳としたDUPは11.1カ月であり，これは海外の先行研究と類似した結果であった。平均値が非常に大きく，かつ標準偏差値も大きいことは，平均から大きく外れた値があることをしめしている。今回対象者のうちで最長者は施設Bにおいて33歳女性の87カ月であった。対象者の受診時の平均年齢はLoebelら[3]の研究において24.7歳だったのをはじめとして，いずれも20代であったのに対して，今回の調査では30.0歳であった。これらの結果からは，日本において精神科外来を受診した初発分裂病患者の発症年齢が，欧米に比べて遅いことが示唆される。この理由としては，欧米の初発精神病者にはかなりの割合で薬物依存が見られるのに対し，今回の調査では1例も見られなかったこと，日本では10代に発症した者は小児科など他科を先に受診し薬物療法を受けている可能性が考えられる。

受診経路については，開業医の紹介で受診した例が1例もなかったことが特徴として挙げられる。また，A，B間には受診経路に明らかな違いがあり，施設の特徴によって，そこへ至る経路にも違いが出てくることが示唆された。

文　献

1) Beiser, M., Erickson, D., Fleming. J. A., et al. : Establishing the onset of psychotic illness. Am. J. Psychiatry, 150 ; 1349-1354, 1993.
2) Birchwood, M., McGorry, P., Jackson, H. : Early intervention in schizophrenia. Br. J. Psychiatry, 170 ; 2-5, 1997.
3) Loebel, A. D., Lieberman, J. A., Alvir, J. M. J. et al. : Duration of psychosis and outcome in first-episode schizophrenia. Am. J. Psychiatry, 149 ; 1183-1188, 1992.
4) McGorry, P. D., Jackson, H. J. : The Recognition and management of early psychosis. A preventive Approach. Combridge University Press, 1999.（鹿島晴雄監修，水野雅文，村上雅昭，藤井康男監訳：精神疾患の早期発見・早期治療．金剛出版，東京，2001.）
5) Sartorius, N., Jablensky, A., Korten, A. et al. : Early manifestations and first-contact of schizophrenia in different cultures. Psychological Medicine, 16 ; 909-928, 1986.

---

*慶應義塾大学医学部精神神経科
Mizuno Masafumi, Yamazawa Ryuko, Miura Yuta, Watanabe Koichiro, Yamashita Chiyo, Murakami Masaaki, Kashima Haruo : Department of Neuropsychiatry, Keio University school of Medicine.

沖縄県における精神分裂病の未治療期間 (DUP)に関する予備的調査

A preliminary survey of the Duration of Untreated Psychosis(DUP)in Okinawa

村上　忠* 　福治　康秀* 　宮里　洋* 　平松　謙一* 　小椋　力*

I. はじめに

近年，精神病性障害の予防の可能性，早期発見・早期治療の重要性が議論される中で，陽性症状が出現してから適切な治療が開始されるまでの期間(Duration of Untreated Psychosis；DUP)が注目されるようになってきている。主に精神分裂病においてDUPが数週間から数年と様々であり，DUPと予後の間に相関が認められることなどが，すでに多くの先行研究により示唆されている。一方で我が国におけるDUPの調査報告は未だ少なく，沖縄県においてもDUPの実態把握は十分になされていないのが現状である。そこで今回我々は予備的調査として，沖縄県におけるDUPの予備的調査を行った。

II. 対象

2000年10月1日～2001年3月31日の6カ月間に琉球大学医学部附属病院精神科神経科を初めて受診し，DSM-IVにより精神分裂病と診断された全症例33名(男性17名，女性16名)を対象とした。対象の平均年齢は31.7±8.4歳であり，病型分類の内訳は妄想型5例，解体型3例，鑑別不能型17例，残遺型2例で，緊張型は1例もなかった。病型分類が保留とされているものが6例あった。

III. 方法

診療録調査により，陽性症状が初めて出現した時期と，精神科医療機関を初めて受診した日を特定し，DUPを算出した。その上で，DUPに影響を与えうる要因として，陽性症状発症時における同居家族の有無や就学・就労状況，精神科医療機関初診時における受診発動者(本人の同意の有無)などを想定し，DUPとの関連を検討した。なお，DUPの定義については，Figure 1に示す概念(Larsenら，2001)に従った。

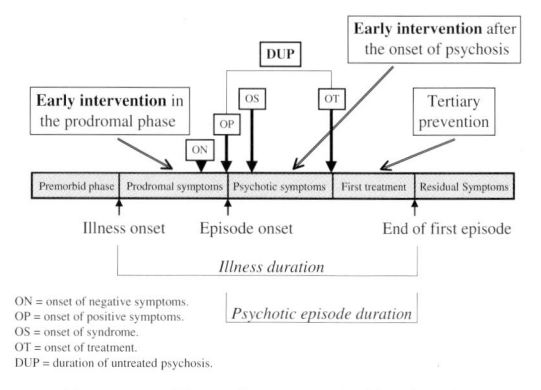

Figure 1　The early course of schizophrenia (Larsen et al., 2001)

IV. 結果

DUPは0～78カ月と広い範囲に分布しており，中央値は12カ月，平均19.6±21.5カ月であった。Figure 2に示すとおり，1カ月未満及び1年以上2年未満にそれぞれ全体の4分の1以上が集中していた。DUPに影響を与えうると想定した各要因については，いずれも有意性は認められなかった。

V. 考察

今回の我々の調査結果と，主な先行研究の結果との比較をTable 1に示す。対象数が30と少ない点は否めないが，先行研究と近似した結果が得られていると言える。表中には示していないが，DUPが3カ月付近および2年付近にピークを有する二峰性の分布を示すとする指摘(McGlashan,

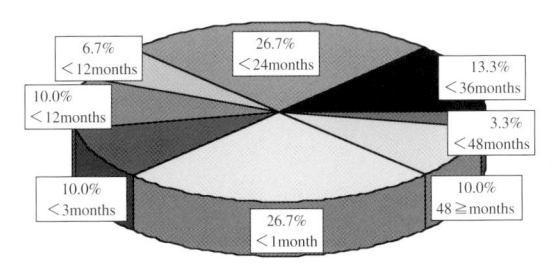

Mean DUP=19.6±21.5, Median=12, Range=0〜78
(months)

Figure 2　Distribution of the DUP

Table 1　DUP in First Episode Schizophrenia (McGlashan, 1999)

	n	Median (wks)	Mean (wks)	SD (wks)
Murakami et al(this study)	**30**	**52**	**83**	**93**
McGorry et al., 1996				
PreEPPIC(1989-1992)	200	30	227	714
EPPIC(1993-1995)	147	52	83	385
Moller and Husby, 1998	18	18	32	35
Hafner et al., 1992, 1994	165	-	109	-
Larsen et al., 1996	43	26	114	173
Moscarelli et al., 1994	20	-	76	92
Loebel et al., 1992	70	39	52	82
Haas and Sweeney, 1992	71	-	99	-
Birchwood et al., 1992	71	-	30	-
Beiser et al., 1993	72	8	56	148

1999)とも類似した傾向が認められている。

　一方，DUPに影響を与える要因については有意な結果が得られなかったが，発症時に同居家族のいなかった場合（平均5.5±9.4カ月）で，同居家族がいた場合（平均24.0±22.9カ月）と比較してDUPが短い傾向が見られており，家族の精神障害に対する構えなども視野に入れていく必要性が感じられた。今後はIRAOS（Interview for the Retrospective Assessment of the Onset and Early Course of Schizophrenia, Hafner et al., 1993）などを用いてDUP算出の正確性を向上させるとともに対象数を増やし，さらにDUPと予後との関連などについても調査を続けていきたい。

参考文献

1) American Psychiatric Association : Diagnostic and Statistical Mannual of Mental Disorders. 4th ed., American Psychiatric Association, Washington, D.C., 1994.
2) Hafner, H., Maurer, K., Loffler, W., Riecher-Rossler, A. : The influence of age and sex on the onset and early course of schizophrenia. Br. J. Psychiatry, 162 ; 80-86, 1993.
3) Larsen, T. K., Friis, S., Haahr, U., Joa, I., Johannessen, J. O., Melle, I., Opjordsmoen, S., Simonsen, E., Vaglum, P. : Early detection and intervention in first-episode schizophrenia : a critical review. Acta Psychiatr. Scand., 103 ; 323-334, 2001.
4) McGlashan, T. H. : Duration of Untreated Psychosis in First-Episode Schizophrenia : Marker or Determinant of Course? Biol. Psychiatry, 46 (7) ; 899-907, 1999.
5) McGorry, P. D., Jackson, H. J. : The Recognition and Management of Early Psychosis : A Preventative Approach. Cambridge Press, Cambridge, 1999.

---

*琉球大学医学部精神神経科学講座
Tadashi Murakami, Yasuhide Fukuji, Hiroshi Miyazato, Ken-ichi Hiramatsu, Chikara Ogura : Department of Neuropsychiatry, School of Medicine, University of the Ryukyus.

分裂病の早期発見・早期治療
―ハイリスク児追跡研究の経験より―

Early detection and early intervention of schizophrenia
——based on our experiences in schizophrenic high-risk follow-up study

原田　誠一[*]　　岡崎　祐士[*]

I．はじめに

　筆者らは，岡崎が中心となり精神分裂病患者の子弟，いわゆる分裂病ハイリスク児の追跡研究を行っている[3,5]。この研究結果の概要は本学会のシンポジウム（1A-10）で発表したので，本論ではハイリスク児2例での早期発見・早期治療の経験を述べる。

II．症例提示

症例1：1976年生まれ　女性
既往歴：アトピー性皮膚炎があり治療中。
家族歴：母親が分裂病で通院・服薬継続中。
生活歴：2人兄妹の第2子長女として出生。幼少時から家の中での一人遊びを好み，友人は少なかった。学業成績は中位で，高校卒業後短大に入学した。
病前性格：内気で控えめ。大人しく無口。友人は少ない。神経質で心配性。
MMPI検査所見（顕在発症2年前に施行）：基礎尺度のF値が高値。追加尺度のR尺度（抑圧尺度）とOH尺度（敵意の過剰統制尺度）が低値。この結果から，表面的には「内気で控えめ」であるが，実際には情動面の不安定さが強くコントロールが困難になりがちであると推測された。
現病歴：X年春の短大の入学式で「おならをしてしまい，まわりの人に聞かれた」という体験があり，その後「自分のニオイで，じろじろ見られてつらい」と家族に訴えるようになった。この時点で母親が筆者の1人に電話で相談したため，精神科受診をすすめたが，本人が拒否して受診に至らなかった。

X年10月から，登校せずに転校のための受験勉強を開始し，X+1年1月に幻覚妄想体験が出現した。
治療歴：幻覚妄想体験が出現して約1週間後に母親が異常に気付き，その翌日筆者の外来を受診した。薬物療法を開始し（bromperidol 3 mg/日），筆者らが考案した「幻覚妄想体験に対する認知療法」[1]を施行した。患者はきちんと服薬し，認知療法の理解も良好であった。
　初診後約1カ月で寛解状態に入り，デイケアに通所後，X+2年4月に復学した。現在，短大を卒業して就労している。
本症例へのコメント：本症例は自己臭妄想，忌避妄想が出現した時点で受診できず1次予防は実現できなかったが，2次予防は実現でき現在までの経過も良好である。診断は，精神分裂病を考えている。顕在発症2年前に，すでにMMPIで異常所見が認められた点[2]は，興味深い所見と思われる。

症例2：1976年生まれ　女性
既往歴：特記すべきことなし。
家族歴：父親が分裂病で不完全寛解状態。母親もうつ病に罹患し，通院・服薬継続中。
生活歴：2人姉妹の第1子，長女として出生。学業成績は上位で友人も多く，小学校～高校を通じて学校への適応は良好であった。
病前性格：社交的で友人が多い。活動的で凝り性。几帳面，心配性で気分転換は苦手。
現病歴：X年9月（高校3年），大学入試の重圧に加えて父親が再発し，母親の精神状態も不安定になった。X年10月，「両親の声がぼんやり聞こ

表 ハイリスク児研究から見た「分裂病の早期発見と早期治療」

(1)現状では，1次予防の実現には困難が伴う。
　　特に，遺伝負因に加えてリスク因子（候補）が加わった個体・状況の危険性
　　　病前の顕著な陰性行動特徴
　　　MMPIでの異常所見
　　　強い家庭内葛藤
　　　ストレス因となるライフイベント，など
(2)「早期発見・早期治療」の有効性
(3)「早期治療」の要点
　　・寛解導入まで「薬物療法，個人精神療法，家庭療法」を統合して，集中的に実施。
　　・病前の陰性行動特徴が顕著な場合，寛解導入後に，集団療法によるリハビリテーションの併用を考える。
　　・寛解導入後も長期間経過を追い，適宜相談にのる。
　　　(特に，根気よく家族の相談にのる必要性と重要性)

えてくる」「昔の厭な記憶がどんどん出てきて止まらない」という幻聴，自生記憶想起が出現。母親がそれを知り，翌日に筆者の外来を受診した。

治療歴：初診時から薬物療法(fluphenazine 1 mg／日)を開始し，幻覚妄想体験への認知療法も行った。患者はきちんと服薬し，認知療法の理解も良好であった。約2週間で，幻聴と自生記憶想起は消失した。

X＋1年4月に大学に入学。経過順調なため大学2年の時に投薬を中止したが，現在まで再発していない。現在，大学を卒業して就職している。

本症例へのコメント：本例は，「大学受験，父親の再発，母親の情動不安定」というストレス因が重なり一過性に精神病状態となったが，治療が奏効して経過順調である。現在までのところ，1次予防に近い早期の治療介入が成功している，とみなしてよい症例と思われる。診断は，急性一過性精神病性障害を考えている。

Ⅲ．おわりに

分裂病ハイリスク児の追跡研究の中で，早期発見・早期治療を実現できた2症例を報告した。筆者らのハイリスク児研究の結果からみた「分裂病の早期発見，早期治療」に関連する事項を表に示した。なお，今回提示した2症例のいずれにおいても認知療法が有効であった点は，初発エピソード症例の精神療法の方略[4]を考える上で参考になるところがあろう。

文　献

1) 原田誠一，吉川武彦，岡崎祐士ほか：幻聴に対する認知療法的接近法(第1報)．精神医学，39；363-370，1997．
2) 原田誠一，岡崎祐士：日常臨床における精神分裂病の早期発見と早期治療—ハイリスク児の追跡研究から．精神神経誌，101；916-922，2000．
3) 原田誠一，岡崎祐士：ハイリスク児研究からみた分裂病の病因と予防．臨床精神医学，29；367-374，2000．
4) 原田誠一：病識の乏しい初発分裂病患者で認知療法が奏効した2症例．臨床精神医学，30；1417-1421，2001．
5) 岡崎祐士：精神分裂病ハイリスク児．精神医学，39；346-362，1997．

*三重大学医学部精神神経科学教室
Seiichi Harada, Yuzi Okazaki : Department of Neuropsychiatry, Mie University School of Medicine.

児童青年期発症精神分裂病患者の発症様式の検討
Clinical characteristics of schzophrenic patients with onset in childhood and adolescence

中谷　英夫[*]　　金田　　学[*]　　柳下　杏子[*]　　下田　和紀[*]
武藤　宏平[*]　　棟居　俊夫[*]　　越野　好文[*]

Ⅰ. はじめに

近年，精神分裂病に対する早期発見・早期治療の必要性・有効性が指摘されている。早期治療のためには前駆症状・初期症状の把握が重要である。児童青年期発症の精神分裂病は予後が不良であると報告されており，また，心理的・社会的発達の途上であること，発症以降の経過が長いことを考えると，特に児童青年期では早期の治療が大切である。今回われわれは，児童青年期に精神分裂病と診断された症例の発症年齢，未治療期間，社会適応などについて調査した。

対象は1993年から1998年の5年間に金沢大学医学部附属病院神経科精神科を初診した18歳以下の患者のうち，初診時あるいは経過観察中にDSM-Ⅳの精神分裂病の診断基準を満たした40例である。

Ⅱ. 方　法

診療録から，性別・年齢・精神病症状出現時からの未治療期間（Duration of Untreated Psychosis：DUP）・前駆症状出現時からの未治療期間（Duration of Untreated Illness：DUI）・初診時診断・発症様式・前駆症状および精神病症状の種類・社会適応の各項目について調査した。また，全体を発症が12歳以前の群（学童群）とそれ以降の群（青年群）とに分け，両群間で比較を行った。

Ⅲ. 結　果

学童群は6例，青年群は34例で，性別は男子17例，女子23例，受診時の年齢（平均±SD）は16.6±2.0歳，前駆症状出現時の年齢は14.7±2.4歳（5.0～18.3歳），精神病症状出現時年齢は16.1±

表1

性別	男2例, 女4例	男15例, 女19例
年齢		
受診時	14.0±2.9歳	17.1±1.4歳
前駆症状出現時	10.4±2.7歳	15.5±1.4歳
精神病症状出現時	13.6±3.2歳	16.5±1.5歳
	学童群(n=6)	青年群(n=34)

2.1歳（11.3～19.7歳）であった。（表1）

DUPおよびDUIはいずれも両群間に有意差は認めなかったが，学童群では6例中3例が受診までに12カ月以上を要し，うち2例で5年以上を要していた。（表2）

初診時に精神分裂病と診断されていなかったのは学童群で2例，青年群で5例あった。

発症様式は，潜行性（前駆期1年以上），亜急性（前駆期1年以内），急性（ほとんど前駆期なし）の3つに分類した。学童群では亜急性または潜行性が80％以上を占めていた。（図1）

前駆症状を，行動上の問題や性格変化を示す型，無為・自閉や不安・希死念慮を示す型，これらの混合型，および偽神経症や離人感・注察感などを示す型の4タイプに分類した。学童群では全例に前駆症状がみられ，行動異常―性格変化型を示すものが多く，無為自閉―気分変動型は認められなかった。青年群では無為自閉型が目立った。（図2）

精神病症状については幻覚，妄想，思考障害，行動障害，感情の障害を検討した。学童群では思考障害を示すものの割合が低く，また全例で行動障害を認めた。（図3）

社会適応は，良好なもの，精神症状が存在しても何とか適応している半適応，適応が困難なもの，入院中のもの，自殺の転帰をたどったものの

表2

未治療期間
DUI　42.5±59.4カ月　19.1±16.5カ月
DUP　5.8± 2.7カ月　 9.3±13.0カ月

　　　　　　　　学童群（n=6）　青年群（n=34）
　　　　　　　DUP : Duration of Untreated Psychosis
　　　　　　　DUI : Duration of Untreated Illness

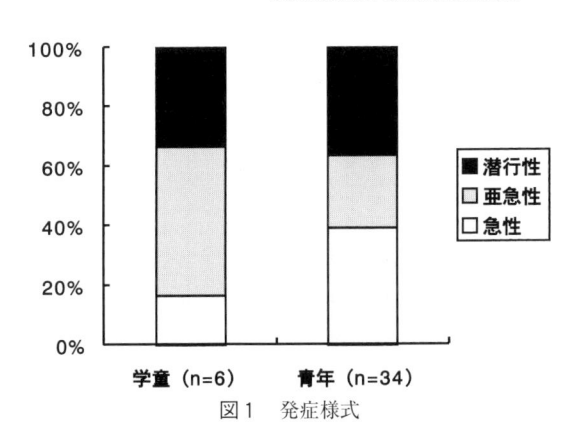

図1　発症様式

図2　前駆症状

図3　精神病症状

図4　社会適応（初診時から平均1.8±2.0年後）

5つに分類した。学童群では良好に適応している例は認められなかった。自殺した例も認められなかった。（図4）

IV．まとめ

　児童青年期に精神分裂病と診断された症例の臨床特徴を検討した。学童群と青年群との間に未治療期間，発症様式，前駆症状・精神病症状の種類，社会適応において違いが認められた。
　学童群では未治療期間の長い例がみられたが，精神分裂病では未治療期間の長短が長期経過に影響することが指摘されており，早期治療を実現するためには一般者に対し疾患について啓発活動をし，早期受診を促すさらなる努力が必要である。

＊金沢大学医学部神経精神医学教室
Hideo Nakatani, Manabu Kaneda, Kyoko Yagishita, Kazuki Shimada, Konhei Muto, Tashio Munesue, Yoshifumi Koshino : Department of Neuropsychiatry, Kanazawa University School of Medicine.

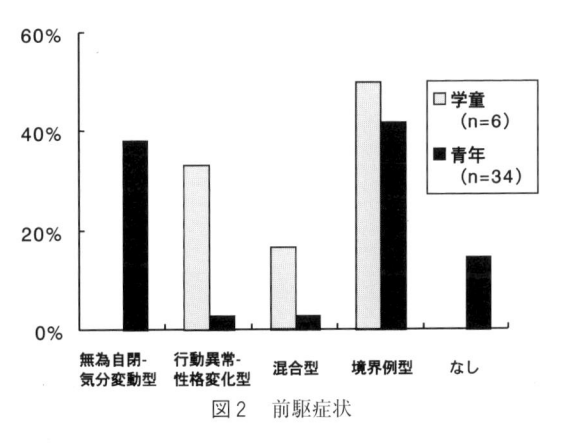

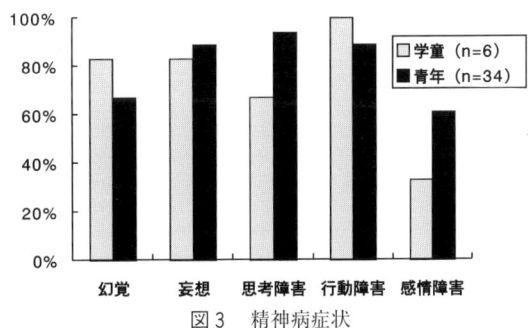

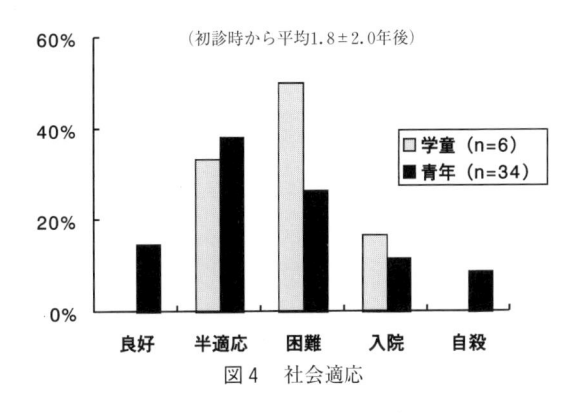

The family attitude scale の日本での妥当性の評価
The family attitude scale in measuring criticism in the relatives of patients with schizophrenia in Japan

藤田　博一* 　下寺　信次* 　三野　善央** 　井上　新平*

I. 背　景

家族の感情表出（Expressed Emotion；EE）は，批判的言辞（Critical Comment；CC），敵意（Hostility；H），情緒的巻き込まれ過ぎ（Emotional Overinvolvement；EOI），温かみ，肯定的言辞から構成され，そのうち CC，H，EOI が再発を促進する因子として知られている。そして治療的には，家族への心理教育などにより，EE の程度を低下させることで分裂病の再発を予防する試みが開始されている。ところが EE の測定は，Camberwell Family Interview（CFI）という労力を要する方法が用いらなければならない。今回我々は，EE を質問紙形式で評価する Family Attitude Scale（FAS；Kavanagh ら）を日本語訳し，日本での CFI への妥当性を検討した。

II. 方　法

対象者は，入院治療を受け，退院時に ICD-10 により精神分裂病または分裂感情障害と診断された41名の患者とその家族57人である。FAS は「ここにいて欲しくない」や「本当にお荷物だ」等，30項目の質問紙票で，「毎日ある」から「ない」までの5段階で回答し，患者に最も否定的な回答をすると4点となり，以下0点までで評価する。原版は英語のため日本語に訳し，バックトランスレーションを行って妥当性を確認した。EE の評価は CFI を基に行い，従来通り CC が6個以上又は H スケールが1点以上の場合 HCC とし，それ以外の場合 LCC とした。また，CFI の簡略版として既に使用されている Five Minute Speech Sample（FMSS）を同時に実施し，EE 評価の精度を FAS と比較した。また，EE と家族の健康度の関連が指摘されているが，FAS がどの程度家族の健康度を反映しているかを，GHQ（General Health Questionnaire）を用いて調査した。

III. 結　果

41家族のうち High-EE と判定された家族は12家族であった。12家族のうち，4家族が HCC，7家族が High-EOI，1家族が HCC + High-EOI だった。また，High-EE と Low-EE 家族の属性（性別，年齢，罹病期間，入院回数，BPRS，SANS，診断分類）に有意な差はなかった。

CFI による全般評価での High-EE 群と Low-EE 群，及び HCC と LCC の2群で，FAS の平均得点を比較した。どちらの比較も有意な差はみられたが，HCC と LCC の比較の方がより鋭敏な有意差がみられた。（表1）

CFI での CC 分類に対する FAS の妥当性を検討するため，FAS のカットオフ値を決定した。ROC 曲線を描くと FAS の得点が60点の時に最も感度が高く，偽陽性率（1−特異度）が最も低い組み合わせとなった（図）。FAS が60点以上を High-FAS，60点未満を Low-FAS と定義すると，感度は100％で特異度は88.5％であった（表2）。また，CFI での CC 分類に対する FMSS との妥当性は，感度は40.0％で特異度は90.4％であった。

GHQ の得点は，High-FAS 群の方が高く，下

表1　FAS 得点の結果

	FAS得点 平均 ± S.D.	
全家族員	39.9 ± 20.4	
HighEE (n=13)	52.8 ± 18.5	p=0.009
LowEE (n=44)	36.1 ± 19.5	
HCC (n=5)	69.6 ± 19.5	p=0.002
LCC (n=52)	37.0 ± 18.8	

表2 CFIに対するFASの妥当性

		overall(CFI)	
		High	Low
FAS	High	5	6
	Low	8	38

感度 5 / 13 = 38.5%
特異度 38 / 44 = 86.4%
PPV 5 / 11 = 45.5%
NPV 38 / 46 = 82.6%

		CFI	
		HCC	LCC
FAS	High	5	6
	Low	0	46

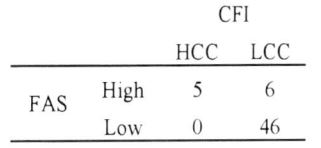

感度 5 / 5 = 100%
特異度 46 / 52 = 88.5%
PPV 5 / 11 = 45.5%
NPV 46 / 46 = 100%

位項目の身体症状では有意にHigh-FAS群の方が高かった。

IV. 考　察

今回の報告は，FASのカットオフ値をROC曲線を用いて求め，感度，特異度を用いてCFIへの妥当性を検討した初めての研究である。FASはCFIでのCC分類に，高い妥当性を示し，FMSSの妥当性と比較すると優れていた。批判的態度の強い家族のEE判定を簡略に行えることが示された。これは，EE判定を実際の臨床場面に応用することに道を開くものである。今後の課題として，前向き調査を行い，FASでのEEと再発の関係を調べる必要がある。

High FAS群では，GHQの得点が高く，身体症状の項目では有意差がみられた。FAS得点が高い家族には，特にメンタルヘルスに注意を払う必要があるだろう。

FASは，感情的巻き込まれ過ぎを判定できないという限界点があるが，家族の批判的態度を簡便に評価する方法として，有効であることが確かめられた。

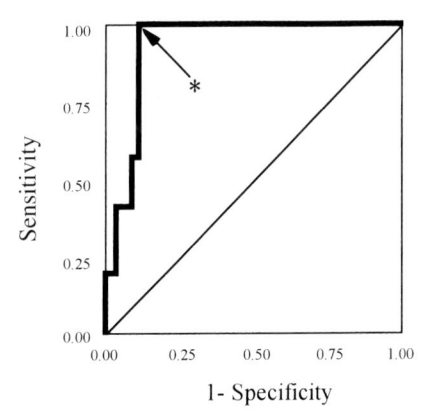

＊FAS60点を示す

FAS得点	感度	1-特異度
48	1	0.288
50	1	0.231
52	1	0.212
55	1	0.173
57	1	0.154
60(＊)	1	0.115
63	0.6	0.115
65	0.6	0.096
67	0.4	0.077

図　ROC曲線を用いたFASのカットオフ値の検討

＊高知医科大学神経精神医学教室
　Hirokazu Fujita, Sihnji Shimodera, Shimpei Inoue : Department of Neuropsychiatry, Kochi Medical School.
＊＊岡山大学医学部衛生学教室
　Yoshio Mino : Department of Mental Health, College of Social Welfare Osaka Prefecture University.

精神病性の初発状況と早期介入
The first psychotic onset and early intervention

仲本　晴男[*]

I. はじめに

　精神病性疾患は，いまだ病因解明の見通しは困難な状況にあり，したがって現時点では第1次予防は容易ではない。そこで臨床医にとって必要なことは，発病状況に早期介入し，精神病性の発動過程を抑制することにあると考える。

　事例を呈示するが，事例1は精神病性の発動に至っていないケース，事例2および事例3は幻覚妄想を呈したが早期に鎮静し維持療法へ導入したケース，事例4は精神病性の発動は起こったが幻覚妄想への拡大を抑制したケースであり，それぞれ発病状況の異なった青年期から成人期にかけて4事例である。

II. 経過と治療，考察

　発病状況と期間を(表1)に，発症様式と治療を(表2)に示した。

　事例1は地元のA小学校を優秀な成績で卒業して有名進学校のB中学へ入学した。ところが父親が病気で入院したため地元のA中学へ転校せざるを得なくなり，そこで上級生のいじめにあい，その対応をめぐって先生への不信感をつのらせた。そして受験2カ月前になって落ち着かなくなり，虫垂炎の手術で4日間入院したことが「受験勉強に遅れてしまった」と急激な焦りとなり，妄想観念の引き金となった。誘因から発症まで2〜3日，発症から当院受診まで2週間と早く，薬物療法も抗不安薬のみclotiazepam 10mg/日と少量で，6回の通院で回復した。しかし高校へ進学した1年後の2月17日に再発し，当院を再受診した。診断としてはICD-10でSchizotypal Disorder，いわゆる思春期妄想症レベルの病態と考えられた。このケースの支援上で最も大切なことは精神分裂病への発展を防止することにある。治療上は抗精神病薬をいつの時点で開始するか，環境要因としては県内唯一の公立進学校である現在の学校環境に耐えられるのかの評価と助言が課題である。

　事例2及び事例3の発症様式は妄想や幻覚，精神運動興奮など比較的明確な精神分裂病性のものであった。事例4では精神分裂病圏の症状は入院中に1週間ほど「何かざわざわする音が耳元で聞こえる」という要素性幻聴のみであり，潜在する精神運動興奮に由来すると思われる当惑した不安げな表情が特徴的で，精神分裂病の診断基準は満たさなかった。誘因から当院治療までの期間は，事例2はいわゆる破瓜型にみられる慢性経過，事例3と事例4は急性発症から2週間以内で治療を開始しており早期介入に導入できたが，これは県内で精神科救急システムが確立し，当院がその中核医療施設として機能していることが大きいと思われた。

　治療では入院した3事例のいずれも閉鎖的治療環境を必要とした。事例3と事例4は入院後1週間で急速に症状が消失したため，一過性の精神病性エピソードも考えられ退院させたが，2〜3週間で再燃し，2事例とも開放病棟に再入院し，約2カ月の入院治療の後，安定した通院治療に至った。入院中の薬物療法は事例2と事例3はhaloperidol 8〜12mg/日と中等量であり，事例4は初回入院はchlorprmazine 100mg/日と少量であった。第2回入院の当初はhaloperidolを21mg/日まで漸増して使用したがAkathisiaの副作用のため中止し，最初に使用したchlorprmazineを800mg/日まで漸増し，内的不穏は鎮静した。

　介入の要点として，事例2は家庭内暴力が以前からあり母親への暴力行為をいかに止めるかが肝要であった。面会時に母親を殴る場面もあり，そ

表1　発病状況と期間

	主な誘因	家族員の察知	誘因から発症までの期間	発症から精神科治療までの期間
事例1 (16歳)	虫垂炎手術のため4日入院 高校受験1カ月前	姉は2カ月前から落ち着かない様子に気づいていた	2～3日	2週間
事例2 (17歳)	妄想の誘因は不明 小学5年から不登校 中学1年から家庭内暴力	受診6カ月前からプレハブで1人で生活するようになった	5年	3カ月
事例3 (21歳)	新しい職種(ネズミ講)への傾倒 職場の人間関係の悪化 夜のライブの過労	初発症状の不眠の翌日から気づいていた	1週間	12日
事例4 (36歳)	他県での季節労務から帰郷	帰沖後は何となく表情が暗いと思ったが,行動に問題はなかった	16日	9日

表2　発症様式と治療

	発症様式	急性症状	治療経過	薬物療法(抗精神病薬のみ最高与薬量)
事例1 (16歳)	抑うつ気分が妄想観念に発展	集中力・持続力低下 抑うつ気分 関係念慮,被害念慮	①X年2/21～3/21(計6回通院) ②X+1年2/17～2/27(計3回通院)	clotiazepam 10mg/日 同上
事例2 (17歳)	閉居後3カ月して被毒妄想が顕在化	被毒妄想,被害妄想 醜形妄想,関係妄想 注察妄想 幻覚なし	①X年3/2～4/24(53日)任意入院・閉鎖 ②それ以後通院治療を継続	haloperidol 12mg/日 haloperidol 4mg/日
事例3 (21歳)	不眠から1週間で幻覚妄想に発展	精神運動興奮,幻聴 誇大妄想,自生思考	①X年2/11～2/21(10日)任意入院・閉鎖 ②X年3/12～5/15(64日)任意入院・開放 ③それ以後通院治療を継続	haloperidol 8mg/日 同上 haloperidol 6mg/日
事例4 (36歳)	突発的な激しい自殺企図が出現	幻覚妄想なし 入院中に一過性の要素性幻聴のみ出現	①X年2/25～3/5(8日)任意入院・閉鎖 ②X年3/20～5/25(61日)任意入院・開放 ③それ以後通院治療を継続	chlorpromazine 100mg/日 haloperidol 21mg/日は中止 chlorpromazine 800mg/日 chlorpromazine 800mg/日

のためケースの頻発する退院要求については,主治医がそれを制止する矢面に立ち,母親はケースの気持ちを代弁する側,すなわちケースと一緒に退院を要求する役を演じさせ,暴力は消失した。事例3はこれまでの過度の労働と葛藤から解放してあげる意味でも,退院後もまだ就労を含めた活動は勧めていない。事例4はchlorprmazine 800mg/日という大量の抗精神病薬で鎮静し,安定した状態へ回復したが,再発予防では精神分裂病を念頭において,今後幻覚妄想に発展させない関与が大切であると考えられ,通院治療ではデイケア療法を併用している。

Ⅲ．まとめと課題

呈示した4事例はいずれも当院を緊急に受診したケースである。事例1のように軽症例で外来治療のみで早期介入が可能な例もあるが,多くの場合は入院治療,とくに事例2,3,4のように閉鎖的な治療環境を要する場合が多いと思われる。したがって早期介入を受け入れる病院側は,初発ケースの病態や発病状況,環境要因を迅速かつ的確に評価し,治療へ導入できる高いレベルの医療チームの確立が必要である。

地域との連携では,家庭訪問による早期介入チームを県総合精神保健福祉センターなどの相談機関で実施できれば,発症から精神科治療までの早期発見・早期治療への導入を短縮させるための第2次予防,さらに同チームの質を向上させ誘因から発症までの第1次予防も可能になると考えられる。以上4事例に対する病院における早期介入を呈示し,今後の地域を含めた予防の可能性についても言及した。

---

*沖縄県立精和病院
Nakamoto Haruo : Okinawa prefectural Seiwa Hospital.

単回エピソード分裂病

Single episode schizophrenia

小林　聡幸* 　　加藤　敏* 　　西嶋　康一*

Recently, we conducted a survey on the course and outcome of 62 cases (29 females and 33 males, average age at first admission, 25.2) with schizophrenia (traditionally diagnosed at admission and retrospectively using DSM-IV criteria) that underwent their initial hospitalizations in the Department of Psychiatry, Jichi Medical School Hospital (JMSH) and were consecutively discharged between June 1983 and May 1988. Within this subject group, the discontinuation of treatment was confirmed in 8 cases. Notably, 6 of these cases have experienced a single episode of schizophrenia, and appeared to make up a characteristic group that could be called "single episode schizophrenia." The characteristics of this group were a favorable outcome, a short period between hospital discharge and the discontinuation of treatment (maximum of 14 months), and a relative young age at the time of first admission (20.3 years). Little attention has been focused on such cases, but "single episode schizophrenia" is worth investigating since they may reveal useful information regarding treatments for first episodes of schizophrenia and the psychopathology of early psychoses.

Case 1 : An 18-year-old girl with delusions of being pursued and of guilt developed a substupor and was hospitalized at the JMSH. Nine serial treatments of electroconvulsive therapy relieved her from her symptoms. She was discharged after 7 months. She discontinued treatment 14 months after leaving hospital. At the time of our survey, she was 34 years old, single and employed.

Case 2 : A 17-year-old high-school girl heard a bad rumor about her future employer and developed auditory hallucinations and confusion. Her symptoms disappeared after 3 months of hospitalization, leaving avolition. Four months after her discharge, she discontinued treatment. At the time of the survey, she was a 31-year-old mother with an elementary school child.

Case 3 : A 19-year-old man who had graduated from high-school and worked for one year began to suffer from delusions of being pursued and started to wander. After 4 months of hospitalization, he continued attending the hospital for 13 months before discontinuing treatment. He returned to work soon after leaving the hospital. He married at the age of 32.

Case 4 : A 24-year-old man who had experienced a short period of auditory hallucinations one year earlier began to experience auditory hallucinations again. The hallucinations only occurred when the man was inside his room. An attempted violence in response to the hallucinations required 2 months of hospitalization. The patient was then seen as an outpatient for 11 months before discontinuing treatment. At the time of the survey, he was 38-year-old father.

Case 5 : A 14-year-old girl developed a substupor and was admitted to the JMSH. She was hospitalized for 2 months and discontinued her treatment 9 months after her discharge. At the time of the survey, she was a 26-year-old married woman with a baby.

Case 6 : A 30-year-old woman began to experience auditory hallucinations, a delusion of reference, and a delusion of being poisoning. She developed a stupor and was hospitalized. Both her brother and her sister had schizophrenia. One month of hospitalization was followed by 6 months as an outpatient. At the time of the survey, she was 42 years old and single. She was a house keeper, living with her parents and her schizophrenic siblings.

Schizophrenia is a heterogeneous syndrome as is "single episode schizophrenia." In Cases 1, 3, and 6, transverse clinical conditions were not distinguished from typical schizophrenia. Case 2 may possibly be diagnosed as atypical psychosis or a schizoaffective disorder. Case 4 differed from typical schizophrenia in that the characteristics of the auditory hallucination were situation-dependent. The clinical condition in Case 5 was characterized by the absence of florid schizophrenic symptoms. "Single episode schizophrenia" is considered to be an example of acute-phasic-remitting schizophrenia (Kato, 1999) or abortion of schizophrenia.

＊自治医科大学精神医学教室
Toshiyuki Kobayashi, M. D., Ph. D., Satoshi Kato, M. D., Ph. D., Koich Nisijima, M. D., Ph. D. : Department of Psychiatry, Jichi Medical School.

複雑系における精神医学
―カオス理論からみた思考障害の発生メカニズム―

Psychiatry in complex systems—The mechanism for thought disorder from the chaos theory

佐藤　武*

I. はじめに

　脳機能は何らかの機構で制御されている。しかし，ある場面や出来事の出現によって，「ずれ」が生じると，全く異なる構造が出現する。例えば，数学の場合，$X_{n+1} = a X_n(1-X_n)$のaをほんの少し変えるだけで解は無数となり，全く複雑な構造となる。このようにパラメータのわずかなずれがシステムの構造を大きく変えてしまう現象は「構造不安定性」と呼ばれている。すなわち，初期状態の少しのずれが，指数的に拡大する結果へと至ることを意味する。このわずかの時間の後に初期状態に関する情報が全く得られなくなる。言い換えれば，初期状態を決定するために必要な情報量は大きいといえる。

　カオス理論における初期状態を臨床精神医学に置きかえると，患者に思考障害をもたらす場ということになろう。すなわち，患者を包み込む環境の変化とでも言えようか。この微妙な変化から生じる何らかの身体および精神的変調（初期状態）をきたす場から離れることが可能であれば，全く混沌とした思考障害への発展を予防できるのではないかと思われるが，この初期状態に適応できずに不眠などの身体症状を合併すると，比較的短い期間にとてつもない思考障害へ発展する症例を経験したので，精神障害の予防医学的観点から発病メカニズムを考察する。

II. 症　例

症例1：15歳・女性・中3（図1）
　両親は離婚し，母親と祖母と妹の3人暮しの複雑な環境に育った。中学3年頃より，不眠，自分が教室にいても浮いたように思える，聞こえてく

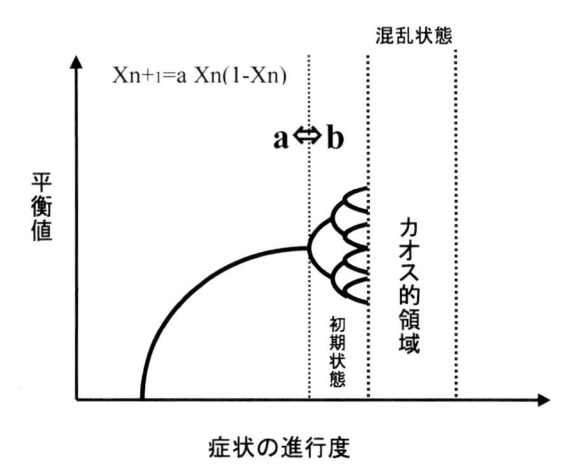

図1　症例1における症状発展過程

る現象が出現し，平成8年12月に総合外来を受診した。教室に入ることが出来ない，成績の低下などの問題が明らかになり，担任の教師より，教室に無理に入るように指示した方がよいのか，しばらく集団から離れて，保健室での対応がよいのか，相談を受けた。抗精神病薬の投与（sulpiride 200mg/日）の投与ならびに当分の間教室に入らず，保健室での対応を指示した。その結果，幻聴などの異常体験は速やかに消失し，外来治療による支持的な精神療法で対処可能であった。

症例2：37歳・男性・教師（図2）
　平成6年4月に職場の転勤が決定した。同年12月頃より，転勤した始めの頃より，気にかかっていた同僚の人間関係が複雑化し，夜何か聞こえる現象（幻聴）が出現し始めた。さらに，担任を持っているために，平成7年2月に修学旅行の引率を担当した。この頃より，「自分が陥れられる」「部屋に盗聴器が仕組まれている」の異常体験が出現

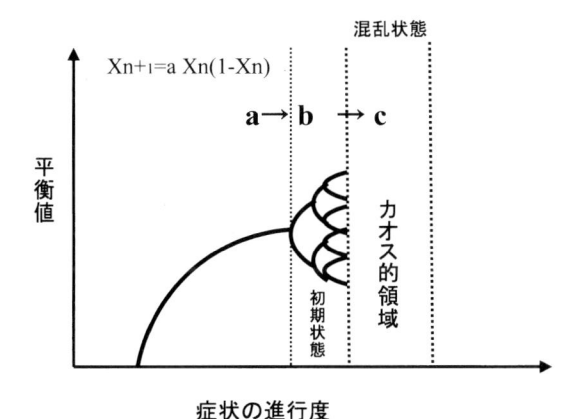

図2　症例2・3における症状発展過程

し，自宅にひきこもりがちの生活となった。総合外来を受診し，抗精神病薬(sulpiride 300mg/日，haloperidol 2.25mg/日)の投与を開始した。しかし，中学3年の担任という役割を辞することは不可能と指示され，最終的には出勤できない状態となり，同時に聞こえる現象(幻聴)がさらに増悪したため，入院治療に至った。

症例3：31歳・女性・主婦(図2)

平成11年6月20日まで分裂病の診断にて，定期的に通院していた。同年4月18日に結婚となり，平成12年1月に出産と子育てのストレスが重なった。平成12年4月に服薬を中断しはじめ，不眠が再燃した。子育ての状況に家族はうまく対応できず，次第にまとまらない行動がみられるようになった。同年5月には昏迷状態となり，食事もできない状態となったため，緊急入院となった。

III. 考　察

精神病の発病初期である初期状態では，主として幻覚妄想状態として症状が表出されるが，この時期に適切な処置を施さないと，カオス的領域へと発展する。カオス的領域に入り込むと，一般には昏迷状態，自殺企図，暴力，引きこもりなどの深刻な事態に発展する。症例1では，環境から早い時期に開放されるという処置をとったため，入院という事態を予防することができたが，症例2と3では，いずれも環境から離れることができず，結局緊急入院という事態に発展した。

初期状態からカオス的領域への進行を高める危険因子として，これまでの著者の経験では，構造不安定性(精神構造の高いフラクタル次元，認知機能の構造的複雑性)，対人関係が複雑な環境(精神機能の次元を高める環境)，精神機能の次元を低下させる薬物(向精神薬)の中断などがあげられる。すなわち，本来の構造的な精神的脆弱性に，回避できない環境要因が重なり，全体として，複雑性の次元が高まり，発病に至るという仮説が考えられるだろう。

そこで，カオス的領域から脱出し，初期状態に戻るにはどのように対処すればよいのか。まず，現在の環境から早期に逃げ出すこと，情報および感覚刺激の遮断，服薬の重要性についての再認識，患者にかかわる人々の理解をあげることができる。思考障害のレベルが発展しないためには，患者の置かれている環境からなるべく早い時期に回避してあげることが治療上，重要であると思われる。

IV. おわりに

症例を通じて，思考障害の発生メカニズムをカオス理論から考察した。思考過程が制御システムの機能不全状態に陥ったカオス状態から脱するには，初期状態のレベルで患者を包み込む環境から速やかに回避できるように計らうことが，精神障害の予防につながるものと思われる。

---

*佐賀大学保健管理センター
　Takeshi Sato : Health Care Center, Saga University.

精神分裂病患者の子供に対する治療的関わりについて
Therapeutic approaches to children of schizophrenic patients

皆川　恵子*　　横山富士男*　　山内　俊雄*

I. はじめに

埼玉医科大学神経精神科の児童・思春期外来に受診し，思春期危機や神経症圏の不登校と診断された子どもの中で，親が精神分裂病患者である「分裂病ハイリスク児」の3名について検討し，精神分裂病症状の顕在化に関与すると考えられた因子について考察した。なお，この3名のうち2名はその後，精神分裂病症状が顕在化したが，残りの1名は現在も分裂病症状はなく経過している。

II. 症例の概要

[症例1] 初診時11歳　男子

3歳年上の兄と2人兄弟。既往歴に特記すべき事項はない。家族歴では父親がうつ病，母親が精神分裂病。本児の出生まで母親は未治療で，出産直後に病状が悪化し，入院。このため本児は出生直後より乳児院で生育。生後6カ月目からは父方祖父母の家で生育し，3歳時から父親と兄と同居。母親と生活した経験はない。母親の治療に関しても母の実家と本児の父とで意見の相違も有り，家族間に葛藤が認められた。また10歳時に母親が退院し，突然本児の学校を訪ね，クラスに現れたことで強いショックを受けた経験があった。当科には本児が大好きだった祖父が急逝した11歳時に「祖父の死後口をきかなくなり，学校にも行かない」ことを主訴に受診。この緘黙・不登校状態は通院により1カ月ほどで改善したが，初診から11カ月後に被害・関係妄想や幻聴が出現し，精神運動興奮状態となり，分裂病症状が顕在化した。

[症例2] 初診時17歳　女子

兄弟はなく一人っ子。既往歴に特記すべき事項はない。家族歴では両親ともに精神分裂病。両親はともに精神分裂病の発病後に結婚し，本児を出産したものの養育することはできず，生後すぐに本児は乳児院へ預けられた。両親はその後も現在まで入院を継続している。本児は3歳時から児童養護施設へ入所。施設内では周囲の子にも好かれ，特に問題もおこさず，おとなしい子であった。親戚などとの交流もなく，高校1年の時に里親に預けられたが馴染めず，3カ月で施設へ戻り，以降は高校卒業まで施設で生活。高校生になるまで両親には会ったこともなかった。当科には17歳時に「施設の職員に幼児のようにまとわりつき，学校に行かなくなった」という主訴で受診。高校2年に進級した後から友人関係がうまくいかなくなり，そのことを悩むうちに幼児のように施設職員にまとわりつき，担当職員が不在だと過剰に不安がり，登校もできなくなるという退行状態であったが，通院後1カ月ほどで改善し，その後何とか高校は卒業。高校卒業後は就職して独立することになり，施設を退所。自分が希望した職場ではあったが，3カ月ほどで退職してしまい，以後定職には就けず当科への通院も中断。その2年後に精神分裂病と診断され，他院へ入院となった。

[症例3] 初診時14歳　女子

兄弟はなく一人っ子。喘息があり，現在も加療中。家族歴では母親が精神分裂病。父親は本児の出生直前に交通事故で死亡。出生時から母親の妄想の影響で，一切外に出ることは許されず，3歳までは自宅に閉じこもりきりの生活であった。3歳時に母親の病状が悪化し，殴る蹴るの暴行を受

けた。母親が入院してからは，母の実家に預けられていた。6歳からは退院してきた母親と再び同居。近所に住む母の弟の一家から援助を受けて生活していた。中学2年までは目立った問題もなく，成績も優秀であった。当科には14歳時に「微熱や頭痛が続き，夜もよく眠れない」という主訴で，小児科から紹介されて受診。その後，症状のうち不眠傾向以外は改善したものの，中3時には生活の雑音がやたらと大きな音に聞こえるという聴覚の過敏を訴えたり，リストカットによる自傷行為が目立つことがあった。高校に進学後は概ね症状は落ち着いており，成績も学年でトップを維持していたが，分裂病の母親と2人暮らしのため，母親の病状が悪化して困ったり，進級や進路問題，修学旅行などの日常生活上の変化の際に不定愁訴や自傷行為が認められたり，拒食傾向による急激な体重低下，過食傾向による肥満が目立つことがあった。高校卒業後は私大の工学部に推薦で合格して進学。現在まで通院は続けているが，明らかな分裂病症状は認められていない。

III. 検討と考察

精神分裂病症状の顕在化した2例と，認められない1例を比べると，性格傾向は3例とも無口で内向的，遠慮深いという傾向があり，いわゆる分裂気質と考えられた。また，家庭的にも両親が不在か片親家庭であった。更に，いずれの症例も支持的精神療法や日常生活への指導のほかに，薬物療法が併用されていた。しかし，症例3は知能検査で正常域上位，他の2例は正常域下位という結果であり，分裂病症状の顕在化していない症例3は他の2例よりやや知的に高いことが目に付いた。そして最も異なる点は，症例3に対する周囲のサポートの状況であった。家庭面では精神分裂病の母親と同居し，母親の症状を目の当たりにしている環境に生活しながらも，一方で母方の実家からの援助や近所に住む叔父夫婦からの親のような関わりが得られた。学校面では，中学・高校とも担任教師とクラブの顧問教師がきめ細やかで臨機応変な対応をとってくれたことに加え，高校では養護教諭が親身になって母親の気付かない女性同士の相談に乗り，世話を焼いてくれた。病院においてはこれらの人達と担当医がことある毎に連絡を取り合うことを心がけ，その結果，家庭－学校－病院で一貫した対応をとることができた。しかし，症例1・2では分裂病症状の顕在化以前の段階では学校面や家庭面での子どもへのサポートが症例3ほどには十分に行われておらず，また子どもに関わる者同士の情報交換も綿密には行えていなかった。

このように分裂病症状の認められていない症例3では，今までのハイリスク児研究から報告されている発病予防に必要とされるポイントのうち，知的に高いことによる「問題処理能力の高さ」が本人にあることや，親から得ることができない日常生活上の配慮やライフイベントに関する問題をクリアする援助が周囲の人達から得られており，本人にかかる負荷が回避・軽減されたことが分裂病の発症予防という点に関連しているがのではないかと考えられた。しかし，症例3は現在まだ分裂病の好発年齢にあるうえ，大学生のため学校教員の援助は得られにくいこと，異性問題等のこれまでにはなかった問題があがっていることなどから，さらに工夫した形での援助を今後も続けていく必要性があると考えている。また今後はハイリスク児に対し，分裂病症状が顕在化していない段階で，十分な子どもへのサポート態勢を築き，家庭－学校－病院などで一貫した対応が取れることが重要であると考える。

参考文献

1) 原田誠一，岡崎祐士：精神分裂病の予防の現状と課題．最新精神医学，3；47-53，1998．
2) 仲本晴男：精神分裂病の発病予防を目的とした介入．最新精神医学，3；39-45，1998．
3) 岡崎祐士：精神分裂病の発症予防．精神科治療学，10；361-369，1995．
4) 岡崎祐士：精神分裂病の高危険者研究の動向．懸田克躬，島薗安雄，大熊輝雄他編：精神医学大系年間版'89A，中山書店，東京，277-320，1990．

---

*埼玉医科大学神経精神科
Keiko Minagawa, Fujio Yokoyama, Toshio Yamauchi : Department of Neuropsychiatry, Saitama Medical School.

分裂病の母と難聴の父から生れ
中学生になって異常行動が出現した一女性例
―分裂病高危険児の予防的介入をめぐって―

A case of the odd behavior in a fourteen-year-old girl born from schizophrenic mother and hard of hearing father : The importance of early intervention for high risk children

田中　晋[*]　三杉　篤[*]　二木　志保[**]　平松　謙一[*]

　精神分裂病の病態は十分に解明されていないが，「脆弱性ストレスモデル」が提唱されている。分裂病に罹患しやすさを持つ者にストレスが加わって発症するとの仮説である。発症を予防するには危険因子とストレスを減弱させ，個体側と環境側の防御因子を強化することであるが，精神障害の発症予防についての有効性を定量的に確認することは困難であり，その効果の医学的評価・限界・倫理的側面についての論議もまだ一定の見解を得ていない。しかし，国内外の予防精神医学の発展とともに，精神障害に対する早期介入と予防については一定の関心と評価を受ける時期に来ている。

　これまでの研究から，環境や成長過程における体験的な要因に加え遺伝要因が分裂病の発症に関わってきているとされており，分裂病の親から産まれた高危険児に対する積極的な地域療法や家族教育が発症を予防できる可能性を大きくするといわれている。精神分裂病の高危険児への介入研究も一定の評価を受けてきているが，報告はまだ少ない。

　今回我々は，分裂病の母と難聴の父から生れ，中学生になって異常行動が出現した一女性例を経験したため，その経過を分裂病高危険児の予防的介入という観点で報告した。

　本例の母親は16歳発症の分裂病で結婚前に3回の入院，結婚後と長男出生後に一回ずつの入院があった。本例の母親は自分の病気のことを隠して結婚したため，夫に対して負い目を感じていた。そのため，夫に逆らうことはほとんどなかった。また，病識がないこともあるが，内服していることを夫に知られないようにしていたりするため，結局服薬を中断しがちで再燃を繰り返していた。調子の良いときには家事を行っているが，調子の悪いときは寝込みがちで，本例が家事を行うことも多かったようだ。子育て，長男や本例の学校への不適応の問題にうまく対処することができず，母親は情動が不安定になりがちだった。母親の結婚と2度の出産のいずれもが外来治療中断中に行われたこともあり，その後の養育のときにも医療関係者を含む地域でのサポートが行われていなかった。母親の通院している病院の方から訪問看護を行うことも提案されたが，父親とその親戚の方から反対され，導入されなかった。

　父親は高度の難聴で，ほぼ文盲。頑固で家族に対しては威圧的な態度で接しており，本例の母親の通院している病院や本例の主治医に対して会おうとせず，通院をやめるように指示することも多かった。

　本例の出生は帝王切開であった。4歳年上の長男と比較すると発育・発達はやや遅いほうで，学校の成績は中の下。内向的で友人は少なかった。小学生のときに喘息とアトピー性皮膚炎がみられ，喘息で一度入院したこともある。母親は自身の精神科治療を子供たちにも秘密にし，子供達に「家の中のことを絶対に他人に話しては駄目だ」と繰り返し，自分の主治医や子供の担任教師にも家庭内のことは一切話そうとしなかった。本例は，小学6年と中学入学時にいじめにあうが，母親は「いじめにあうのは自分が弱いからだ」と言うのみで，やがていじめは自然に無くなった。本例が中学3年生の5月から再びいじめにあい，そ

れをきっかけに不登校となり，緘黙，自傷行為，遊園地の檻によじ登る奇妙な行動がみられ入院となった。

　入院時，分裂病の診断基準を満たすには至っていなかったが，対人場面での緊張感，自発性の乏しさ，抑うつという症状に加え，分裂病の発症につながりかねない自我構造の脆弱性が認められていたため，本例を分裂病の高危険因子を負うものと位置づけ治療的介入を行った。本例の不安定な精神状態を受け入れる器として入院環境を提供し，家族との環境調整，学校関係者との密な連絡を行いつつ当科病棟からの中学校通学を継続した。中学卒業と高校受験というイベントを通過した後，退院となった。退院後約一年間経過しているがその間も関係者間の連絡と，当科外来での面接を定期的に行ってきている。本例は情緒的・対人的発達が十分に行われない養育環境で成長し，思春期になり社会的に一度破綻したが，介入を行うことにより精神状態の安定と卒業・入学試験・進級というイベントを通過することができた。本例の退院後も父親は治療に対して非協力的で本例や母親を責めるだけであり，母親も家庭内のことは話そうとしなかった。娘の病気に関して自分と同じようにならないか心配する反面，病院で治療されることに反対したり，薬を飲まないように指導したりすることもある。

　本例は分裂病高危険児であり，養育環境にも大きな問題がある事は容易に想定されたはずであるが，15歳で精神病症状が出現し入院するまで，具体的な援助がなされなかった。このようなケースの場合は，子供に対する育児環境の保証や育児支援を通した家族教育や地域ネットワークの活用をすることが顕在発症する以前から重要であったと思われた。

＊琉球大学医学部精神神経科学講座
　Shin Tanaka, Atushi Misugi, Ken-ichi Hiramatsu : Department of Neuropsychiatry University of the Ryukyus.
＊＊東京都立梅ヶ丘病院
　Shiho Futaki : Tokyo Metropolitan Umegaoka Hospital.

子どもを持つ分裂病利用者に対する
作業所を中心とした地域トータル・サポート
―利用者の再発予防と子の養育環境保障による発症予防の試み―

Total support through sheltered workshops for schizophrenic patients and their children : Support in parenting as protective measure against relapse and reduction of the children's risk for psychosis

友田奈津美[*]　小島　幸太[*]　鈴木　裕美[*]　石川英五郎[*]　平松　謙一[*,**]

　グループ・オアシスでは精神分裂病患者の再発予防には社会の中で彼らが自らの人生を再発見し実現していくことが重要であるという考えをもって約18年間に渡り地域の精神障害者を支援してきた。

　グループ・オアシスでは単に利用者の作業所での労働活動のみならず，利用者の地域生活を全体として多側面から支援することを重視してきた。それは利用者をとりまく環境や状況は様々であるためその生活課題も目標も多様であるからである。

　作業所の利用者の多くは独身者だが，今回は特に，年少の子どもを持つ母親の分裂病利用者に焦点を当てる。

　これまでグループ・オアシスでは子どもを持つ男性分裂病2名，女性分裂病5名，母と子ともに分裂病の1組の支援を行ってきた。特に年少の子どもを持つ分裂病の母親は育児が十分にできない，母親として思い描く理想像に近づけないという問題を抱え，その子どもは母の入院等で幼い時期に離別の悲しみを経験する，親が病気であることの罪悪感を持つ，十分な養育環境が得られないなどの問題を抱えている。本報告ではこのような利用者の地域生活支援について具体的な症例を挙げて検討・考察する。

　今回取り上げる事例D.Kは夫，息子3人の5人家族で，事例が作業所通所開始当時のそれぞれの年齢は事例42歳，夫53歳，長男13歳，次男12歳，三男6歳。このころには長男，次男はすでに中学生だったが，三男は小学校一年生でそれまで乳児院で育った。その後長男は住み込みの仕事のため家を出た。翌年以降から次男は家に寄りつかなくなり，現在まで三男，夫，事例の三人暮らしである。

　事例は23歳で結婚するが，姑とうまくいかず2年半で離婚，そのころが初発と思われる。27歳で現在の夫と再婚し，長男，次男を出産するが，拒薬傾向があるため再発・再入院を繰り返した。このような状況の中三男を出産したため，三男は小学校入学まで乳児院で過ごした。そして事例が42歳の時作業所利用開始となり，この同時期に三男（小1）は家庭に戻ることとなり，母親と三男への援助はほぼ同時に開始された。作業所利用開始までの事例は，病気だからこんな夫としか結婚できなかったという不満を抱え，そのためか見知らぬ男性とすぐに関係を持ち，家に連れ込んだりしていた。また家庭の中で母親の役割を全く果たせていなかった。

　家族の概要は夫は軽い知的障害があるが，まじめでよく働き家庭のことをほとんどやっていた。しかし問題解決能力が乏しく困っても助けを求めることができず問題は深まるばかりだった。長男も軽度の知的な遅れがあり，父に似てとてもまじめ。しかし学校ではいじめられることが多く殴られることもあった。次男は家庭の中で一番事例に対し不満，反発が強く，非行グループに入るなど不適応が多いようだった。三男は繊細で賢く優しい子で学校では頭も良く他の子どもからうらやましがられるような存在だった。

　事例と三男への具体的な援助についてだが，子どもが小学校低学年の頃は母親へはまず医療へつなげることを確立し，母親の役割とはどういうも

のなのか示した。また地域支援者(保健婦,病院,児童相談所,小学校の担任教師)とのネットワークを作った。三男へは作業所との関係をつくり生活空間の拡大をはかった。

子どもが小学校高学年の頃は母親へは家庭の中で母親の役割が果たせるように調理実習をして家庭に持ち帰られるようにしたり金銭管理の訓練を行い,家庭の状況把握に努めた。三男へは母との生活上のマイナスイメージを軽減させるような援助をした。

子どもが中学生の頃は,母親へは自立しようとする子どもとの関係について援助し,その後のお互いのありかたについて考え始める必要を示した。三男へは自立に向けての援助,彼の人生が否定されないような支援をした。

これまでの援助をまとめると本事例に対し作業所では多くの地域支援者と連携を取り,事例だけでなくその子どもを含む家族もトータルに援助してきた。これによって事例はある程度の役割を家庭で担えるようになり,通所も安定し作業にも集中できる時間が増えた。また何より作業所利用を開始してからは再発・再入院していない。三男は高校生になった今でも作業所と関わりがあり,とても有意義な学校生活が送れているようである。

この事例が再発見し実現したい人生の主な舞台は家庭に置かれていた。その中で良き母良き妻でありたいと強く思うものの,なかなか実現できないでいた。作業所では事例の抱える辛さはこのような所にあると考え援助してきたのである。また一般的に幼い子どもと母親の関係は深く密接であり,事例も例外ではなかった。よって事例を援助するにはその子への援助は欠かせないものであった。こうした包括的な援助によって母と子どもを含む家族の成長と健康を守ることができたのである。

考　察

分裂病利用者への地域生活のサポートは,本人だけを対象に行うだけでは不十分である。その分裂病利用者を含んだ家族システムへのトータルな援助が必要である。

特に家庭生活で多くの役割を期待される母は子どもを含む家族との良好な関係があってこそ地域生活が成り立ち,本人の生活の質も向上する。育児ができないことを理由に幼い子どもを母から引き離す事だけが対処の方法ではない。母子分離は本人が家庭生活の中で最も期待されている母親としての役割の実現を妨げるばかりか,本人が希望する「母としての人生の再発見」を阻むことにつながると考えるからである。

分裂病利用者に対する援助は本人にとってどんなに困難が多くとも,利用者自身が希望する人生(生き方)を選択・再発見できるように,トータルに援助することが重要である。利用者の生活の場に拠点を置く作業所だからこそ本人と家族を包括的に援助し希望する人生の実現に向けて丁寧な働きかけが可能となった。

作業所が行った本人への援助は母としての自覚を強化し,家庭という場での自己実現を促進した。それが本人への3次予防へとつながった。同時に家族への長期に渡るトータルな援助は子どもの1次・2次予防にも繋がったのである。

最後に本報告を振り返り,子どもを持つ分裂病利用者の再発を予防するのに必要なことは,本人だけではなくその子ども,家族ともに援助すること。親としての役割を果たせるように援助すること。子どもの成長とともに本人も一緒に成長できるように援助すること。親子ともなった成長の上に,お互いが自立し,それぞれの人生を歩めるように援助すること。その家族を守る地域の支援ネットワークづくりをすること。という5点だと考えられる。

---

*東京都江東区グループ・オアシス
　Natsumi Tomoda, Kota Kojima, Hiromi Suzuki, Eigoro Ishikawa, Ken-ichi Hiramatsu : Group Oasis Koto Ward Tokyo Metropolitan.
**琉球大学医学部精神神経科学講座
　Ken-ichi Hiramatsu : Department of Neuropsychiatry, Univeristy of the Ryukyus.

精神分裂病患者の再入院調査
Study of readmission of schizophrenic patients

岡　　　敬[*1]　東間　正人[*1]　大野　耕嗣[*2]　平尾　直久[*3]　武田　　務[*1]
越野　好文[*1]　浜原　昭仁[*4]　中村　一郎[*4]　澁谷　禎三[*5]

I. 序　論

　われわれは，精神分裂病の再燃・再入院の要因を明らかにすることを目的に，再入院患者の通院・服薬状況，支援者の有無，日常活動などの特徴を調査した。今回，得られた結果から，再燃再入院の最も重要な原因と考えられている服薬状況に焦点をしぼり，服薬遵守の患者と中断した患者の特徴を比較した。

II. 対象と方法

　対象は平成12年6月から平成13年5月までに，金沢大学医学部附属病院精神科，公立精神科病院2施設，公立総合病院精神科1施設，民間精神科病院2施設に再入院したDSM-IVにて精神分裂病と診断された57名（男性33名，女性24名）。年齢は38.7±13.9(15〜67)歳，前回までの入院回数が5.1±4.7(1〜21)回であった。方法は，医師が，同意を得た患者と家族を面接し，以下，16項目の内容の質問をし，服薬状況により患者を3群に分け，t検定またはχ^2乗検定を用いて，特徴を比較した。

1) 外来通院は誰がしているか？
2) 通院間隔
3) 症状の悪化時期
4) 生活状況
5) 通院に要する時間
6) 薬物の投与法，1日の処方回数
7) 服薬コンプライアンス
8) 減薬・断薬の理由
9) 服薬をする理由
10) 医師からの服薬説明の有無
11) 患者と家族の服薬に関する理解度

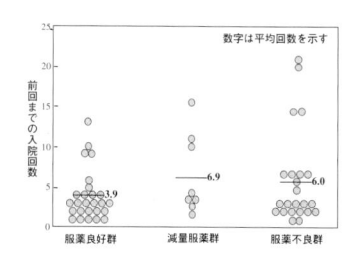

図1　服薬状況と前回までの入院回数

12) 服薬の支援者の有無
13) 作業・デイケア等の利用の有無
14) 入院の原因となった症状
15) 初発および再燃時の症状の既往
16) 入院前6カ月間のライフイベント

III. 結　果

　1) 今回の入院の原因となった症状では，幻覚・妄想及び興奮が最も頻度が高かった。
　2) 服薬状況は，全て服用が45.6%，3分の2以上毎日服用が8.8%，3分の1以上毎日服用が5.3%，不規則が7.0%，全く服用しないが33.3%であった。再入院患者の半数近くが，服薬遵守していたが，この中で，全て服用を服薬良好群(26名)，3分の2以上と3分の1以上毎日服用を減量服薬群(8名)，不規則と全く服用しないを服薬不良群(23名)とし，各々の要因を各群間で比較した。
　3) 過去の入院回数が服薬に与える影響を図1に示した。個々の入院回数を各群ごとに示したが，t検定の結果，服薬状況において過去の入院回数の差は無かった。入院を何回へても，服薬が良好とならなかった。
　4) 医師の服薬の必要性に関する説明に対して

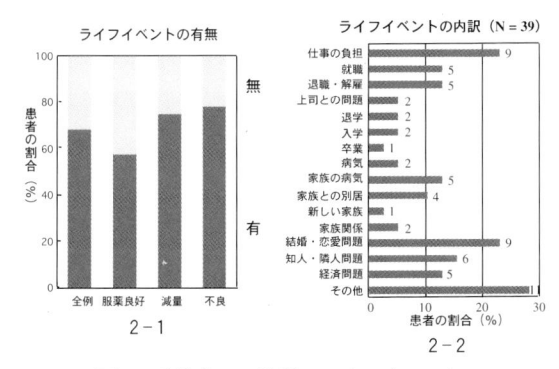

図2　入院前6カ月間のライフイベント

の理解度が服薬コンプライアンスに与える影響を示す。χ2乗検定の結果，服薬不良群が良好群と比較し，服薬説明に関する理解が乏しく，納得していなかった。

5) 服薬を支援してくれる家族等の存在が，服薬遵守に繋がるかどうかを調査した結果，服薬良好群も不良群も約8割が家族と同居していた。また，患者からみて，家族等が服薬を何らかの形でサポートしていると感じているか否かを検討したが，服薬援助者がいる患者は，52.6%であり，服薬不良者が良好者と比較して少ない傾向にあったが，有意差はなかった。

6) 断薬および減薬する理由として，65%の患者が副作用を，36%が「服薬の必要を認めない」をあげた。副作用として，「何となく調子が悪い」が40%，眠気が25%だった。

7) 活動性と服薬状況の関係では，仕事・学業，作業所・デイケア，家事，何もしていないと回答した患者がほぼ同じ割合だった。又，生活状況は，服薬良好と不良群で差は無かった。

8) 図2-1は，入院前6カ月間のライフイベントの有無に関するもので，有りが全体の68%であり，服薬良好群と不良群では差はなかった。図2-2は，その内訳を示す。上から，仕事，学業，家庭内の問題，恋愛などの対人的問題の割合を示す。特に，就業問題，恋愛結婚問題が多く，19%は，服薬遵守し，ライフイベントを認めなかった。

IV. 考察とまとめ

1) 入院した精神分裂病患者57例の調査より，服薬遵守している患者と中断した患者の特徴を比較検討した。

2) 調査した57例のうち，26例が服薬良好，8例が減量服薬，23例が服薬不良であった。

3) 入院回数の増加は，服薬を良好にする要因とはならず，むしろ服薬中断による入院を頻回に繰り返す患者が多かった。

4) 服薬不良者に，医者の服薬説明が不十分であるか説明内容に納得がいかないとする患者が多かった。

5) 服薬をサポートする家族の有無は，服薬状況に影響しなかった。

6) 服薬良好群と不良群で仕事など活動性に差がなかった。

7) 減薬及び断薬の原因として副作用が多く，なかでも眠気の訴えが多かった。

8) 以上より，服薬遵守のため，医師の十分な説明と副作用に対する適切な対応が必要と考えられた。

9) 入院前6カ月間のライフイベントでは，就業問題と恋愛結婚問題が多く，これらの問題に対する支援が必要と思われた。

10) 一方，服薬遵守し，ライフイベントが無いにも関わらず，再入院した患者が2割を占めたことから，他の再発要因を検討する必要がある。

[*1] 金沢大学医学部神経精神医学教室
Takashi Oka, Masato Higashima, Tutomu Takeda, Yoshifumi Koshino : Department of Neuropsychiatry, School of Medicine, Kanazawa University.
[*2] 川田病院
Kouji Ono : Kawada Hospital.
[*3] 福井県立病院精神・神経センター
Naohisa Hirao : Fukui Center Hospital for Mental and Nervous Disorders.
[*4] 石川県立高松病院
Shouni Hamahara, Itirou Nakamura : Ishikawa Prefectural Takamatsu Hospital.
[*5] 十全病院
Teizou Shibutani : Juzen Hospital.

精神分裂病患者の再入院因子についての考察

Factors of readmission in patients with schizophrenia

福田　耕嗣* 　西村　克彦* 　小川美菜子* 　鈴木　節夫** 　村上　弘司*** 　石田　孜郎*

I. 目　的

　精神分裂病(以下，分裂病)の経過・予後に対する予測因子に関する研究は，これまでに数多くなされている。しかしながら，これらの因子を再入院に関する予測因子として検討した報告は稀である。今回我々は，分裂病の再発予防および社会生活を維持する要因を明らかにするために，分裂病の再入院に関する予測因子(再入院因子)について検討した。

II. 対象および方法

　1) 1997年1月から1999年12月までの3年間に，分裂病の診断で，静岡県立こころの医療センターに初めて入院し，同期間内に退院した患者を対象とした。分裂病の診断はICD-10に準拠した。また，これより以前に精神科に入院歴のある者は，対象より除外した。2) 同期間内に，1回の入退院歴のあるものを単回入院者，2回以上の入退院歴のあるものを再入院者とした。対象の内訳は表1に示した。3) 再入院因子として，表2に示す検討項目について調査した。再入院因子は，これまでに分裂病の予後を予測する因子として検討されてきた項目を参考に，今回我々が独自に作成した。4) 再入院因子の有無は，診療録より調査した。診療録の調査は4名の精神科医によって行った。診療録から情報が得られないものに関しては，当該項目を調査不能とした。5) 再入院因子の各項目について有意差検定を行った。間隔尺度に関してはt-testを，分類尺度に関してはFisher's exact probability testをそれぞれ用い，$p<0.01$を有意差ありとした。

III. 結　果

　静岡県立こころの医療センターにおいて，精神分裂病の診断で初回入院した患者73人(単回入院者61人，再入院者12人)を対象に，表2に示した再入院因子について，調査，検討した。その結果，いずれの項目に関しても，単回入院者と再入院者の間に有意差は認められなかった。ただし，生活歴に関わる因子として検討した項目のうち，転居・転校歴の有無に関しては，有意差は認められなかったものの，再入院者に多くみられる傾向があった(Fisher's exact probability test, $p=0.011$)。

IV. 考　察

　1) 精神分裂病患者の初回入院時点で，その患者の再入院の有無を予測することは，困難であると考えられた。

　2) 再入院因子のうち，転居・転校歴の有無に関しては，有意差は認められなかったものの，再入院者に多くみられる傾向があった。この理由に関しては不明であり，今後の検討を要する。

　3) 再入院因子として，決定的な因子が見いだせなかった理由として，以下のことが考えられた。①症例数が少なかった(特に再入院症例)。②再入院には多くの要因が関与していると考えられるため，再入院に対して単一要因のもつ影響力が相対的に低い。③本研究では，分裂病の予後を予測する因子を参考にしつつ，独自の再入院因子を検討した。今回検討した項目以外に，再入院因子となりうる因子が存在している可能性がある。

表1 対象

	対象数	年齢（平均±標準偏差）	性別（男：女）	入院形態		
				任意	医療保護	その他
単回入院者	61人	30±15歳	21人：40人	29人	32人	0人
再入院者	12人	31±18歳	4人：8人	2人	10人	0人

表2 検討項目（再入院因子）

病型分類	
生活歴に関わる因子	発症に関わるストレスの有無
	発症前，6カ月以上継続しての就学，就労の有無
	教育年数（高校卒業以下または以上で分類）
	単身生活歴の有無
	結婚歴の有無
	転居／転校歴の有無
家族歴に関わる因子	精神医学的遺伝負因の有無
	High Emotional Expressionの有無
身体合併症の有無	
初回入院時の経過に関わる因子	初回入院時の入院日数
	初回入院時の保護室利用の有無
	初回入院時のECTの有無
	初回入院後の拒薬の有無
初回退院後の経過に関わる因子	初回退院後の抗精神病薬服用量（haloperidol換算量）
	初回退院後の通院頻度（1カ月当たりの通院回数）
	初回退院後の主な受診者（本人受診の有無）
	初回退院後の社会適応の有無

表3 結果

生活歴に関わる因子	単回入院者	再入院者
発症にかかわるストレスがあった（％）	38	50
発症前，6カ月以上継続しての就学／就労があった（％）	57	67
教育年数（高校卒業以上の割合，％）	39	25
単身生活歴があった（％）	16	25
結婚歴があった（％）	31	17
転居／転校歴があった（％）	31	67

家族歴に関する因子	単回入院者	再入院者
精神医学的遺伝負因がある（％）	39	42
High Emotional Expressionがある（％）	23	17

身体合併症に関する因子	単回入院者	再入院者
身体合併症がある（％）	18	42

初回入院時の経過に関わる因子	単回入院者	再入院者
初回入院時の平均入院日数（日数）	121	102
初回入院時の保護室利用があった（％）	44	75
初回入院時にECTを施行した（％）	7	15
初回入院後の拒薬があった（％）	18	0

初回退院後の経過に関わる因子	単回入院者	再入院者
初回退院後の抗精神病薬服用量（haloperidol換算量，mg／日）	13	13
初回退院後の通院頻度（1カ月当たりの通院回数，回／月）	1.6	1.8
初回退院後の主な受診者（患者本人の受診率，％）	87	75
初回退院後の社会適応が良好である（％）	16	0

---

*静岡県立こころの医療センター
 Koji Fukuda, Katsuhiro Nishimura, Minako Ogawa, Shiro Ishida : Shizuoka Prefectural Mental Care and Rehabiritation Center.
**静岡県精神保健福祉センター
 Setsuo Suzuki : Shizuoka Prefectural Mental Health and Welfare Center.
***藤枝駿府病院
 Koji Murakami : Fujieda Sunpu Hospital.

三次予防のための精神分裂病の治療を展望する
―福間病院の分裂病統計から―

Review of the treatment of Schizophrenia for secondary and tertiary prevention
―From statistics of Fukuma Hospital―

梅田　征夫*　　高柴哲次郎*

　福間病院は表1のように，1955年に開院して以来，一貫して精神分裂病を中心とした治療を展開してきた。1959年から72年まで作業療法主体の分院「希望が丘村」を設立，61年には福岡市内にサテライト・クリニック開設，74年には精神科デイケアの保険診療施設として認可を受けた。89年に社会復帰施設「緑の里」（援護寮と授産施設）を，95年からSSTを導入しSSTの治療スタッフ養成に取り組み，96年，精神科急性期治療病棟（開放46床）の承認を受け，グループホーム2棟を設置，98年から訪問看護部門をスタート，更に99年には精神科急性期病棟（閉鎖40床）の認可を受けた。

　このような治療システムの構築により精神分裂病の再発の防止（三次予防）に力を注いできた。その他地域における精神障害に関する相談事業，啓蒙活動を行っている。今回は特に当院における精神分裂病統計資料を基に最近の当院の分裂病治療の現状を述べ，再入院までの期間の動向，そして地域ケアの主体となるデイケアの観点から再入院予防（三次予防）について検討してみた。

I．当院の分裂病患者の入院の変遷

　図1は開院から2000年までの46年間の入院件数の変遷である。開院後5～6年まで増加しその後は平均約160件を中心に増減しながら経過している。また開院10年頃まで初回入院が再入院を上回るがその後は逆転し再入院が上回っている。再入院件数の減少は見られない。

表1　福間病院の分裂病治療の経緯

1955年	開院（開放療法）
1974年	デイケア認可
1984年	外来担当ナース制，3カ月未来院のチェック開始
1989年	「緑の里」（援護寮，授産施設開設）
1995年	SST導入
1996年	精神科急性期病棟認可（開放46床）グループホーム開設
1998年	訪問看護開始
1999年	精神科急性期病棟認可（閉鎖40床）デイホスピタル試行

II．年間に何人の分裂病者を治療しているか

　表2に示すように，当院で2000年の1年間に治療した分裂病者は1218名であった。このうち1年間入院継続した者が306名，外来のみで治療した者が686名，その他226名が入院したり退院したりした者である。入院した者が延べ183件，退院が延べ186件であった。外来を利用した者が895名で，そのうち95名が新患であった。デイケアの利用者は206名で外来利用者の23.0％であった。分裂病者の地域ケアを重視するならば，この23.0％という数字は少なすぎるのではないか。患者のニーズにマッチした地域ケア・プログラムが用意されているのかどうか更に検討を要するところであろう。

III．再入院のインターバルについて

　1988年，93年，98年と5年毎にその1年間に退院した分裂病者の再入院までの期間を調べた。図2に示すように全体では退院後2年以内の再入院

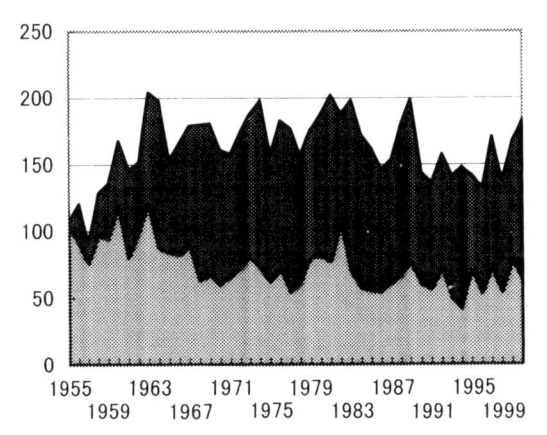

図1 福間病院における精神分裂病入院患者の推移
（1955～2000年）

表2 当院の精神分裂病統計（2000年）
―ICD10でF20と診断された者―

・治療総数／年　1218名
　―1年間入院継続中　306名（25.1%）
　―入退院の異動のあった者　226名（18.6%）
　　・入院者数／年　117名
　　・退院者数／年　173名
　―外来のみで治療した者　686名（56.3%）
・外来利用者数／年　895名
　―外来新患登録者数／年　95名
　―再来登録者数／年　800名
・デイケア利用者数／年　206名（外来利用者の23.0%）
　―デイケア新規入所者数／年　32名
　―デイケアからの再入院／年　10名

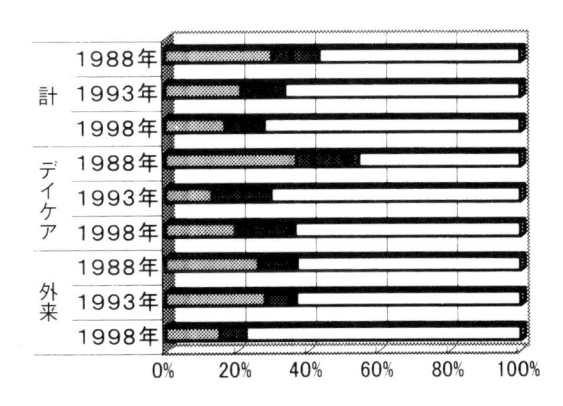

図2 再入院までの期間（1983, 1993, 1998）

表3 デイケア入所後の再入院（81例）

	外来から入所	退院後入所
入所後の再入院 1年後	19.8%	(8.6%, 28.3%)
2年後	29.6%	(20.0%, 37.0%)
3年後	37.0%	(28.0%, 47.8%)

永松ら（1991）

表4 デイケアにおける医学的管理の強化の影響
（デイケア初回入所分裂病について）

	1年目までの再入院率
強化前（56例）	23.2%
強化後（60例）	6.7%

米澤ら（1993）

の割合は減少していると言えよう。デイケアを利用している患者でも再入院率は必ずしもよくはないのである。デイケアに所属する患者の中にはかなり重症な一群がいて度々再発再入院を繰り返している。表3は永松らが当院デイケア患者について調べたものである。外来から入所した群と退院後入所した群ではその後の再入院率が大幅に違う。ではどうすれば再入院が防止できるのであろうか。当院デイケアでは93年にスタッフがチームを作り，服薬管理など医学的管理の強化を図った。その結果を米澤らがまとめたものが表4である。医学的管理をする前と後とでは1年までの再入院率が16.5%も低下する。当院では最初に述べたようにデイケア，SST導入，援護寮，グループホーム，急性期治療の強化に加え，最近，服薬の勉強グループ，家族塾（心理教育）も展開されており，これらが分裂病者の2年以内の再入院の減少に関与しているのではないかと推測する。

今後更に分裂病者の地域ケアの促進を図り，再発・再入院の防止するための努力を積み重ねていきたい。

*福間病院
Yukio Umeda, Tetsujiro Takashiba : Department of Psychiatry, Fukuma Hospital.

再発予防
―拒薬の服薬指導を通して―

Prevention of relapse : Compliance instruction
—A Solution of refusal to take medication due to lack of insight about the illness—

中村　靖* 　浦崎　政枝* 　下地　泉* 　名城　真治* 　久場　兼功*

I. はじめに

　一般的な症例においては正常な部分と病的な部分が混在しており，処方箋の中からは正常な部分は見えない。服薬指導に入るには，まず正常な部分を把握しなければならない。そのためには，症例の内面から入り信頼関係を構築することが重要である。つまり，白衣の薬剤師ではなくチームスタッフの1人として自分を受け入れてもらうためにエネルギーを注ぐことが必要になる。個々の症例の情報は看護記録やカンファレンスなどから収集し，実際に病棟で患者と接して動き回ることで真の症例が見えてくる。そこから服薬指導の手がかりを掴むことができる。薬剤師の立場から患者の服薬指導を通して信頼関係が構築されると，病識，薬識が正しく理解され，レベルの高い退院が実現し，再発予防も可能になる。本日は，特に拒薬の症例を取り上げ議論を深めていきたい。

II. 服薬コンプライアンスを左右する主な素因

① 患者さん側の素因
・病状の悪化　思考障害，自我障害，被毒妄想，病識・病感・薬識の欠如
・薬物乱用　　アルコール依存との合併
・患者の心理　心理的側面を十分に配慮した接し方が必要不可欠
・生活形態　　単身者のコンプライアンス
・経済面　　　精神保健法32条他の活用
② 家族側の素因
・家族，周囲のサポート
　患者と同様に，服薬に対する教育が前提になる。患者の服薬自己管理がうまくできるように，患者とその家族を教育することがコンプライアンス向上につながるとされている。

III. 症　例

精神分裂症（被害関係妄想・幻聴）
40歳　男性　　性格：易怒的，攻撃的
（経過）
S61年　　初発，本土の病院に措置入院
　　　　　幻覚，妄想状態
　　　　　薬剤による不快反応，厳しい処遇を経験　処方不明　入院3回
H5年
5/21　　当院へ医療保護入院　服薬拒否（詰所）
　　　　　主治医から，患者へ服薬指導の告知
5/25　　「薬は，いらない」「自分は，病院の人は信用しない」（病室）
5/26　　意識的に興味を引くように，ホールやサンルーム等で服薬指導を見せる。
5/27　　スタッフは，「4時半の男が来てるよ。どうしますか？」と毎日アプローチ
5/28　　自己紹介（詰所）
　　　　　「中村です。薬についての不安や不満な事を，一緒に相談して解決していきたい。どうですか？」うなずいて，詰め所から出ていく。
　　　　　看護記録，スタッフとの話し合いで，一日の動きを知る。
　　　　　患者の「安心する部分」「誇りたい部分」を探す。

患者に「言ってはいけない」「訊いてはいけない」ことを把握する。

6／1　面談室にて　（面談室）
過去の経験，重機の免許の事など，自慢話を聞く。「他の患者さんには，こんな話は出来ないけど，あなたなら理解できますね」
血中濃度の話をする。

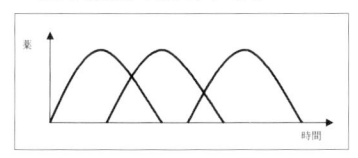

6／4　服用開始
「脳が働きすぎているので，少し休ませてあげましょう」

6／7　OT活動に参加　（面談室）
ボールペンを使って，ドパミンの話をする。

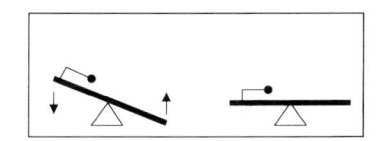

6／11　病棟スタッフからの依頼で，家族と面談　（DI室）
複雑な家族関係で，しかも全くの病識欠如であった

6／18　スタッフから，服用確認の報告

6／25　自分自身をコントロール　（サンルーム）

6／30　母親の面会あり。デポ剤終了，内服のみで　（ホール）

7／2　主治医より，表情に活気あり，妄想否定の報告

7／8　自ら，家族の事，特に父親にたいする思いや精神病院との関わりを語る。（ホール）

7／12　母親が面会，父親と電話で口論

7／16　父親と電話で口論

7／23　主治医より，拒絶傾向（－）。（DI室）
「自分はもう薬が必要のないくらい，良くなっているのでは」（笑顔で）

8月上旬の主治医の評価
・幻覚，妄想はほぼ改善（あったとしても表面化する事はなし，病的体験に左右された行動はない）
・服薬及び作業状況も良好

今後の方針
・服薬の継続
・飲酒はしない事→本人の心構えしだい（二度と失敗しない事）
・仕事について　→運送屋に勤めたい
・家族の受け入れ体制作り→受け入れ体制が確立したら退院へ

外来での，フォローを記入する。

「予防の服薬」
1）社会の中で，仕事や家庭の喜びは，大きいですね。入院中のつらかった事，苦しい思いは二度とさせません。
2）薬が環境の変化やストレスがかかった時，クッションの様な働きで，あなたを守ってあげます。

H13年5／16現在の状況
現在も外来で通院中であり，予防の為の内服続けながら，結婚をして土木関係の仕事を頑張っているとの事。時々，母親が薬をもらいに来院する。

Ⅳ．総　括

病棟スタッフとの協力のもと，患者との信頼関係を構築する事が肝要である。

また自らを受け入れてもらうよう力を注ぎ，病識，薬識を易しい表現でわかりやすく患者に説明し，段階的に理解度のレベルを上げていく。『私自身が薬です。』

次に，家族の方々には病識や退院後の服薬の必要性を認識してもらい，継続して病院との連携を図り，受け入れ体制を維持し協力することに努める。

以上のことを踏まえて，予防の為における服薬の必要性をポジティブな角度から助言し外来での服薬を生活の一部として理解してもらい，そうすることによって社会復帰が可能となり，再発予防が可能になる。

---

*沖縄中央病院
Yasushi Nakamura, Masae Urasaki, Izumi Shimoji, Shinji Nashiro, Kenko Kuba : Okinawa Chuoh Hospital.

精神科病院薬剤科の機能と役割
―薬剤事故防止のための調剤支援システムを導入して―

Function and role of the mental institution pharmacy
―Introducting a dispensation support system for preventing accidents with drugs―

石田　保美*　木藤　弘子*

I. はじめに

精神科病院薬剤師業務の業務割合は日病薬の調査によると調剤が約70％を占めていることがわかった。当院薬剤科では平成8年4月より調剤支援システムを一部導入し，その合理化に努めた。（図）

II. 当院薬剤科の特徴

当院薬剤科は外来棟と離れ，別棟に設置されている。患者さんは自ら処方箋を薬剤科窓口へ持参される。すべてオープンカウンターとし服薬指導コーナーでは，退院患者のほぼ全員に退院時服薬指導を行っている。また，薬剤情報提供は外来患者全員に実施している。実績は次の通りである。

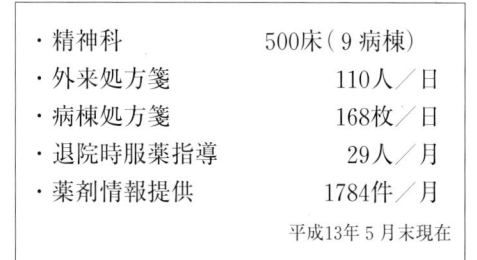

・精神科	500床（9病棟）
・外来処方箋	110人／日
・病棟処方箋	168枚／日
・退院時服薬指導	29人／月
・薬剤情報提供	1784件／月
	平成13年5月末現在

III. 調剤支援システム導入の経緯概略

平成8年4月　調剤支援システムを一部導入し，業務の合理化を実施した。

平成11年8月　前任者2人の退職後，薬剤師6名プラス事務員1名体制となる。

平成12年5月　薬袋発行機導入および外来医事とパソコンを連動し，外来患者の薬待ち時間の短縮を図る。

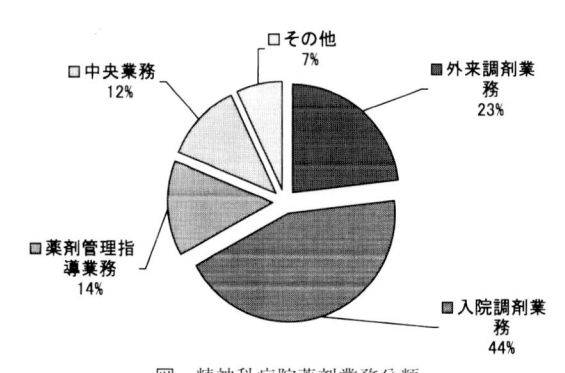

図　精神科病院薬剤業務分類

引用文献　日精協誌　第19巻　第2号　2000年2月　精神科薬剤業務について

当薬剤科での事務員は調剤以外の種々の業務（システム管理や事務統計処理・薬歴打ち出しなどパソコンを利用しての業務）を担っている。

IV. 調剤支援システム導入の利点

この導入で薬剤師の手による分包作業がなくなり，スピードアップと各種チェック可能となった。調剤業務に深みを増し，精神科薬物療法への大いなる貢献と薬剤過誤防止対策として大役を担うことになった。

各種チェック機能としての重複投与（日数・薬効）・相互作用（併用禁忌）・散薬実測量の印字（倍散の計算）などが1回の処方入力で可能となる。

V. 調剤支援システム導入の問題点

高額な設備費がかかり，診療報酬では採算が見込めないため，民間の精神科病院での導入は少ない。包括病棟での薬剤管理指導業務報酬が算定できないのも原因の一つとなっている。さらに，精

神科ではマンパワー不足もあって，薬剤師が日々の業務に追われ導入に積極的になりにくい。

VI. 精神科薬剤師の役割

精神科薬剤師には調剤以外の役割としては積極的な病棟活動をあげる。長期になる服薬期間への理解や説明などで職能を発揮すれば，怠薬などを予防できると考える。副作用発生時の対処法指導は重要な役割である。薬物療法において，院内におけるセカンドオピニオン的存在になれるのが薬剤師である。病識のない患者や認知機能障害がある患者への対応も精神科特有なのかもしれない。

これらの業務への拡大のためには普段の日常業務（主業務の調剤）をいかに効率よく行うかである。機械で賄えることはできるだけ機械にまかせ，捻出できた時間を患者さんへの服薬指導業務へ注がねばならないと思う。

VII. まとめ

精神科病院の現配置基準で薬剤業務を遂行するには調剤支援システムに頼らざるをえない。調剤が主業務の精神科病院薬剤科では最も必要とされるシステムである。

導入することで薬剤過誤防止にも寄与できたし，人手ではできなかったチェックが数多く可能となり，調剤業務の向上にもつながった。システムを利用して，調剤中心業務から患者中心業務への転換の可能性がみえてきた。服薬指導の実施により，患者さんの身近な存在となり，患者教育にも参加し，効果的な薬物療法の一端を担えるように変化してきた。

VIII. 終わりに

調剤支援システムを利用し，多くの施設で薬剤業務の拡大を図り，多くの患者さんの肉声を聴く薬剤師が増えることを期待する。薬剤師の頑張りで病院の質が上がるだろう。

---

*(医)恵愛会　福間病院薬剤科
Yasumi Ishida, Hiroko Kito : Department of Hospital Pharmacy, Fukuma Hospital.

地域住民の精神障害者観に関連する要因の分析

Analysis of factors concerning the views of the community about the people with mental disorders

田中　悟郎* 　木崎　晴美** 　菊池　泰樹* 　稲富　宏之* 　太田　保之*

Introduction

Prejudice against people with mental disorders limits their social participation and impedes the promotion of community psychiatric services. The prejudice is not only making their social participation difficult, but also delaying their visit to psychiatric settings and worsening their condition. If we can reduce such prejudice, they can seek psychiatric help more easily and consequently we can expect higher therapeutic effects through psychiatric care. Considering such circumstances, it is extremely important to study factors relating the attitudes toward people with mental disorders of the community and searching for strategies to reduce prejudice.

In Japan, some investigations have been conducted on attitudes toward people with mental disorders and on the effects of people having contact with them[1,2]. However, no study has yet been conducted on the effects of awareness campaigns by administrative bodies such as a community health center.

Using a questionnaire, we have conducted an investigation of residents living within the jurisdiction of the Nagasaki Prefecture Central Health Center (two cities and eight towns) in order 1) to check understanding of people with mental disorders, 2) to evaluate the success of awareness campaigns and 3) to design an effective intervention aimed at changing attitudes.

Subjects and methods

With the cooperation of the administrative staff of the cities and towns, we distributed anonymous questionnaires to 2632 people who resided in the investigation areas and were considered as major targets of awareness campaigns, such as members of the Chamber and Commerce, district welfare commissioners, health promoter, town office staff, social adjustment training staff and participants of mental health welfare volunteer training classes. Of them, 1586 replies were given (reply rate : 60.6%). The investigation period was from August to November in 1999. The investigation included a prejudice scale against people with mental disorders[1], a social distance scale[2], contact with people with mental disorders, welfare activities (volunteer experience), participation in awareness campaigns, knowledge of schizophrenia and other basic attributes.

Results and discussion

Of the 1596 replies, 1211 were valid (valid reply rate : 75.9%). The main characteristics of the subjects were as follows, 72.9% was female, the average age was 51.3 ± 13.3, main occupations were office worker (27%) and housewife (26.2%). Factor analysis (varimax rotaion) of the prejudice scale revealed three components (cumulative proportion of variance 48.5%) : Factor 1 (proportion of variance 20.8%) ; rejection, Factor 2 (15.5%) ; peculiar views to mental disorders and Factor 3 (12.2%) ; neglect of human rights of people with mental disorders. The Cronbach α coefficient of prejudice scale, which was 0.91, and was found quite reliable. In order to analyze factors related to attitudes towards people with mental disorders, we practiced multiple regression analysis with setting prejudice scale as a dependent variable and sex, age, education, resident area, degree of contact, degree of participation in welfare activities, participation in awareness campaigns, misunderstanding of schizophrenia as a independent variable. As a result, age ($\beta = -0.27$, $P<0.001$), residing in the city ($\beta = -0.09$, $P<0.01$), degree of contact ($\beta = -0.12$, $P<0.001$), degree of welfare activities ($\beta = -0.13$, $P<0.001$), degree of active involvement in solution of community problems ($\beta = -0.07$, $P<0.05$), participation in awareness campaign ($\beta = -0.08$, $P<0.05$), and misunderstanding of schizophrenia ($\beta = 0.14$, $P<0.001$) had significantly independent effects on the prejudice scale. These results suggested the followings as effective and important factors for reducing prejudice, 1) the diffusion of knowledge, 2) contact with people with mental disorders, and 3) participation in volunteer activities and the effectiveness of awareness campaigns.

Various suggestive descriptions which are useful when considering future awareness campaigns were also given voluntarily in 341 replies, and some of them are reported here. If we come to see mental and psychiatric disorders as more common and familiar diseases, there is possibility for a change in attitudes. For example, there were descriptions such as, "If we think that everybody could have mental disorders as catching colds, we see such disorders without prejudiced eyes", "In such times as today, I could have some mental problems, and even if I don't know anybody with problems around me, it is important to learn and understand", and "These days I see people who have depression for interpersonal problems, but when they are someone close or friends, I don't know how I should deal with them and so I tend to avoid them. I wish I have some chance or information leaflets to learn about mental disorders and how to deal with people with disorders." There are self-agonizing opinions as such, "When it has to do with those relating to my own situation, I reject people with mental problems, but when it concerns others, I can be very tolerant. I realize that I am very self-oriented", "I was annoyed myself talking a principle against my true feelings", and "Without any person with such problems close to myself, I can speak out that we should help people with mental disorders to adjust socially, but if they come into my life, I am afraid I would look at them with prejudiced eyes and attitudes. I feel I faced my own foolishness for having such thoughts". These opinions showed that it is necessary to understand these feelings and include methods to bring relief to such anguish in those replying to awareness questionnaires, when we try to build 'relationship' with community people. One person said in a voluntary reply, "Answering this questionnaire, I had a chance to think about mental disorders which I have not given much thought about." It is important to create an opportunity in which people could exchange their opinions freely, not only having lectures. It is important to recognize that people in the community are not mere subjects for awareness activities, but partners to work together in creating a secure and tolerant community.

References

1) Machizawa, S., Sato, H., Sawamura, M. : The measurement of attitude toward psychiatric disorder : A comparison among patients, patients' family and general resident. Jpn. J. Clinical Psychiatry, 19 ; 511-520, 1990. (in Japanese)
2) Zenkaren Health and Welfare Research Institute : The attitude toward people with mental disorders 1997. Zenkaren, 1998. (in Japanese)

---

*長崎大学医療技術短期大学部
Goro Tanaka, Yasuki Kikuchi, Hiroyuki Inadomi, Yasuyuki Ohta : School of Allied Medical Sciences, Nagasaki University.
**長崎県県央保健所
Harumi Kisaki : Nagasaki Prefectural Central Health Center.

精神障害者支援のための健康教育を実施して

Health education campaigns to support the people with mental disorders

木崎　晴美*　　田中　悟郎**　　松尾　文子*　　大川　嘉子*　　古賀　敏治*

I. はじめに

県央保健所では，平成11年度から，「精神障害者が地域で生活していくための支援をすることは，自分たちが生活しやすい地域づくりにつながる」というメッセージを住民に伝えるための健康教育を実施してきた。

その中で，地域の人たちが精神障害に対する理解を深める健康教育（普及啓発活動）のあり方について検討し，その結果をもとにさらに平成12年度健康教育を実施したので報告する。

II. 対象と方法

平成11年度にモデル地区を一地区設定し健康教育を行い，同時に「精神障害に対する意識調査」を実施した。その結果をもとにプログラムを再検討し，平成12年度2地区で健康教育を実施した。対象及び内容については，表1，表2のとおりである。

III. 結果及び考察

平成11年度，健康教育を行うにあたって，モデル地区を設定し，地域のリーダー的な役割（地域の人たちの相談役を担っている人）が期待できる人たちに，精神保健福祉に関する普及啓発のためのプログラムを組んで実施した。

平成12年度の実施にあたっては，「意識調査」や，A地区参加者のフリートークをもとに，精神障害者のイメージを良くするキーワードの，「正しい知識の理解」，「良い触れあい体験」などを考慮し，①当事者・家族から地域のみんなに何をして欲しいのかというメッセージを伝えてもらう，②一緒に活動するというプログラムを取り入れた。

プログラムの最終日のグループワークの中で出された意見は，①精神障害を理解することができ，他の人にも伝えて行きたい，②精神障害者と交流することで，学び，自分のできるところで力になりたい，③精神障害者が集まるような場所が近くにあれば，交流がしやすい等の意見が多く出された。この内容については，3地区とも同じであった。

また，平成12年度健康教育の前後に実施した意識調査の結果，早くから障害者を受け入れてきたB地区では，偏見度が終了後改善され，閉鎖的なC地区では，終了後もほとんど変化は見られなかった。このことから，今まで種々な活動として障害者が地域で一緒に過ごせるような「地域づくり活動」が行われているか，または，その考え方が地域の中に浸透しているかが，今後の活動の展開へ大きく影響すると考える。

よって，健康教育の内容だけでなく，地域の特性をいかに活用するかが課題と考えられる。その良い例として，2年目を迎えたA地区では，精神障害者との交流を積み重ねながら，代表者会議を組織し，第1回『A地区町民による精神障害を考える保健福祉大会』が開催された。その中に当事者との交流を目的にバザーを実施するなど，広く町民の理解を得る啓発活動を展開することができ，当事者の要望から2年目には，町内に活動の拠点を確保することができた。また，C地区では，地域のリーダーより動かされて行政側が家族の支援を実施するための検討を始めた。

IV. おわりに

地域での教育活動は，精神障害者が地域の中で生活していくための地域住民間での支援ネットワークを作って行くことが重要と考えられるので，

表1　モデル地区及び健康教育の対象者

	A 地区	B 地区	C 地区
選定理由	・当事者の集いの開始。 ・当事者が活動の拠点を要望。 ・活動の中心となるボランティアの存在。 ・町がその支援を検討中。 ・町内に利用可能な社会資源が少なく，近隣市町を利用する人も少ない。	・町の事業として当事者の集いを「心のリハビリ事業」として実施していた。 ・町が管内でも，早くから家族へ支援を実施していた。 ・町内に利用可能な社会資源はないが，近隣市町の資源の利用は多い。	・保健所が実施していた当事者の集いが町内に定着できなかった。 ・町内に専門の医療機関はあるが，他の社会資源の利用は，圏域外に頼っている。 ・家族会は，広域で設置されているため利用がしにくい。
対象者	町職員・教育委員会・小中学校教諭・児童民生委員・福祉施設関係者・ボランティア等	町職員・教育委員会・小中学校教諭・町議会・児童民生委員・食生活改善推進員・母子推進員・ボランティア等	町職員・児童民生委員・婦人会・食生活改善推進員・ボランティア等

職種別参加状況	参加職種	実数	参加職種	実数	参加職種	実数
	町職員	22	町職員	18	町職員	18
	教育委員会・学校教諭	13	教育委員会・学校教諭	2	教育委員会・学校教諭	2
	児童民生委員	12	児童民生委員	17	児童民生委員	21
	ボランティア	17	食生活改善推進員	4	食改・婦人会	35
	福祉施設関係者	16	母子推進員	9		
			ボランティア	8		
			町議会	1		
			その他(学校・一般)	10		
	合計	80	合計	69	合計	76

表2　健康教育の内容

平成11年度健康教育内容			平成12年度健康教育内容		
ねらい	内容	担当者	ねらい	内容	担当者
精神疾患を理解し身近なものとしてとらえる。	幼児期～青年期の精神疾患	精神科医師	ライフサイクルから精神疾患を理解する。	幼児期～青年期の精神疾患	精神科医師
	成人期～老年期の精神疾患			成人期～老年期の精神疾患	
精神障害者の生活のしづらさを理解する。	生活障害の援助について	作業療法士	当事者・家族のおかれている状況を理解する。	当事者・家族からのメッセージ	当事者
				スポーツ交流会	家族会会員
当事者・家族のおかれている状況を理解する。	施設見学を通しての当事者家族との交流	家族会会長 地域活動所	精神障害者の生活のしづらさを理解する。	生活障害の援助について	作業療法士
			精神障害者の地域での活動状況を理解する。	施設見学	地域活動所
町内において自分がどう精神保健福祉に関与できるか。	フリートーク(グループワーク)	精神科医師	精神障害者を地域で支えていくのに必要な事を考える。	フリートーク(グループワーク)	保健婦

地域の関係者と一緒に，地道な活動を続けていきたいと考える。

*長崎県県央保健所
Harumi Kisaki, Fumiko Matsuo, Yoshi Ookawa, Toshiharu Koga : Nagasaki Kenou Health Center.

**長崎大学医療短期大学部
Goro Tanaka : School of Allied Medical Scoences, Nagasaki University.

三次予防のための療養病棟における
コミュニティミーティングの試み

A trial of community meeting in a sanatorium ward

庄司　恵美* 　古井　博明*

I．はじめに

　精神医療を取り巻く政策の変化に伴い，患者中心の医療提供の視点が導入されつつある。そのひとつとして，入院中心主義からの脱皮を目指すこと，つまり，リハビリテーションにより社会復帰を促進することが望まれており，私たち医療スタッフは具対策を模索している。

　当院は精神分裂病が主体の定床500床の病院である。2つの急性期治療病棟を中心に，治療病棟・療養棟がある。療養棟のひとつである当病棟は，定床60床，男女混合の開放病棟であり，平均年齢51才，平均在院期間は6年7カ月である。

　平成12年4月，新しい病棟医長を迎え，難しい症例を抱えた開放療養病棟で何かできることはないか，と投げかけられた。そこで5月より，患者の主体性を重んじた治療関係を作り上げることを目標に，患者・看護婦・作業療法士・医師といった多職種で構成されるミーティングを開始した。

　試行錯誤を重ねながら1年が経過し，ミーティングに参加することで，スタッフや患者の，意識や取り組みに少しずつではあるが変化が見られてきた。

　今回，長期入院患者の退院事例を通し，ミーティングのもたらした影響について考える。

II．ミーティングについて

　平成12年5月より，従来の回診に代えてミーティングを開始した。

　進め方は，司会役の看護婦から患者1人ずつに声をかけ，その日の申し送りや，この2週間の治療的取り組みなどについて，看護婦の考えを伝え，患者の意見を聞いた。一巡した後，自由に討論している。

　ミーティング開始当初，患者にとってミーティングに参加すること自体，不安や緊張が強かった。中には，ミーティングを被害的に捉える患者も見られた。スタッフにも，問題点・気になることをどう患者に投げかければよいのかといった戸惑いが見られた。次第にミーティングに慣れてくると，参加スタッフは，各患者の話に共感し，スタッフの意見を患者に伝えることができるようになるなど，介入に余裕がでてきた。各患者は，他の患者の発言に耳を澄まし，理解しようとする意識が芽生えてきた。今では，患者同士でアドバイスしあい，意見交換するようになっている。

III．症例報告

　ミーティングの中で退院に対する思いを表現したことが一つのきっかけとなり，他患者からのフィードバックを受けながら，9年5カ月ぶりに退院し単身生活になったケースについて報告する。

　Y氏　51才　男性。病名は精神分裂病。20歳代で発症し，当院4回目の入院である。幻聴や対人関係による不安・緊張状態を自覚はしていたが言語化できず，器物破損や大声を出し，後悔しては苛々するといったことを繰り返していた。最近では，激しい行動化はなくなったものの，外泊日程や小遣い管理に関しても細かな指示を受けなければ不安・緊張を呈するようになっていた。もともと単身生活で持ち家もあるY氏には，これまでの間何度か退院の話が出ていた。しかし，具体的に退院の話が持ち上がってくると，いつかは退院したいという本人の願いとは裏腹に，生活の寂しさや金銭・食事管理に対する不安が強くなり，いまひとつ退院に至るきっかけがなかった。

ミーティングの中で他患者より「Yさん，随分良くなったよ」「近頃落ち着いているね」「年を取ってしまわないうちに，一度退院したほうが良いよ」との声掛けがあった。これに対し，「今，外泊を繰り返して退院への準備を考えている」等の経過報告をしたり，「姉さんに上手く気持ちが伝わらない」「一人生活は気ままで良いけど，問題は孤独との付き合いだ」「病院にいたら結構楽しいけど，年をとって退院するのは不安。だめもとで退院するっていうのも一つの方法ですね」と，退院に関する思いをメンバーの中で言語化できていた。

　そして平成13年5月，入院期間9年5カ月目にしてY氏は退院し，病院外来・訪問看護部を中心として，保健や福祉，支援センターが連携したサポート体制のもと，単身生活をはじめることになった。

Ⅳ．考　察

　精神障害予防戦略の三次予防では，障害の軽減と社会復帰・再発予防があげられている。療養病棟の中でも患者にとって，長期入院生活の中で引きこもって他者に依存している状況から，いかに周囲のサポートを受け入れ，自立していくかが大きな課題になっている。

　私たちが行っているミーティングは，いわゆるコミュニティミーティングの一つの形態として位置付けられるものと考えている。私たちは病棟を治療共同体としてとらえ，患者一人ひとりが自立した形で，病気との付き合い方等を身につけていくことに病棟活動の焦点を当てている。

　ミーティングでは，集団の中でサポートを受け，情報交換を行い，自己を振り返るなど，様々な体験がなされる。いずれ地域というコミュニティで生活していくことを前提に考えると，サポートを受け入れ有効利用することが必須であり，その疑似体験としてミーティングの場は意義がある。

　Y氏のケースでは，自分の置かれている状況をミーティングの中で表現し，退院が実現可能かどうかを検討することから，社会復帰への準備が始まった。Y氏自身は他者から「状態が良い」という評価を受け，自分の社会復帰への思いを言語化していった。同時に，他患者の意見を聞くことで自分の現実を見つめなおし，自分一人が悩んでいるのではないことを実感した。そうした病棟コミュニティの中でのやりとり自体が，他者の援助を受け入れ自立していくという，社会復帰を考える上での疑似体験になっていったと思われる。

Ⅴ．終わりに

　療養病棟で患者一人ひとりにとって納得のいく療養生活を送ってもらう為には，工夫が必要である。入院期間が延長するほどに，スタッフに対する依存が高まってしまい，本人・家族に対し，社会復帰を目指したリハビリテーションを展開するには多くのマンパワーが必要となる。療養棟においてもスタッフの充実を図る政策がとられることを強く望みつつ，今後さらに，療養生活での患者さんの生活の質を高め，その人らしく生きていけるような援助を目指したい。

＊福間病院
Shoji Megumi, Furui Hiroaki : Fukuma Hospital.

精神医療におけるインフォームド・コンセントについて
Informed consent in psychiatric practice

古井　博明*

I. はじめに

現在，我が国では，情報化，国際化の流れで，情報開示を求めることを一つの権利として確立しようとする動きがある。情報開示はインフォームド・コンセントと切り離せない関係にある。こうした欧米で発達した医療倫理の考え方は，文化的背景が異なるので理解されにくく，我が国の精神医療の中でまだ十分に消化されていない。しかし，「治療者患者関係はパターナリズムの時代からパートナーシップの時代へ」と言われ，特にインフォームド・コンセントの実践は当然のこととみなされるようになってきた。精神科の予防医学を発展させる上でも，医療倫理に基づいた研究や実践が必要であり，私はこうした精神医療の新しい流れの中でのインフォームド・コンセントの現状と問題点および実践について述べたい。

II. インフォームド・コンセントの現状と問題

最近，カルテ開示の運動が高まり，それに対応して，2000年に，日本精神病院協会（以下，日精協）から「診療情報提供について」という文書が出された。この文書は，我が国のインフォームド・コンセントの現状を如実に示しているものと考えられ，ここで取り上げたい。この文書でも冒頭にインフォームド・コンセントが謳われているが，患者に情報提供を細かく制限している具体的内容との間に一貫性を欠く。まだ我が国では診療情報を提供するにもとまどいがある。アメリカでは，カルテは法的文書としていつ開示されてもよいように整備されているが，日本はまだカルテ開示のシステムは緒についたばかりで，今後，患者に堂々とカルテを開示するようになることが望まれる。日精協の指針はその一里塚であろう。その文書は患者への配慮や用語使用に問題があると思われ，私は，日精協に私見を送付したことがある。以下にその要点を示したい。

1. インフォームド・コンセントの視点

精神医学事典には，インフォームド・コンセントは「十分に説明を受けた後の承諾」とされ，患者は事前に自己決定の為に治療の情報を得る必要がある。説明が先であるはずだが，日精協の文書は既に行われた診療行為に対する情報提供についての条件を述べている。したがって，インフォームド・コンセントについて説明した序文と情報開示の条件を述べた内容との間に矛盾が生じている。診療情報提供という用語が，インフォームド・コンセントと混同されるところがある。

2. コンフィデンシャリティの視点

アメリカの教科書，「Psychiatric Ethics Third Edition」（1999）では，「コンフィデンシャリティ(Confidentiality)とは秘密を守られるものと期待し他者を信用して情報を与えることで，信用(confidence)，告白(confession)，信任(trust)，信頼(reliance)，尊重(respect)，安全(security)，親密(intimacy)，プライバシー(privacy)という用語と密接に関連した言葉である」と定義されている。コンフィデンシャリティという言葉は日本では守秘義務と訳されているが，アメリカではもっと幅広い信頼関係という意味で使われているようだ。当然のことだが，患者の秘密を守るからこそ医師患者間に信頼関係が生まれ，お互い自由に情報交換ができる。日精協の文書は患者のプライバシーを第三者から守るという視点が曖昧だ。患者のプライバシーは徹底して守るという「患者側に

> 資料：患者へのミーティング勧誘文の一部抜粋
> 2病棟の患者さんへ
> 　現在，情報化社会といわれる中で，医療にも新しい動きが見られるようになりました。…インフォームド・コンセントという言葉で表されているように，医師は患者さんが治療の方向性を自分で決定できるように，十分に情報を伝えることが大切だと言われています。そこで，この度，2病棟におきましても，皆様と一緒に治療に取り組むスタイルをとることを目的としたグループ（HPSミーティング）を発足することになりましたので，その主旨をご説明したいと思います。
> 　HPS（Humanistic-Patient-Staff）ミーティングは，患者さんが，自分の病気のことや，治療のこと，入院生活で感じたり考えたりしていることなどを治療スタッフと共に語り合う集団療法です。………ミーティングの主な目的は患者さんが自分の治療について隔週毎に振り返ることです。自分自身の治療プログラムを確認し，それが病棟生活で活用できているかどうかを報告し合います。スタッフは各患者さんの治療プログラムを確認し，2週間の経過を報告します。患者さんはそれに対する意見を述べ，自分の治療目標についてスタッフと相談します。治療情報をスタッフと患者さんが出来るだけ共有し，協力して治療の方向性を決めます。治療スタッフは患者さんがインフォームド・コンセントに基づいた治療を受けられるように援助をします。患者さんは他者から見た自分を知り，「等身大の私」に気付いていきます。そして，このHPSミーティングに出席を重ねていく過程で健康を回復していくことを実感していきます。…………

立つ」姿勢を明確にすべきだろう。

3．カルテの開示の視点

　精神科の場合，カルテ開示は他科と同じにいかない特別の事情がある。「Law and Ethics in the Practice of Psychiatry」（1981年）によると，カルテの中身には時に患者にショックを与える内容もあり，精神科の場合カルテを開示しないこともある。メニンガー・クリニックのDean T. Collinsは「患者の記録は，患者についての情報が記載されているのであるが，必ずしも患者のものとは言えない。その情報は，家族や近所の人など患者以外のところからも集められ，また，医師や看護婦などのスタッフの主観も述べられている。患者が読むことで治療の障害になることもある。しかし，私はできるだけ患者にも読んでもらえるようにしているし，患者の求めがあったらできるだけ開示することにしている」と述べている。患者本人にカルテを開示する場合は，治療を促進するために開示するというというポジティブな姿勢が必要であろう。

III．精神科予防医学における実践

1．一次・二次予防におけるインフォームド・コンセント

　山本はバイオエシックスの4つの基本的原理，①自律尊重原則，②無危害原則，③仁恵原則，④正義原則を紹介しているが，精神疾患の予防もこうした考え方に沿って実践する必要がある。一次・二次予防では，特に病名の告知は難しい問題を引き起こすだろう。精神疾患は，決してガンと同じような悪性の疾患ではないが，偏見の問題がある。私は精神疾患の告知においても，主にガン告知等で用いられるBreaking Bad Newsの方法（文献：古井博明：WHOがすすめる Breaking Bad News．精神療法，23；459-467, 1997）は有用であると考える。

2．三次予防におけるインフォームド・コンセント

　我が国の精神医療の課題に，長期入院がある。私は，沈殿化した患者を中心とした開放療養病棟の担当となり，従来主治医と別に行われていた病棟医回診にかえて，インフォームド・コンセントをその主旨にうたったコミュニティミーティングを始めた（資料）。三次予防では，患者の自律性を促進することが，再発を防止することにつながるであろうし，患者への啓蒙も必要となる。

IV．おわりに

　インフォームド・コンセントを中心にした医療倫理を確立することは，予防医学の発展にも不可欠である。治療者患者関係のパートナーシップが成立すれば，患者が自律的に治療に取り組めることで二次，三次予防が円滑化するだろう。医療倫理の確立が，精神疾患に対する偏見を少なくし，「精神障害の予防」を現実のものにすることが出来ることを期待する。

---

*福間病院
　Hiroaki Furui : Psychiatric Department, Fukuma Hospital.

精神分裂病患者の自殺企図因子の検討
―中井の寛解過程モデルによる事例分析を通して―

An examination about risk factors for suicical attempt in schizophrenic patiens
―Using of the Nakai's Remitting Process Model―

松村みゆき*　堤　由美子**　白澤　彰子*

Ⅰ. はじめに

精神科において，患者の自殺を予防することは看護の中で重要な役割であるが，精神分裂病（以下，分裂病と略す）患者においては時に唐突に自殺は行われ予防の困難さが指摘されてきた。しかし，高橋は"従来の報告では，病的体験に支配されて自殺行動に走るといった例が強調されたが，最近の報告では，自殺する症例が幻聴や妄想に支配されて行動を起こすばかりでなく，慢性の経過中に直面するごく現実的な問題が自殺の契機になっている"[2]と述べている。

したがって，分裂病患者の自殺を病的体験の観点からのみ捉えるのではなく，生活上の様々な苦悩の表現として捉えていく必要がある。

そこで今回，分裂病の寛解過程を重視している中井のモデルを用いて，自殺は状況の様々な変化の中で経過によって特有の現れ方をするのではないかという観点から，入院中自殺企図のあった5事例より自殺企図前後の行動について分析し，自殺企図因子について検討したので報告する。

Ⅱ. 研究方法・結果

1）研究対象

平成9年1月から平成10年12月まで分裂病でK病院に入院した86名中，自殺企図のあった5名

2）データ収集

①事例の中井の分裂病寛解過程モデルによる分類

②各事例の自殺企図前後の行動・症状

事例A〜Eについて看護記録より収集した。なお収集項目は，阿保[1]の行動観察項目（1）精神症状，（2）身体症状，（3）特異な言動，（4）日常生活行動，（5）対人関係の5項目であった。

③各事例の自殺企図因子の抽出

中井の分裂病寛解過程モデルへの分類と自殺企図前後の行動・症状に関する記述データを分析し自殺企図因子を抽出した。

3）結果：表1〜表4参照

表1　各事例のプロフィール

	年齢	性別	企図行為
事例A	50歳代	男	窓ガラス割り
事例B	10歳代	女	絞首
事例C	20歳代	女	絞首
事例D	30歳代	女	柵上がり
事例E	20歳代	女	リストカット

Ⅳ. 考　察

事例Aは，幻聴や妄想の内容が直接企図に結びついている。急性期は，幻覚妄想が活発であり特に命令性の幻聴から自殺に到ることから，患者の表情の変化や行動を十分把握し危険防止に努めていく必要がある。事例B・Cは，分裂病による異常体験を多少とも自分という存在に対するもの，苦しみをもたらす症状として捉えるようになった段階で企図が生じた。我々看護者から見れば，精神症状が落ち着いてきてとりあえず急性期を脱したということに一安心してしまいがちである。しかし，この時期の患者の心理状態は，病識とともに不快な身体症状まで出現し心身ともに不安定な状態であることを念頭に置かなければならない。そのために，患者の状態に合わせ身体的苦痛をできるだけ軽減しながら支持的に接し，安心感が持てるように援助していく必要がある。事例Dは，多少とも現実認識ができる段階まで回復したが，逆に自分の置かれている立場への絶望を感じたことから企図が生じた。事例Eは，外泊によって現実的な生活に直面し将来に対する不安が

表2　中井の寛解過程モデルへの分類

	自殺企図発生時の状態	寛解過程モデル
事例A	看護者の問いかけに反応はなく,自分の世界に閉じこもり空笑したり鋭い目つきになり異常体験に左右された行動が著明に見られた。	急性期
事例B	独語があり支離滅裂な多弁状態で,幻聴による不穏が持続し,度重なる幻聴の煩わしさをイライラすると訴えるなど表出行動が認められた。	急性期から臨界期への移行期
事例C	幻覚妄想が持続して,自分は何の病気かと不安を表出し,幻聴の煩わしさから頭痛等身体症状の訴えの表出があった。	臨界期
事例D	身体症状の訴えは見られなかったが,臥床傾向が多く倦怠感を訴えていた。また,他者との積極的な交流は見られなかった。	寛解前期
事例E	部屋で臥床している姿や一人で行動することが見られたが,自ら他者と交流をしたり自発的な行動も見られた。	寛解後期

表3　各事例の自殺企図前後の行動・症状

	収集項目	自殺企図前後	自殺企図後
事例A	精神症状	落ち着きがなく疎通も悪く表情が硬い。空笑がある。	妄想(家がつぶされた)や命令性の幻聴(脱出しろ)を訴えた。
	身体症状	睡眠は中途覚醒がある。	不眠が出現する。
	特異な言動	靴を並べたり,もって歩き回る。眉間にしわを寄せ一点凝視している。	窓の外をにらみつける。もうだめだと訴える。
	日常生活行動	更衣はせず,同じものを着ている。食事は自分で食べるが中断する。	食事は自分で食べるが時間がかかる。個室になり行動制限がある。
	対人関係	看護者の問いかけに返答はせず,同室患者との交流はなく,気にとめることもない。	妄想に関した質問だけして,看護者の質問には曖昧な対応をする。
事例B	精神症状	幻聴(バカバカ),妄想(目が寄らない),独語が持続する。表情はおびえている。	幻聴(口が臭い,豚鼻),妄想(飲むと口が臭くなる),独語は持続している。目は一点凝視している。
	身体症状	不眠　便秘　嘔気	ふらつき　便秘　嘔吐
	特異な言動	大声を出したり泣いたりを繰り返す。イライラする。拒薬が始まる。	大声を出した後泣くことは少なくなる。死にたい,迷惑をかけた,殺してと訴える。
	日常生活行動	食事は徐々に中断し途中で下膳するようになり,拒食が始まる。	食事は付き添い,自分で食べるようになる。個室になり行動制限がある。
	対人関係	看護者に泣きながら抱きつく。	じっと見たまま黙っている。
事例C	精神症状	幻聴(タバコを吸え)や,妄想(神様の試験に落ちた)　独語空笑	幻聴(呪う)や妄想(皆が悪くなったのは私のせいです)　離人感を訴える。
	身体症状	不眠　便秘　頭痛	便秘　頭痛
	特異な言動	頭を叩いたり押さえる。私は何の病気?と訴える。	私は何の病気?の訴え続く。
	日常生活行動	洗面,更衣は声かけで行う。作業療法は集中にかけ途中中断する。	企図前後と変化なかった。
	対人関係	臥床が多く一人こもりがちであった。	企図前後と変化なかった。
事例D	精神症状	幻聴(子供の声がする)	幻聴は持続する。
	身体症状		便秘
	特異な言動	子供が心配です。私がこんな病気だから一緒にいてあげられなくてかわいそう。早く帰りたい。私はいつまでここに居るの,良くなったから帰してと訴える。夜中に洗髪や清拭を始める。	皆に迷惑をかけるから死のうと思ったと話す。
	日常生活行動	倦怠感を訴え臥床が多い。食事は皆に遅れて取りにきた。一人部屋で過ごすことが多く見られた。	設備の都合で転院となる。
	対人関係	話し掛けると曖昧に返答する。	
事例E	精神症状	初回の外泊後からそわそわし,落ち着きがなくなった。	幻聴(〜した方が良い)を訴えた。
	身体症状	嘔気　便秘	不眠　嘔気
	特異な言動	前の夫に会って言返してやりたいと思ったけど会えなかった。母が監視している。	うつ状態です。今後どうなるんだろう。
	日常生活行動	作業療法は自分から参加していた。	作業療法への参加が減った。
	対人関係	過干渉で他患者より拒否されることがあった。	一人で臥床していることが多くなった。

表4　各事例の自殺企図の因子

	寛解過程	自殺企図の因子
事例A	急性期	・被害関係妄想の持続による恐怖・絶望感 ・命令性の幻聴
事例B	急性期から臨界期への移行期	・批判的な幻聴 ・幻聴の持続や身体症状の出現に伴う苦痛
事例C	臨界期	・幻聴妄想による無力感 ・病識の出現に対する不安感 ・身体症状の不安感
事例D	寛解前期	・将来に対する不安感 ・罪意識 ・長期入院生活による焦燥感
事例E	寛解後期	・現実生活への直面による不安感 ・将来に対する不安感

増したことから企図が生じた。"分裂病の自殺のうち65%が寛解期に生じた"[2)]と報告があるように看護者の注意が必要な時期であると言える。

以上,5事例の自殺企図の生じる背景を検討して,患者の苦悩が減少するにつれ逆に社会的存在としての苦悩が増大し,そのいずれの苦悩も患者にとっては耐え難いものであるということがわかった。看護者は,どちらかと言えば患者の病的苦悩のほうばかりに関心が奪われやすい傾向があるように見受けられる。しかし,患者は回復過程の各段階における症状の変化と生活現象との相互作用の中で常に激しい不安や絶望,無力感,孤独感を体験しているという事実を認識し,それらに対する看護者としての感受性を発揮しながら患者にかかわり自殺予防に努めていく必要がある。

V. まとめ

各期の自殺企図の発生因子は,①急性期は幻覚妄想など異常体験によるもの,②臨界期は病識の出現によるもの,③寛解前期は将来に対しての不安によるもの,④寛解後期以降は社会的出来事によるものであることが示唆された。

したがって,分裂病の自殺は,回復過程における生活上の様々な苦悩の結果として生じており,看護者は回復過程のそれぞれの段階で自殺に到ろうとする苦悩を了解しながら予防していく必要がある。

引用文献

1) 阿保順子:精神科看護の方法,医学書院,東京,p.71-78, 1995.
2) 高橋祥友:自殺の危険,金剛出版,東京,p.61-73, 1992.

*鹿児島大学医学部付属病院
　Miyuki Matsumura, Shouko Shirosawa : Kagoshima University Hospital.
**鹿児島大学医学部保健学科
　Yumiko Tsutsumi : School of Health Science, Faculty of Medicine, Kagoshima University.

仙台市精神保健福祉総合センターの電話相談における精神医学相談の実態について

Actual condition of telephone counseling carried out by Sendai City Mental Health and Welfare Center

林　みづ穂*　　滝井　泰孝*

I. はじめに

仙台市精神保健福祉総合センターでは，平成11年6月から専用回線による電話相談を開始した。このうち毎週金曜日の午前10時から正午を「精神医学相談」と設定し，精神科医が相談に応じている。全国の精神保健福祉センターのうち，電話相談に精神医学相談専用の時間帯を設け，医師が担当することを広報しているのは，当センター以外には3か所のみである。開始から約2年を経たこの「精神医学相談」の実態を調査したので報告する。

II. 対象・方法

当電話相談中「精神医学相談」につき，記録や聞き取りにより件数及び内容を調査した。

III. 結果及び考察

1) 月別相談件数

月別相談件数は3件から23件にわたり(平均11.5件)，市政だよりや情報誌などにおける広報が行われた後増加する傾向が認められる。

2) 相談者の性別

相談者の性別は，男性が42%，女性が52%と，女性の方が若干多い。何も語らずに切れ，性別の判別が困難であった場合は「不明」とした。電話相談の相談者の性別は女性が多いとの報告が石原らをはじめ多く認められているが，当相談でも同様の結果が得られた。これは，相談時間帯が，主婦をはじめとする女性に利用されやすいためと考えられる。

3) 相談者の年齢

相談者の年齢は10歳代から60歳代にわたり，30歳代をピークに20歳代，40歳代の順となっている。20歳代から40歳代が相談の7割を占めていたのは，青年期における自我同一性の確立のための模索や，中年期の自己の再構築，更に，子育てに際し，親としての自分自身の問題や子供の問題行動などが，相談を利用する動機となりやすいためと推察される。

4) 相談種別件数

相談件数は254件で，そのうち特に疾病・医療についての精神医学的知識を要するものを対象とする医学相談は約7割の168件，それ以外の一般相談は71件であった。

5) 対象者

相談対象者及びその中の医学相談の対象者とも，本人が約7割，家族が約3割であった。また，その他として友人やメル友などに関する医学相談もみられた。

6) 加療歴

医学相談168件中，加療中及び加療歴のあるものは約6割を占めていた。このうち，加療中の症例は80件(うち通院74件，入院6件)，加療歴のある症例は17件であった。

7) 相談時間

相談時間は，10分から20分をピークに10分以内，20分から30分の順となっているが，原則として相談員側からは電話を切らないため，60分以上に及ぶ相談も6件みられた。

8) 対応内容

対応内容としては「助言」が一番多く約4割を占めており，次いで「傾聴」が約3割，「情報提供」が約2割となっている。「情報提供」71件中，医療機関に関する情報提供を行ったのは34件であった。

9）医学相談の内容

医学相談の内容としては，医療的関わりのある例では，主治医に話を聞いてもらえない・医師の診断が間違っていると思う（精神分裂病と言われているが鬱病ではないかなど）・薬が合わない・治療の意味合いがわからないなどの医療に対する不満や，入院中の処遇に対する不満，患者に対する対応法を知りたい・再発かと不安であるなどといった医学的観点に基づく説明の希望が聴かれた。また，医療的関わりがないと推察された例では，病気かどうか知りたい・病院に行きたいので情報が欲しいなどの医療に関する情報提供の希望や，精神病の遺伝について知りたい・問題行動のある家族や知人に対する対応法を知りたいといった，医学的診断や医療・対応の実際に関する説明の希望が聴かれた。

10）当電話相談の特徴

電話相談の特徴として，簡便性，匿名性，一回性の3点がしばしば指摘される。すなわち，いつでもどこからでも，プライバシーを守ったまま，相談者に主導権のある1回限りの関わりを展開することができる。これらに加え，当相談では，現在の主治医との関係性を損なうおそれがないという特徴が挙げられる。加療中の症例では，疑問を投げかけると主治医との関係が損なわれるのではないかとのおそれが多く聴かれるが，疾患や治療などに関して疑問や不安を抱きながらも主治医に尋ねるのがはばかられるとき，主治医との関係性を損なうことなく質問が可能であることは，当相談の大きな利点といえよう。

11）当電話相談の役割

医療的関わりがない例では，医療に関する種々の情報提供の希望が聴かれ，また，対応内容の中の「情報提供」では，医療機関に関する情報提供すなわち医療への「つなぎ」が約半数を占めていた。このように，当相談は医療への窓口としても機能している。更に，相談員が医師であるため，電話による情報の限界を考慮しながらも，疾患の可能性や緊急性などを推測し，医学的情報として伝えることができる利点がある。医療の必要性を相談者に再確認させる役割も当相談は果たしており，これは一般の相談にはないものといえよう。また，疑問を投げかけることで主治医との関係を損なうのではとの相談には，不安や疑問を主治医に伝えても関係性は損なわれない旨を伝え，不満の原因や疑問点などを整理して主治医への伝え方を考える援助をすることで，不安が軽減されているようである。また，加療歴の有無に関わらず医学的知識に基づいた情報に対する需要は多く，その提供も当相談の大きな役割の一つと考えられる。更に，簡便性，匿名性，一回性，主治医との関係性を損なわないといった特徴から，医療側からは見えにくい相談者の不安や不満や疑問を知ることができる面もある。

今後も，精神科医が担当しているという特徴を生かした，精神保健福祉センターにおける精神医学電話相談の役割を果たしていきたいと考えている。

---

*仙台市精神保健福祉総合センター
Mizuho Hayashi, Yasutaka Takii : Sendai City Mental Health and Welfare Center.

電話相談による自殺予防活動に関する統計的評価
―日本における自殺急増前後の比較―

Statistical assessment of telephone counseling service for suicide prevention in Japan

影山　隆之*

Introduction

Telephone counseling (TC) is one of the typical approaches for suicide prevention. In the case of Japan, Inochi No Denwa (IND) is the most popular, nationwide TC service for this purpose ; i.e. 46 telephone centers of IND received 624,558 calls in 1998, and 4.6% of them were suicidal calls[1]. However, only a little evidence for the effectiveness of TC has been available. The effectiveness of TC has been measured with suicide mortality, counselor performance, counselor satisfaction, caller satisfaction, change in callers' knowledge or behavior, caller compliance with counselor recommendation, utilization and reutilization rates, change in callers' suicidal thought during the calls, etc.[2,4]. The author proposed a new method to statistically assess the activity of TC service[3], and concluded that little effect of IND on suicide prevention for middle-aged/elderly men can be expected because IND was mainly working for suicidal calls from the young women.

Then, the suicides in Japan suddenly increased in 1998, and the high suicide mortality has continued for three years. We therefore applied the above method to the statistics in 1998, comparing the IND activity in 1998 with that in 1995.

Method

Suppose that the annual number of suicide deaths among a gender-age group in Japan was n_1, and then it decreased to n_2 because IND succeeded to prevent the suicide of k persons per year ; $n_2 = n_1-k$ … (a). On the other hand, we can suppose that the social need for suicide prevention in a gender-age group was proportional to the potential number of suicide deaths (n_1) in this group. If IND received x calls in this year from the suicidal callers belonging to the above gender-age group, therefore, we can assume that the ratio of x to n_1 is an activity index of IND to the need for suicide prevention in this group. Put $p = x/n_1$. If the value of k is sufficiently low (this is true as shown below), p approximates x/n_2 … (b). Based on the vital statistics (Ministry of Health and Welfare, Japan) and the IND statistics[1] in 1998, p value ($= x/n_2$) was calculated for each gender-age group, and compared with the values in 1995. IND workers estimated the age of callers, although this estimation was impossible for 29.1% of all the calls. Since the calls from children aged 9 years or younger are very rare, the callers categorized into "elementary school students" were assumed to be 10 years or older.

Results

As shown in Table, activity index (p) exhibited higher values in women than in men regardless of age. Among women, it was particularly high in those aged 49 years or younger. In the case of men, it was relatively high in those aged 39 years or younger. The distribution of p among gender-age groups in 1998 was similar to that in 1995, except for the women aged 10-19 years.

Discussion

The efficiency of suicide prevention per suicidal

call (q) in a gender-age group can be expressed as follows ; $q = k/x$. Substituting $k = qx$ for equation (a), $n_1-n_2 = qx$ ⋯(c). According to (b), $x = pn_2$, ∴ $n_1-n_2 = qpn_2$, Namely $n_2/n_1 = 1/(1+pq)$ ⋯(d). The left side of (d) obviously shows the effectiveness of suicide prevention for this gender-age group. When p shows sufficiently low value, the right side of (d) approximates 1, regardless of q value, meaning no effect on suicide prevention can be expected.

Although the number of suicides in Japanese men is twice greater than that in Japanese women, IND functioned mainly for young women in 1998. This tendency was similar to that in 1995 or before[4], in spite of dramatic increases in suicide among middle-aged and old men in 1998. It was impossible for IND to take responsibility for suicide prevention for men aged 40 years or older or for women aged 50 years or older. If IND continues to aim at preventing suicide, its strategy should be reorganized. First, it should be discussed whether TC is an adequate approach to respond to the mental health needs of middle-aged or old men. Second, it should be decided whether IND focuses on the youths or young women only. Third, the aim of IND (suicide prevention) should be clearly shown to the general public and to callers. The percentage of suicidal calls (4.6%) is too low. Since many kinds of TC are available today, the characteristics of IND should be clarified.

Table Activity index (p) of IND by gender-age group in 1998 and 1995

Gender Age (yrs)	Men (1998)	(1995)**	Women (1998)	(1995)**
10-19	0.70	0.76	2.19	1.44
20-29	1.02	1.00	2.85	3.05
30-39	0.97	1.02	3.41	2.71
40-49	0.27	0.30	1.80	1.10
50-59	0.07	0.10	0.69	0.45
60-69	0.02	0.04	0.24	0.32
70+	0.01	0.01	0.04	0.04
Overall*	0.34	0.40	1.17	0.97

*This category includes the calls from the clients whose age was unreported.
**See ref. 3.

References

1) Federation of Inochi-no-Denwa : Statistics of telephone counseling. 1998. (in Japanese)
2) Hornblow, A. R. : The evolution and effectiveness of telephone counseling services. Hospital Comm. Psychiat., 37 ; 731-733, 1986.
3) Kageyama, T., Naka, K. : A new approach to assess a suicide prevention program by telephone counseling, Inochi-no-Denwa : quantitative analysis based on telephone statistics and vital statistics. Jpn. J. Mental Health, 12(2) ; 23-32, 1997. (in Japanese)
4) Mishara, B., Daigle, M. : Intervention style with suicidal callers at two suicide prevention centers. Suicide & Life-Threaten. Behav., 25(2) ; 261, 1995.

*大分県立看護科学大学
Takayuki Kageyama : Department of Mental Health & Psychiatric Nursing, Oita University of Nursing & Health Sciences.

精神疾患の一次，二次予防を目的としたこころの検診
―ストレスドックより―

Medical examination as primary and secondary prevention in psychiatric disorders
-From the results of "stress dock"-

野田　哲朗* 　谷　美加* 　夏目　誠**

I．はじめに

　急速に進行する社会・産業構造の変化は不適応者の増加をもたらし，従来精神障害者の社会復帰に主眼が置かれてきた精神保健福祉施策において，ストレス対策を含むこころの健康づくりが求められるようになった。こうしたニーズを受けて大阪府立こころの健康総合センターは1994年の開設当初からストレス対策事業を実施してきた。
　事業の一つである「ストレスドック」は個人のストレスを測定し，適切なストレスマネジメント法の援助を行い，精神疾患の一次，二次予防を目的とするものである。
　今回はストレスドック受検者の特性を分析し，意義と課題について論じる。

II．対象と方法

　1994年10月から2000年3月末までにストレスドックを受検した2900名（男性1513名，女性1387名）を対象とした。平均年齢（mean±SD）は40.9±11.4歳（男性41.8±10.4歳，女性40.0±12.5歳）であった。ストレスドックは月曜日・水曜日の午後1時から5時半の時間帯に行う。概要は以下のとおりである。

1．ストレス度測定検査
1）質問票による検査
　ストレッサー：ライフイベント（夏目），日常苛立ち事尺度（宗像），ストレス反応：一般精神健康質問調査（GHQ-60項目），性格傾向・行動パターン：東大式エゴグラム（TEG），タイプA行動パターンスクリーニング（前田）の他に，対処行動（宗像）やソーシャルサポート（Sarason et al），KAST（久里浜式アルコール依存症スクリーニング・テスト）などを用いた。

2）精神生理学的検査
　脳波，眼球運動・顔面表情筋を中心としたポリグラフ，心電図R-R間隔変動係数（CVr-r），事象関連電位である後期陽性波（P300），随伴陰性変動（CNV）を測定した。

3）血液検査
　ライフスタイルに焦点をあて，血中γ-GTP，コレステロール，HDL，尿酸値，血糖値，ヘモグロビンA_1cの測定を行った。

2．心理・医師面接
　心理面接では心理技師，保健婦が受検者の生育歴，家族関係，親子関係，生活環境，職場環境などを半構造化した面接により聴取した。
　医師面接では質問票，精神生理学的検査，心理面接により得られたデータをもとにストレスへの気づきを促すとともに，精神疾患の有無の把握を行い，必要に応じてさらなる検査および治療の勧奨を行った。

3．セミナー
　受検者全員のストレス度測定検査と心理・医師面接の終了後，ストレスについての講義と自律訓練法の実習を行うセミナーを行った。

4．判定会議
　受検者のデータをもとに，従事スタッフ（医師，心理技師，検査技師，保健婦，看護婦）による判定会議を行い，ストレス状態を判定し，検査

表 ドックでの疾患の把握率と精神科・心療内科での未治療割合

ICD-10に基づく診断	把握割合(%)	未治療割合(%)
F0 症状性を含む器質性精神病	0.3	80.0
F1 精神作用物質使用による精神行動障害	2.6	81.1
F2 精神分裂病・分裂病型・妄想障害	1.2	20.0
F3 気分障害	5.9	33.7
F4 神経症性・ストレス関連・身体表現性障害	33.7	59.5
F5 生理的・身体的要因に関連した行動障害	5.4	79.1
F6 成人の人格・行動障害	4.7	41.6
F7 精神遅滞	0.0	100.0
F8 心理的発達の障害	0.1	100.0
F9 小児期・青年期発症の行動, 情緒障害	0.2	50.0

結果を各受検者に郵送した。

III. 結　果

1. 受検者の傾向

ストレスドックで検査可能な人数は年間540名前後で、受検者の性別では、96年度までは女性の方が多いかほぼ同数であったが、97年度以後は男性の占める割合が多くなった。常勤勤労者の割合は、団体のストレスドック利用の増加に伴い、99年度には88.0％となった。

2. ICD-10に従った診断

ICD-10に従って受検者の精神科診断を行ったところ、1625名(56.0％)に診断がついた。「F4神経症性障害、ストレス関連障害および身体表現性障害」が977名(33.7％)と最も多く、「F3気分障害」172名(5.9％)、「F5生理的障害および身体的要因に関連した行動症候群」158名(5.4％)、「F6成人の人格および行動の障害」137名(4.7％)、「F1精神作用物質による精神および行動の障害」67名(2.6％)、「F2精神分裂病、分裂病型障害および妄想性障害」35名(1.2％)、などとなった。

年度毎に疾患を有する受検者の割合を見ると、94年度に受検者の76.4％に疾患を認めたが、団体のストレスドック利用の増加に伴いその後減少し99年度は32.6％となっていた。

3. 精神科, 心療内科治療歴

精神科、心療内科での治療歴が730名(25.2％)に認められた。診断名別にみると「F2精神分裂病、分裂病型障害および妄想性障害」では35名のうち28名(80.0％)、「F3気分障害」172名のうち114名(66.3％)、「F6成人の人格および行動の障害」137名のうち80名(58.4％)、「F4神経症性障害、ストレス関連障害および身体表現性障害」977名のうち396名(40.5％)、「F5生理的障害および身体的要因に関連した行動症候群」158名のうち33名(20.9％)に治療歴が認められた。

IV. ストレスドックの意義と課題

1）「F4神経症性障害、ストレス関連障害および身体表現性障害」が受検者全体の33.7％を占め、そのうち約60％は精神科・心療内科での治療歴がなく、早期発見、治療勧奨が行えた。

2）「F2精神分裂病, 分裂病型障害および妄想性障害」は、全受検者の1.2％であり約80％に治療歴があり、セカンドオピニオンの役割を担った。

3）ストレスドック利用団体の増加に伴い、健康・半健康の勤労者を対象としたストレスマネジメントを援助することによって精神疾患の一次予防の試みが行えた。

4）受検者のストレッサーとして職場の問題、家族の問題、夫婦間暴力、虐待、アルコール問題など、様々な問題が把握され、今後一層受検者の幅広いニーズに応える必要がある。

5）利用団体の増加に伴い、団体の予約でかなり年間予約数が埋まるため、精神科受診に抵抗のある一般受検者層の身近な相談窓口としての機能が低下していることが考えられる。

---

*大阪府立こころの健康総合センター
　Tetsuro Noda, Mika Tani : Osaka Prefectural Mental Health and Welfare Center.
**大阪樟蔭女子大学
　Makoto Natsume : Osaka Shoin Women's University.

U市職員に対するメンタルヘルスケア

Mental health care to the U-city office personnel

衛藤　進吉*

U市役所職員(3,900人，2000年4月現在)のメンタルヘルスケア活動の一つとして，職員が気兼ねなく利用できるように市庁舎外の場所で，1996年1月より月1回ストレス相談室を開いている。個人的な予約により30分から60分の時間枠で面接を受け付けている。

現在のU市職員のメンタルヘルスケア体制は，従来の庁舎外ストレス相談室に加えて，庁舎内ストレス相談室を開き，それにカウンセリングを加えて，いろんな側面から対応できるようにしている。

I．対象と方法

1996年1月より，2000年12月までの5年間に庁外ストレス相談室で行った市役所職員の精神保健相談事例90人(全職員の約2.3%)(相談件数154件)を対象とした。

方法は，対象事例の面接記録，その後，病院での治療につながった事例では，その臨床経過の記録を用いて，職場のメンタルヘルス活動の問題点を検討した。

II．結　果

1．相談者の内訳

相談者は，圧倒的に本人が多く72%を占めていた。問題者の性別(154相談件数)では，男性が66%，女性34%であった。問題者の年齢分布は，20代から30代の若年職員が65%を占めていた。

2．相談者の主訴

相談者の主訴を個人的問題，職場内問題，個人・職場内問題，家庭内問題に分類した。個人・職場内問題が46%(91件)と一番多く，ついで個人的

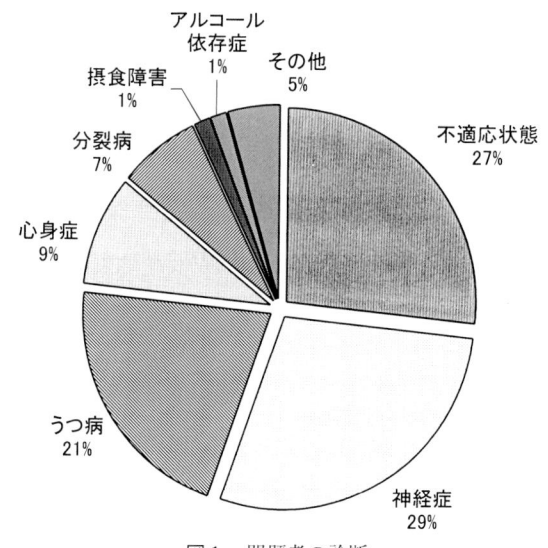

図1　問題者の診断

問題26%(52件)，職場内問題15%(29件)，家庭内問題13%(25件)であった。そのうち，職場内問題と個人・職場内問題の比率は2000年で全体の77%を占め，職場不適応を引き起こす職場側の要因が強まっている。

3．相談者の診断

最も多かったのが神経症圏(29%)であり，次いで不適応状態(27%)，うつ病(21%)，心身症(9%)，分裂病(7%)であった。(図1)

4．相談事例の治療歴

相談者のうち，外来通院歴のある者は，50%と半数を占めていた。通院して服薬しているが主治医がよく話を聞いてくれないので，じっくり話を聞いてほしいという希望で利用する職員が多かった。治療歴のない者は42%で，約4割の相談者は，精神科的相談は初めてであった。

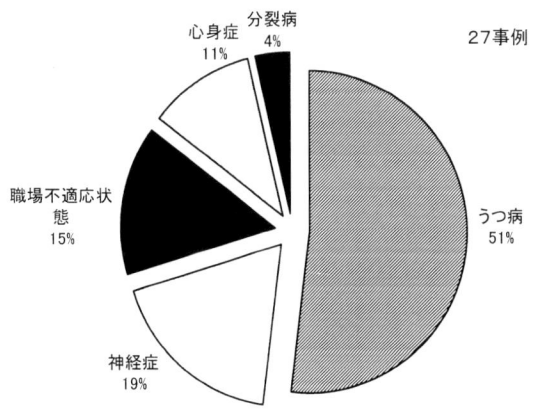

図2　職場異動とメンタルヘルス（27事例）

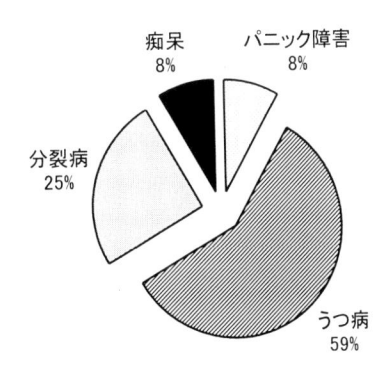

図3　医療機関を診断したケース（12事例）

5．相談事例の来所状況

90相談者のうち，80％（72人）は1回のみの相談で終わっている。2回の相談を行った事例が9人（10％）であった。3回以上の相談を行った事例は9人（10％）いた。これらの事例では精神療法的関与が行われた。

6．職場異動とメンタルヘルス

メンタルヘルス問題が職場異動と関連している職員は，問題者の30％（27人）を占めていて，職場異動が精神保健問題の大きな要因となっている。問題の内訳をみると，うつ病14人（51％），神経症5人（19％），職場不適応状態4人（15％），心身症3人（11％）となっていた。とりわけ，うつ病の発生が一番多い。（図2）

7．相談者への対応

これまで治療歴がなく，医療機関での専門的治療をすすめた相談ケースは全問題者の13％（12人）あり，そのすべてが医療機関を受診し治療を受けるようになった。その内訳は，うつ病7例（59％），分裂病3例，パニック障害1例，痴呆1例であった。（図3）

Ⅲ．考　察

ストレス相談事例では，問題者（90人）の30％（27人）が職場異動と関連してメンタルヘルス上の問題が生じていた。U市役所職員においては職場異動が大きなストレス要因となっている。そのうち，うつ病事例が半数（51％）を占めていることから，職場の精神保健ではうつ病の問題がとりわけ重要である。

5年間で全職員の約2.3％に相当する職員90人が庁舎外ストレス相談室を利用した。そのうち全相談者の13％（12人）は医療機関に紹介し，専門的治療を受けることができた。ストレス相談室が医療機関への橋渡しの重要な機能を果たしていた。とりわけ，うつ病の早期発見・早期治療に役立っていた。

Ⅲ．まとめ

1）相談ケース90事例のうち，メンタルヘルス問題が職場異動と関連のある職員は問題者の30％（27事例）を占め，職場異動が精神保健上の大きな問題となっている。

2）医療機関に紹介したケースは12例あり，全相談者の13％を占めていた。その全てが医療機関を受診し，治療を受けている。このことは庁舎外ストレス相談室が，医療機関での専門治療の必要な相談者に対して，医療機関への橋渡しの役割を果たしている。

3）医療機関を紹介した12例のうち，7例（59％）がうつ病であった。このことはうつ病が職場のメンタルヘルス上重要な問題であり，職員の自発的なストレス相談がうつ病の早期発見・早期治療，自殺予防に役立っている。

---

*上都賀総合病院精神神経科
　Shinkichi Eto : Department of Neuro-Psychiatry, Kamitsuga General Hospital.

全国の自治体職場におけるメンタルヘルス状況と対策の実態
Actual condition of mental health in the local government workshop in Japan

吉岡　伸一[*,**]　　永田　耕司[*,***]　　内田　江里[*]　　上野　満雄[*]

Ⅰ．はじめに

　我が国では最近,自殺者が年間で3万人を超え[1]、また地方公務員の在職死亡原因として自殺は悪性新生物,心疾患に次いで第3位に位置するようになっている。職場内のストレスも増加し,メンタルヘルス対策やメンタルヘルスケアシステムの構築が急がれている。そこで今回,全国の自治体職場のメンタルヘルスの状況や対策,評価等の実態を明らかにし,これからの対策を講じるためにアンケート調査を実施したので報告する。

Ⅱ．対象と方法

　平成11年6月に結成された自治体労働安全衛生研究会職場のメンタルヘルス対策プロジェクトチームにより,88の設問からなる職場のメンタルヘルス対策のための調査票を作成した。平成12年4月に全国3,295単組(全道庁支部14,都庁職局支部・区職労25を含む),及び調査に協力を得た全国消防職員協議会(全消協)168組織に調査票を配布した。回収された調査票をもとに,各職場のメンタルヘルス状況や対策,その評価等の実態について集計・解析を行った。

Ⅲ．結　果

　回収集計されたアンケートは1,495(45.4％),全消協99(58.9％),全体で1,594(46.0％)であった。そのうち団体記載などの記入漏れを除く1,575(45.5％)を有効回答とした。以下の解析には全消協を除いた結果を用いた。
　団体区分別回収数は,都道府県67,政令市18,特別区2,市371,町村779,一部組合117,公社・事業団60,社協20,国保21,民間企業30,市町村共済29,その他30,臨時・非常勤31であった。職員数で記載があったのは1,533で平均職員数は676人,回答組合の職員の合計は1,043,760人であった。
　職場のストレスが「増えている」と回答したのは85.0％で,逆に「減っている」と回答したのはわずかに0.1％であった。職場のストレス要因で「増えているか」で最も高かったのは「業務の量のストレス」78.9％,次いで「業務の質のストレス」77.2％,「人員削減に関すること」68.9％,「職場の人間関係のストレス」50.8％,「賃金カットなど待遇に関すること」50.5％であった。
　職員の健康状況や職場の雰囲気については,「身体疾患以外で長期に休む職員の増加」が36.7％,「体調不良を訴える職員の増加」60.0％,「職場の雰囲気の悪化」43.2％,「自殺者の増加」8％であった。ちなみに記載のあった回答のうち過去5年間の自殺者の合計は431名であった。
　メンタルヘルス対策については20.1％のみが実施し,8割近くが「実施していない」と回答していた。特に民間では9割以上が「実施していない」と回答していた。メンタルヘルス対策の実施主体は,人事関連部課係が40.5％と最も高く,次いで安全衛生(非専門)部課係24.1％,安全衛生専門部課係16.5％,労働組合7.0％,組合・人事一緒に4.3％であった。実施している具体的な内容は,「内部に相談窓口をつくる」133件,次いで「職員の研修会・講習会を実施する」114件であった。メンタルヘルス対策の実施に関する労使間の協議については,「安全衛生委員会等」が24.5％,「団体交渉」が11.9％で,「労使協議は行われていない」が60.7％を占め,多くが協議されていなかった。
　職場のメンタルヘルスケアについて「うまくいっている」と回答したのはわずか5.0％で,「うま

くいっていない」が38.9％，「どちらともいえない」が56.0％であった。メンタルヘルスケアのなかで「うまくいっている」取り組みとしては，「主治医の意見が復帰時尊重」が31.8％，「職場復帰に同僚の理解」28.6％，「管理職が職場復帰に理解」24.6％であった。一方，「うまくいっていない」取り組みとしては「業務量の偏りをなくす」が44.0％と圧倒的に多かった。確保されているメンタルヘルスケアのスタッフは産業医が17.4％と最も多く，次いで保健婦16.4％で，カウンセラーは3.6％，選任職員は2.0％と少なかった。うまくいっているメンタルヘルス対策の最も大きな理由としては，「職員間の交流が活発」34件，「主治医の意見が復帰時尊重される」21件，「復帰について同僚の理解」21件，「キーパーソンになる組合仲間がいる」17件であった。

メンタルヘルスケアのために現在実施しているもので最も多かったのは「相談窓口を設置」が10.7％，次いで「軽減・リハビリ・慣らし勤務など」8.4％，「健診の事後指導でよろず相談」7.6％，「啓発パンフレットの作成」7.0％，「精神科・産業・主治医連携で復職検討」6.9％の順であったが，ほとんどの職場でメンタルヘルス対策は実施されていなかった。

Ⅳ．考　察

今回の調査から，全国の自治体職場の8割以上においてストレスが増加していることが示された。職場のストレス要因としては，業務の量と質がほとんどで，人員削減，職場の人間関係に関するものも多かった。働く者のストレスの増加要因として，職務のOA化，職場構成者の高年齢化，情報化の進展，女性の職場進出，家庭内の変化，企業のリストラ傾向などが指摘されている[2]。今回の調査結果からも，人員削減などによる業務の量のストレスの増大，配置転換やテクノストレス等によって業務の質のストレスや仕事への適正ストレスの増大が引き起こされていると考えられる。さらには職場内の人間関係の悪化も生じてきていると考えられる。

職場でのメンタルストレス対策の実施は約2割で，うまく機能している職場は5％にすぎなかった。具体的な内容としては，内部に相談窓口を作る，職員の研修会・講習会の実施が多かった。うまくいっているメンタルヘルスケアの内容として，復帰時の主治医の意見尊重，同僚や管理職の理解が多かった。メンタルヘルスケアのためには，職場での同僚や管理職の理解の必要性やそのための健康教育や研修が必要と考えられる。

調査したほとんどの職場でメンタルヘルス対策の実施がなく，また対策のために確保されたスタッフとしても産業医，保健婦が多く，カウンセラーや専任職員は少なかった。メンタルヘルスの推進には，上級管理者・人事担当者の理解と関心，職場内でカウンセラーやメンタルヘルス推進のキーパーソンの育成，嘱託に専門医の設置などがあげられている[2]。各組合がメンタルヘルス対策にあたる嘱託のスタッフを専属，もしくは広域で雇用するなどの対策が必要であると考えられる。

今回の調査から身体疾患以外で長期に休む職員や体調不良を訴える職員の増加，職場の雰囲気の悪化に加え，自殺者が増加している回答が多かった。今後，継続的かつ各職場に応じた柔軟なメンタルヘルス対策を進めていくことが重要であることが示唆された。

文　献

1) 厚生の指標，国民衛生の動向，47(9)；(財)厚生統計協会，東京，2000.
2) 藤井久和：職場における精神保健活動．総合臨床，49(12)；3056-3062，2001.

＊自治労職場のメンタルヘルス対策プロジェクト
　Shin-ichi Yoshioka, Koji Nagata, Eri Uchida, Mitsuo Ueno : Mental health countermeasure group of JICHIRO.
＊＊鳥取大学医学部神経精神医学
　Shin-ichi Yoshida : Department of Neuropsychiatry, faculty of Medicine, Tottori University.
＊＊＊長崎大学医学部公衆衛生学
　Koji Nagata : Department of Public Health, Nagasaki University School of Medicine.

児童養護施設における心理学的援助について

Psychological support for abused and school-refusing children in the residential facility

植田　聡美* 　　橋口　浩志* 　　三山　吉夫*

　近年，子どもと家庭を取り巻く環境は大きく変化しており，養護施設への児童の入所理由，児童福祉に対する家庭や社会からの要請は多様化する傾向にある。

　宮崎県では平成10年度から12年度まで「不登校児童特別指導モデル事業」を県立の児童養護施設であるA学園で実施した。児童養護施設に，臨床心理士，精神科医が配置されるのは，本県では初の試みであった。今回，カウンセラーという立場でA学園を訪問した3年間の経験を振り返り，児童養護施設の現状と心理士の活動について考察した。

　主として児童・思春期の子どもを支援する児童福祉施設には以下のようなものがある。

名称	対象・目的	設置数（全国/宮崎県）
児童養護施設	保護者のいない児童，虐待されている児童，その他環境上養護を必要とする児童を入所させて，養護するとともにその自立を支援する	553/9
児童自立支援施設	不良行為を行ない，または行なうおそれのある児童及び家庭環境等の理由により生活指導を要する児童を入所させ，個々の児童の状況に応じて必要な指導を行なうとともに，その自立を支援する	57/1
情緒障害児短期治療施設	不登校児をはじめ情緒障害児の入所及び通所による治療を行なう（臨床心理士が常勤）	17/0（九州では熊本に1施設）

　今回のモデル事業では，不登校児だけでなく被虐待児も対象とした。A学園は定員50名，平成12年9月時の入所児童は46名であった（男子28名女子18名）。そのうち不登校を事由として措置された子どもは12名，虐待を事由として措置された子どもは3名であった。他にも児童相談所やA学園において虐待が確認されたケースが13例あった。

　A学園はこのモデル事業の目的として「養護施設は不登校への対応という点で有効な資源であり，さらに専門性を高め，有効性を明確にすること」をあげていた。環境を変えること（家庭からの分離，施設入所，転校）や，指導員による登校刺激と集団の力（登校する大多数の他児の影響）といった従来の指導法が通用しない子どもがあらわれたことで，入所児に対する心理的ケアの重要性が認識され，外部の専門家の導入に至ったようである。さらにカウンセラーには，「子どもの心に寄り添う」というスタンスやその上での子どもへの関わり方，集団生活で問題となる行動をどのように理解し援助するかについてなど，指導員の資質向上における役割も期待されていた。

　カウンセラーは臨床心理士3名（筆者を含む），精神科医1名で，基本的には週1回あるいは2週に1回，2時間程度A学園を訪問し，施設側が選定した対象児に個別のカウンセリング（年齢によっては遊戯療法）を行なった。対象児の両親に学園まで足を運んでもらって家族面接を行なったケースもあり，対象児と担当指導員の同席面接という形も試みられた。また，年に2～3回，カウンセラーと指導員によるケース検討を行ない，対象児の面接場面での状態や変化，生活場面における行動などについて情報交換を行なった。カウンセラー，児童相談所，学校，学園指導員など，関係機関合同のケース検討が予定されていたが，全ての関係者が顔を合わせることは困難であった。

　今回カウンセリングを行なったケースは，家族面接も含めて26例であった。継続期間は2カ月～3年と幅があった。筆者が担当したケースは8例で，女性カウンセラーが筆者のみであったため

か，全て女児であった。8例中，施設入所，転校によって不登校が解消され，高校受験にも合格してスムーズに家庭復帰できたのは1例のみであった。言語面接によって自己洞察が進み，成長が感じられたケースも1例あった。その他の不登校事例(3例)では，カウンセリングに導入した後も無断外出や無断外泊といった問題行動が繰り返され，登校できず，不適応状態が続いた。無断外泊からそのまま措置解除となり家庭に戻ったケースもあったが，カウンセラーには事後報告となることが多く，カウンセラーの力量不足と同時に，その機能が有効に活用されなかったと残念に感じることもあった。このようなカウンセラーと学園側とのコミュニケーションのまずさは，初期にはお互いに遠慮があったり，あるいは指導員の勤務体制や事務的な手続きの煩雑さのためであったりとその背景は様々であったが，完全に解決されることはなかったように思う。

不登校ではなかったが個別面接を行なうことで生活場面での行動に変化が見られ，情緒的にも安定したという評価を得たケースもあった。児童養護施設で生活し，行動上大きな問題はない子どもであっても，心理的援助がその子の成長を助けられる部分が多分にあることをあらためて教えられた。大人がその子自身をそのまま尊重し，受け入れ，自己表現する場を確保することの大切さを再確認した。

虐待ケースでは，就学前から遊戯療法を開始したが，小学校入学後，学校場面で落ち着きのなさや衝動性，攻撃的な行動など被虐待児特有の問題行動が出現し，学園でも過去の虐待の再現ともとれるような，年長児から「生意気」と攻撃される立場に自らをおいてしまう不適切な対人関係が見られるようになった。個別面接だけで状況を改善することは難しく，担当指導員に説明や指導を繰り返し行ない，1度は母親と面談する機会ももつことができた。学校の担任へのコンサルテーション的関わりをもてなかったことが不十分であった。

施設指導員の感じたカウンセラー配置による効果として「個別心理面接を行なった児童の問題行動が減少し，情緒的にも安定した」「問題行動の意味や理由，理解するための考え方がわかった」「入所児童に発達障害があったことが初めてわかった」「器質的あるいは精神的な障害についてすぐに相談できる」「同僚には言えない悩みを打ち明けることができた」というものがあった。

筆者が感じた反省と今後の課題としては「カウンセラーと職員との間で十分に意思疎通を図る」「十分に守られた面接室の確保」「対象児の選定，導入の仕方」「大きな問題を示していない児童へのかかわり」「子どもが自分から相談できるシステム，雰囲気作り」「指導員へのコンサルテーション，カウンセリング」「外部機関との連携，外的資源の有効活用」などがあり，これらの課題について臨床心理士が果たせる役割は大きいと考える。

最後になりましたが，貴重な機会を与えてくれたA学園の子ども達，指導員の皆さんに感謝いたします。

---

*宮崎医科大学精神医学講座
Satomi Ueda, Hiroyuki Hashiguchi, Yoshio Mitsuyama : Department of Psychiatry, Miyazaki Medical College.

総合精神保健福祉センターにおける児童虐待家庭への取り組み
Preventive approach to parents with child abuse in a comprehensive mental health center

小川　一夫* 　前田　智子* 　金井　祐美* 　赤松　寛子* 　江畑　敬介**

Ⅰ．目　的

　中部総合精神保健福祉センターにおける相談，特にアルコール・薬物相談においては，児童虐待の問題を併せ持つ事例が少なくない。当センターでは，こうした事例に対して，児童虐待という視点から見直し，特に，親への専門的相談体制を中心とした取り組みを行ってきた。本報告は，これまでの取り組みについて述べるとともに，その意義や今後の課題を明らかにすることを目的とする。

Ⅱ．対象と方法

1．予備調査

　予備調査として，平成10年度における，アルコール・薬物関連問題を主訴とした面接相談者を対象とし，その相談記録を調査した。そのうち児童虐待が認められた事例について，その特徴と虐待の状況を明らかにするとともに，事例の相談開始後の経過・転帰を整理した。

2．新たな取り組み

　予備調査を基に新たな取り組みとして，平成11年度から相談事例検討会を定例化した。平成12年度からは母親を対象として「子育て支援講座」を開始した。また，虐待に悩む親を対象として「医師による専門相談」を実施するとともに，ネットワークによるサポート体制の整備を図った。

Ⅲ．結　果

1）予備調査での児童虐待事例の特徴

　予備調査から，児童虐待事例は安定した家庭生活を送るうえで障害になりうる，以下のような問題をいくつも併せ持っている多問題家族であることがわかった。①予期せぬ妊娠や不本意な出産，②不良な夫婦関係と夫婦間暴力，③親自身の被虐待体験，④借金，頻繁な転職，等である。

2）予備調査での事例の転帰

　予備調査で把握された平成10年度における児童虐待事例は5例であった。このうち，当時虐待として対応できていた事例は2例に限られていた。2例のうち1例はセンターだけでの援助であり，他の1例は関係機関との連携を組んでの対応であった。後者の方が虐待を防ぐためのより効果的対策につながっていた。

3）相談事例検討会

　相談事例検討会における検討事例数は，平成11年度4例，平成12年度8例で，合計12例である。事例の特徴を見てみると，まず相談者については，虐待者本人が4例，虐待者の伴侶が4例，関係機関2例，そして被虐待児（者）本人が2例である。虐待者が精神障害者である場合が7例認められ，その精神障害はアルコール依存4例，薬物依存2例，うつ病1例であった。これら相談事例の転帰としては，一応の解決を見たものが4例，継続中が6例，中断が2例であった。

　事例検討会には，保健所，児童相談所，児童相談センター，子どもの虐待防止センター，子ども発達センターからの参加があった。

4）子育て支援講座

　子育て支援講座は1シリーズ4講座から成り，平成12年度は2シリーズ実施した。各シリーズのプログラムは，第1回「子育ての悩み（1）〜子どもとの暮らしを楽にするには〜」，第2回「子どもの心の育ち」，第3回「子育ての体験から」，第4回「子育ての悩み（2）〜親になるということ〜」のような構成となっている。講座への参加人数は，延べ31人（実人数17人）であった。

5）医師による専門相談

相談事例は2例であった。このうち1例は「子育て支援講座」に参加後，相談を希望したものであった。2例とも生育歴で被虐待体験のある母親であることが共通していた。

6）ネットワークの整備

事例検討会を介して，子どもの虐待防止センター，児童相談所，児童相談センター，保健所，子ども発達センター等と，事例毎に具体的役割分担を明らかにし，ネットワークを整備してきている。

Ⅳ．考　察

総合精神保健福祉センターを訪れる相談者の中には，児童虐待の問題を併せ持つ事例が少なくない。こうした問題を見逃さずに対応するには，相談を受ける際に「虐待の可能性」という視点を持って臨むことが重要であり，このことで早期発見と予防的働きかけの可能性が広がるといえる。虐待が起きていても，当事者は必ずしも虐待であるとの認識はなく，こうした場合相談者の主訴に応えながら，虐待問題を早期に解決していくこととなる。逆に，現に虐待が生じていない場合でも，被虐待体験を持つ親など子どもとの関係に不安を持っている親は少なくなく，心理教育的サポートによって予防的働きかけが可能となる。

児童虐待は多問題家族で起こっていることから，家族を取り巻く多くの関係者（機関）間で連携を組むことが不可欠である。当センターでは，事例検討会を核として関係者（機関）との連携を実践的に図ってきているが，引き続きその整備が必要である。

その際，児童虐待事例の親には精神障害者が少なくないことから，総合精神保健福祉センターの役割としては，特に親の精神面や家族病理に着目した，専門的なアプローチを行うことが重要な役割であると考えられる。これまでに実施してきた個別面接と平行して，グループミーティングの実施も今後の課題である。

---

*東京都立中部総合精神保健福祉センター
Kazuo Ogawa, Tomoko Maeda, Yumi Kanai, Hiroko Akamatsu : Tokyo Metropolitan Chubu Center for Mental Health.
**江畑クリニック
Keisuke Ebata : Ebata Clinic.

中高校生の自尊感情，不安傾向と学校適応状況，親子関係との関連

Self-esteem and anxiety level in junior and senior high school students in relation to school adjustment and parent-child relationships

與古田孝夫* 高倉 実* 赤嶺 依子* 和氣 則江*
名嘉 幸一* 石津 宏* 東風平智江美** 秋坂 真史***

I. Purpose

With a state of mental health and psychosomatic instability, junior and senior high school students are likely to manifest psychological conflicts and school maladjustment[1,2]. The purpose of this study was to examine self-esteem and anxiety level in junior and senior high school students in relation to school adjustment and parent-child relationships.

II. Method

Subjects were 2,903 students who responded to a set of personality questionnaires. Data was collected from randomly selected 6 public junior and senior high schools (3 each) in Naha city, Okinawa, from September to October in 1998. Subjects' self-esteem and anxiety were measured by the Japanese version of Rosenberg Self-Esteem Scale and Spielberger State Anxiety Inventory, respectively. These measures were analyzed by gender, school year, grade, school adjustment, and parent-child relationships using a series of t-test.

III. Results and discussion

The results indicated that self-esteem and anxiety among junior and senior high school students were associated with gender, grade, school adjustment, and parent-child relationships (Table 1). The female students showed lower self-esteem and higher anxiety than the male students (p<.01). High school students showed lower self-esteem and higher anxiety when compared to the junior high school students (p<.01). For junior high school students, the higher the grades, the lower the self-esteem (p<.01) and higher the anxiety (p<.05). In connection with school adjustment (Table 2), low self-esteem and high anxiety were significantly associated with having a negative perception of teacher, no close friends in class, and bad physical conditions. In connection with parent-child relationships (Table 3, 4), positive perception of own

Table 1 Average score of self-esteem and STAI-I among junior and senior high school students Mean (SD)

		self-esteem	STAI-I
Sex	Male	25.32 (4.15)	49.45 (8.60)
	Female	24.08 (0.45)	51.68 (9.16)
School	Junior	24.96 (4.24)	50.07 (8.96)
	Senior	24.19 (3.91)	51.48 (8.95)
Junior high school	1 st grade	25.23 (4.44)	49.70 (9.17)
	2 nd grade	25.10 (4.09)	49.69 (8.50)
	3 rd grade	24.57 (4.17)	50.79 (9.17)
Senior high school	1 st grade	23.85 (3.97)	52.02 (9.08)
	2 nd grade	24.44 (3.88)	50.94 (8.90)
	3 rd grade	24.33 (3.86)	51.39 (8.80)

Mann-Whitney U-test *P<0.05 **P<0.01 ***P<0.001

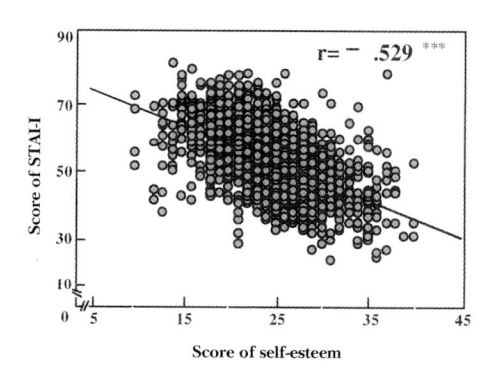

Figure 1 Correlation between self-esteem and STAI-I score

Table 2 Relationship between the consciousness about the school life and self-esteem and STAI-I   Mean(SD)

Contents		Junior high school		Senior high school	
		self-esteem	STAI-I	self-esteem	STAI-I
It is troublesome to go to school	Yes	24.38(4.27) ***	51.69(8.78) ***	23.61(3.84) ***	52.78(8.87) ***
	No	26.08(4.20)	47.05(8.85)	25.16(4.03)	49.25(9.07)
School regulations are strict	Yes	24.78(4.18) **	50.75(8.74) ***	23.65(3.97) ***	52.92(8.83) ***
	No	25.52(4.62)	48.70(9.63)	24.70(4.11)	50.09(9.30)
A teacher forces his thought	Yes	24.67(4.37) ***	51.03(9.29) ***	23.99(3.98) **	52.43(9.38) **
	No	25.89(4.36)	48.05(8.87)	24.56(4.27)	50.15(9.49)
The condition of the body is bad	Yes	23.63(4.21) ***	53.95(8.99) ***	23.14(3.80) ***	55.10(8.76) ***
	No	26.15(4.17)	46.57(8.33)	25.25(4.13)	47.72(8.61)
A good friend is in the class	Yes	25.20(4.23) ***	49.60(8.87) ***	24.27(3.92)	51.35(8.85)
	No	23.70(4.66)	53.71(9.79)	23.85(4.00)	50.90(10.81)

Mann-Whitney U-test **P<0.01 ***P<0.001

Table 3 Relationship between the consciousness about the father and self-esteem and STAI-I   Mean(SD)

Contents		Junior high school		Senior high school	
		self-esteem	STAI-I	self-esteem	STAI-I
Being manly	Yes	25.38(4.07) ***	49.33(8.88) **	24.56(3.89) ***	50.63(9.03) ***
	No	24.00(5.00)	51.86(9.23)	23.40(4.07)	53.32(9.12)
Doesn't stay at home	Yes	24.49(4.16) **	50.67(9.15) **	23.73(4.05) **	52.33(9.00) ***
	No	25.23(4.34)	49.69(8.85)	24.46(4.04)	50.83(9.35)
A promise is kept well	Yes	25.57(4.13) ***	49.20(8.99) ***	24.49(4.10) ***	50.39(9.41) ***
	No	23.95(4.43)	51.97(9.07)	23.86(3.91)	53.07(9.25)
Being understood me very well	Yes	25.66(4.12) ***	48.57(8.99) ***	24.69(3.77) ***	50.43(9.12) ***
	No	23.77(4.49)	52.09(9.08)	23.29(4.06)	53.63(8.96)
Being collected at home	Yes	25.63(4.14) ***	48.51(8.93) ***	24.69(3.77) ***	50.44(9.36)
	No	24.04(4.45)	52.24(9.17)	23.29(4.06)	53.14(9.03)

Mann-Whitney U-test **P<0.01 ***P<0.001

Table 4 Relationship between the consciousness about the mother and self-esteem and STAI-I   Mean(SD)

Contents		Junior high school		Senior high school	
		self-esteem	STAI-I	self-esteem	STAI-I
Being tender	Yes	25.29(4.19) ***	49.44(8.80) ***	24.43(3.92) ***	50.63(9.03) ***
	No	24.04(4.45)	54.27(10.04)	23.40(4.22)	53.32(9.12)
Doesn't stay at home	Yes	24.72(4.39)	51.10(9.21) *	23.67(4.02)	52.33(9.00) ***
	No	25.10(4.29)	49.80(9.12)	24.30(3.98)	50.83(9.35)
A promise is kept well	Yes	25.36(4.14) ***	49.30(9.07) ***	24.42(3.84)	50.39(9.41) ***
	No	24.15(4.93)	52.26(9.08)	23.78(4.29)	53.07(9.25)
Being understood me very well	Yes	25.48(4.11) ***	49.21(8.95) ***	24.47(3.77) **	50.43(9.12) ***
	No	23.39(4.98)	53.75(9.69)	23.29(4.23)	53.63(8.96)
Parents' relationship is very well	Yes	25.47(4.04) ***	49.10(8.89) ***	24.39(3.96)	50.44(9.36)
	No	23.82(4.71)	52.56(9.49)	23.80(4.09)	53.14(9.03)

Mann-Whitney U-test **P<0.01 ***P<0.001

parents was significantly associated with high self-esteem and low anxiety.

A significant negative correlation was found between scores on self-esteem and anxiety (STAI-I) (r = −.529, p<.001, Figure 1).

Thus, the findings of the present study indicated that the mental health for junior and senior high school students need to be promoted by health education and counseling that take account of students' self-esteem and anxiety. In addition, a comprehensive and collaborative support system by schools and families is essential.

References

1) Herd, F. Jr. : Studying mental illness : a student's perspective. J. Psychosoc. Nurs. Ment. Health Serv., 32(6) ; 20-22, 1994.

2) Poikolainen, K. Kanerva, R. Lonnqvist, J. : Life events and other risk factors for somatic symptoms in adolescence. Pediatrics, 96(1) ; 59-63, 1995.

---

*琉球大学医学部
Takao Yokota, Minoru Takakura, Yoriko Akamine, Norie Wake, Koichi Naka, Hiroshi Ishizu : Faculty of Medicine, University of the Ryukyus.

**琉球大学医学部附属病院看護部
Chiemi Kochinda : Department of Nursing, University Hospital of the Ryukyus.

***茨城大学教育学部
Masafumi Akisaka : Faculty of Education, Ibaraki University.

私立中高等学校における精神科校医としての相談業務と役割について

The role of the psychiatrist in the health care office of a private junior and senior high school

中村　道子[*]　　菅原　道哉[*]　　鈴木　二郎[**]　　中根　晃[*]

I. はじめに

近年子供の精神保健，とりわけ学校精神保健が注目されているが，学校現場で精神科医が校医として相談業務を行っている学校は未だ数少ない。筆者は都内にある一私立中高等学校において精神科校医として，相談業務に携わっている。今回は平成6年6月から5年10カ月の期間の相談業務について，特に初回の来談者と相談内容に注目して報告し，学校保健室における精神科医の業務と役割について考察し，検討する。

II. 対象と方法

この中高等学校は1学年の生徒数は250名であり，全校生徒は1500名の男子校である。今回は5年10カ月の期間に精神科校医が相談に当たったケースについて，初回来談者と相談内容について，相談記録をもとに調査した。プライバシーを守るため，個人が特定できるような情報は記載しないよう留意した。

III. 結果

この5年10カ月の期間に実数として，60名の生徒の相談を受けた。各年度毎の初回来談者は平成6年度においては17名，7年度5名，8年度9名，9年度6名，10年度11名，11年度12名であった。延べ来談者数は平成6年度においては32名，7年度39名，8年度51名，9年度42名，10年度37名，11年度42名であり，年平均41.7名であった。初回来談者としては母親が26名（43%），両親が4組（7%），生徒本人が14名（23%），母親と生徒が1組（2%），教師7名（12%），養護教諭8名（13%）であり（図1），初回来談者の約50%が親で

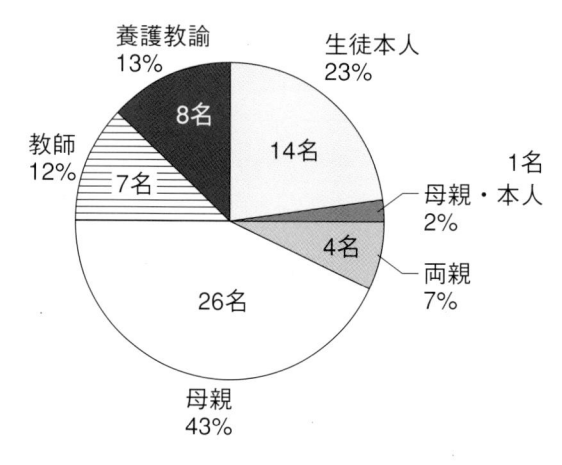

図1　初回来談者

あり，初回から生徒本人が来談したのは25%であった。

初回の相談内容として最も多かったのが，不登校問題であり，24名（41%），腹痛，頻尿，動悸などの心気症状についての相談が6名（10%），人間関係の悩みや対人恐怖についての相談が5名（8%），アイデンティティー，不安についての相談が5名（8%），おちこみ・うつ3名，強迫症状，窃盗，勉強をしない，不眠についてはそれぞれ2名ずつ相談があった。また無気力，眠気，いじめ，集中力低下，けいれん，頭痛，家庭内暴力，過食，成績不振などの相談が各1名ずつであった（図2）。

初回来談時の相談内容を初回来談者別に調べた。生徒本人が来談した14名の相談内容をみると，「周囲の人が恐い」「恐喝を受けた後他人の視線が気になる」「他人が悪口を言っている」など対人恐怖3名（19%），「父親が医師で医学部に進学するつもりで，長時間勉強するが，不安が強

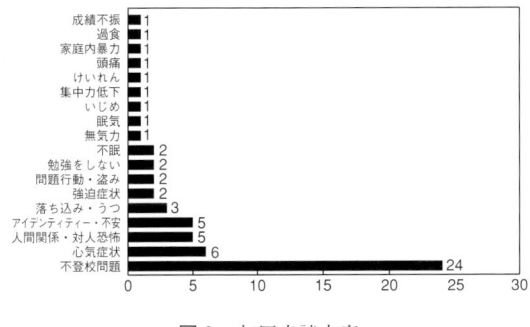

図2　初回来談内容

項目	件数
成績不振	1
過食	1
家庭内暴力	1
頭痛	1
けいれん	1
集中力低下	1
いじめ	1
眠気	1
無気力	1
不眠	2
勉強をしない	2
問題行動・盗み	2
強迫症状	2
落ち込み・うつ	3
アイデンティティー・不安	5
人間関係・対人恐怖	5
心気症状	6
不登校問題	24

い」「試験の時の不安，緊張」などアイデンティティー・不安の相談が2名，抑うつ3名，心気症状，「勉強が手につかない」と集中力低下の相談や，「毎年3月頃になると学校に来たくなくなる」と訴え，不登校問題を相談に来た生徒や強迫症状，不眠，頭痛，けいれんの相談に来た生徒が各1名ずつであった。生徒本人が来談したケースでも，担任教師が予め，養護教諭と打ち合わせを行い，相談を勧め，促してくれたケースが3件あった。次に親が初回来談者であったケース（母親26名，両親4名）の相談内容をみると不登校問題が18名（61%）と多く，次いで心気症状4名，勉強をしないなどの相談があった。不登校で，強迫症状，被害関係妄想が認められたケースは2年の相談の経過のうちに精神科受診し，精神分裂病と診断された。「勉強をしない，部屋がひどく散らかっている，人柄が変わって暗くなった，ゲームばかりしている」という母親からの相談があったケースは本人との面接の中で，幻聴を症状として認め，無断遅刻，欠席，自殺念慮を認めたため入院となり，意欲低下，思考障害，自我意識障害等の症状を認め，分裂病と診断されている。また母親が来談し，「無気力，元気がない，だらしなくなっている，部屋が非常に乱雑，汚い」と言われ，生徒本人とも面談を重ねていくうちに強い不安，対人恐怖，自閉，自己不全感，自殺念慮を認め，病院での治療に導入し，精神分裂病の診断のもとに外来治療を継続している。クラス担任から相談があったケースで，学校を休みがちであり，出席できていても，教室で落ち着かず，不穏な様子がみられ，家庭でも父母をバットで殴るなどの暴力を振るい，入院直前には廊下で突然他生徒の顔面と腹部を殴打し，被害妄想による行動化がみられた生徒は両親に治療の必要性を説明し緊急入院となった。

相談室で面談を重ねていく中で，明らかに精神病圏の疾患を発症していると考えられたケースは60名中10名存在した。その中で病院に受診し，精神病圏の疾患として治療を受けている生徒は9名いた。60名中，病院やクリニックの精神科に受診したケースは18名存在した。2名が入院治療を必要とした。17名は治療を受けながら登校し，頻繁に保健室を利用した生徒は5名であった。

IV. 考　察

中高校保健室における精神科医の業務と役割について考える。1) まず来談した生徒，家族，教師と学業も含んで広く心の問題を話し合う。2) 思春期の生徒達はしばしば，親や教師に心を開かないが，第三者としての専門家の立場で話し合い可能なことが多い。3) まずそのことにより中高校生という思春期の不安と不安定さを支え，自我の成長を助ける。4) 家族と生徒の関係調整の役割がある。5) 生徒の問題や悩みを教師に伝え協力してこれを解決する。6) これらを含んで中根の言うサブクリニカルな対応がある。7) 病的な現象や症状に対しての助言や対応。8) 発病した生徒へのケア。9) 生徒，家族のプライバシーを共有しつつ，守る事自体に深い意味がある。

参考文献

1) 小林司：学校精神衛生の歴史と展望．徳田良仁，小林司編：学校精神衛生の展望．日本精神衛生会，p.9-23, 1975.
2) 中根晃：学校精神保健におけるサブクリニカルな対応について．第40回日本児童青年精神医学会総会抄録集，p.131, 1999.

---

*東邦大学医学部精神神経医学講座
　Michiko Nakamura, Michiya Sugawara, Akira Nakane : Toho University School of Medicine.
**国際医療福祉大学
　Jiro Suzuki : International University of Health and Welfare.

日本における自閉症圏障害の診断告知に対する親の満足度の決定因子

Determinants of parental satisfaction with disclosure of autistic spectrum disorders in Japan

納富　恵子* 　　木舩　憲幸* 　　吉田　敬子** 　　田代　信維**

Introduction

Many studies on process of telling parents about the diagnosis of mental disability in a child have been reported. This process has been described as a crisis event for the parents (Emde and Brown, 1978). It has been suggested that the mode of disclosure may affect later adaptation (Blacher, 1984). As professionals find it difficult to handle the disclosure, a number of studies have recommended a guideline for good practice (Cunningham et al. 1984 : Cottrell and Summers, 1990). The recommendations include early disclosure, with both parents together and with the child present, giving early opportunities for follow-up interviews, providing sufficient information in clear non-technical terms, and handling the interview in a sympathetic and honest manner.

However, most of these recommendations were based on a descriptive survey of parents or clinical impression in western countries. There has been little substantial study of which factors are most important to parents' satisfaction with the disclosure process (Sloper & Turner, 1993), especially on diagnosing autistic spectrum disorders (ASD).

Objectives

In order to elucidate the factors involved in the satisfaction of the parents who had received the diagnosis in which their childeren were found to be suffering from autistic spectrum disorders (ASD), using questionnaire.

Methods

The Questionnaire including demographic data, when and where the diagnosis was disclosed, who reported the diagnosis, general satisfaction of disclosure experience, and factors which may affect the general satisfaction were sent to the parents association of autism, FUKUOKA. Seventy-two parents took part in our survey and mailed back the questionnaire as well as written informed consent (Table 1). The multiple regression analysis was used to examine the significant factors, which influenced general satisfaction of the each disclosure process.

Results

Number of diagnosis : sixty-six parents out of 72 visited another doctor to seek a 2nd diagnosis, 44 parents had a 3rd diagnosis. Percentage of general satisfaction : At the 1st disclosure 9.8%, the 2nd 37.7%, the 3rd 47.7%. Factors which influenced general satisfaction were as follows ; the 1st diagnosis was related to a thorough explanation, the 2nd diagnosis, listening to parents' complaints, less severity of diagnosis, and diagnosis by medical professionals, the 3rd diagnosis, less severity, milder intellectual disability of the child, telling parents what to do, and earlier diagnosis (Table 2, 3, 4).

Conclusions and clinical implication

Very few parents were satisfied with the first disclosure of ASD. The percentage of satisfaction increased as parents had the second and the third

Table 1 Subjects and Characteristics of individuals of ASD in this study

Subjects			
Parents Association of Autism in FUKUOKA 72 parents who agree to participate in this study			
Individuals Characteristics			
Sex	M : 57	F : 14	? : 1
Age range	3 y.o.～36y.o.		

Table 2 Correlation between descriptor variables and parental satisfaction with the first diagnosis

Factor	Standardized Partial Regression Coefficient	Partial Correlation Coefficient
Thorough Explanation	.655	.655

R(Square)　　　　　= .655 (.429)
Adjusted R(Square) = .634 (.402)　$P<0.001$
(N = 72, percentage of satisfaction　9.8%)

Table 3 Correlation between descriptor variables and parental satisfaction with second diagnosis

Factor	Standardized Partial Regression Coefficient	Partial Correlation Coefficient
Listening Parent's Complaint	1.478	.887
Less Severity of Diagnosis	.738	.755
Diagnosis by Medical Professionals	.300	.566

R(Square)　　　　　= .934 (.873)
Adjusted R(Square) = .899 (.809)　$P<0.001$
(N = 66, percentage of satisfaction　37.7%)

Table 4 Correlation between descriptor variables and parental satisfaction with third diagnosis

Factor	Standardized Partial Regression Coefficient	Partial Correlation Coefficient
Less Severity of Diagnosis	1.350	.980
Milder intellectual Disability	.463	.596
Telling Parent What to Do	.455	.813
Earlier Diagnosis	.286	.677

R(Square)　　　　　= .965 (.932)
Adjusted R(Square) = .929 (.864)　$P<0.001$
(N = 44, percentage of satisfaction　47.7%)

professionals opinions. In each disclosure the factors, which affected the parent's satisfaction, changed. It is essential to confirm that parents are actually satisfied with and fully understand our explanation in the first clinical setting. As a professional, we should be aware of the fact that many parents actually ask a second opinion seeking for more information regarding the diagnosis, treatment, or prognosis of their children. It is suggested that in the disclosure of the child diagnosis of ASD, good parent-professional communication is essential for parent's satisfaction.

References

1) Blacher, J. : Sequential stages of parental adjustment to the birth of a child with handicaps : fact or artifact. Mental Retardation, 22 ; 55-68, 1984.
2) Cunningham, C. C., Morgan, P., McGuckn, R. B. : Down's syndrome : is dissatisfaction with disclosure of diagnosis inevitable? Developmental Medicine and Child Neurology, 26 ; 33-39, 1984.
3) Emde, R., Brown, C. : Adaptation to the birth of a Down syndrome infant : greaving and maternal attachment. Journal of the American Academy of Child Psychiatry, 17 ; 300-323, 1978.
4) Sloper, P., Turner, S. : Determinants of parental satisfaction with disclosure of disability. Developmental Medicine and Child Neurology 35, 816-25, 1993.

*福岡教育大学教育学部障害児教育講座
Keiko Yoshida, Nobutada Tashiro : Department of Special Education, Fukuoka University of Education, Munakata.
**九州大学医学部神経精神科
Keiko Notomi, Noriyuki Kifune : Department of Psychiatry, Kyushu University, Fukuoka.

大学生に多発する60項目版 GHQ の異常高値

High prevalence of abnormal values on General Health Questionnaire (GHQ-60) among medical and nursing students

泉　慈子*　久郷　敏明*　竹内　博明*

I. はじめに

Goldberg ら[1]が開発した GHQ(General Health Questionnaire)は、内科受診患者の神経症的傾向を抽出することを意図していたが、最近では全般的な QOL 評価尺度としても幅広く使用されている。

1999年4月、香川医科大学保健管理室が開設され、初期活動として精神保健に関する基礎資料の収集を試みた。活動の一環として、希望者に60項目版の GHQ 精神的健康調査票(GHQ-60)、CMI 健康調査表(CMI)、YG 性格検査(YG)を実施したが、多数の学生の GHQ 総得点が、神経症的傾向を意味する高値を呈していた。

本研究では、GHQ-60総得点の上昇の規定要因を多角的に分析するために、3種類の心理検査の相関および臨床特徴としての学科と性別の影響を検討した。

II. 対象と方法

対象は、心理検査を希望して保健管理室を訪れた学生227名(医学科男子85名、医学科女子89名、看護学科男子1名、看護学科女子52名)である。希望者に回答方法を説明し、3種類の質問紙法検査(GHQ-60、CMI、YG)を持ち帰らせた。すべての質問に回答した学生は、検査用紙を保健管理室に提出した。本研究に際しては、過去1年間に集積した全学生の検査成績と臨床特徴をパソコンに入力し、3種類の検査の相互関連と臨床要因の影響を多角的に分析した。

III. 結果

1. GHQ-60の総得点

GHQ-60(60点満点)の総得点に関しては、16点以下が正常範囲内、17点以上が神経症的傾向と考えられている[2]。全対象の結果を要約すると、総得点の平均は15±10点であり、88名(39%)が正常範囲を超える高値(17点以上)に達していた。

2. 心理検査の相互関連

1) CMI の影響

CMI の結果は、身体的／精神的自覚症得点から領域 I ～IVに区分される。本研究では、神経症的傾向が否定される I 群と II 群(179名)、疑われる III 群と IV 群(48名)という2群間の GHQ 総得点と17点以上の比率を比較したが、GHQ 総得点と異常率は後者が有意に高値であった。

2) YG の影響

YG による性格類型は、A、B、C、D、E 型という5種類に分類される。本研究では、対象症例の性格類型を A+C 群(72名)、B+E 群(49名)、D 群(106名)の3群に区分し、各群の GHQ 総得点と17点以上の比率を比較したが、B+E 群は GHQ 総得点と異常率が有意に高値、D 群は GHQ 総得点と異常率が有意に低値であり、A+C 群は両者の中間に位置していた。

3. 臨床特徴との関連

1) 学科の影響

医学科174名と看護学科53名に区分し、両群の GHQ 総得点と17点以上の比率を比較したが、医学科学生の GHQ 総得点と異常率は、看護学科学生に比較していずれもが有意に低値であった。

2）性別の影響

男子学生86名と女子学生141名に区分し、両群のGHQ総得点と17点以上の比率を比較したが、男子学生と女子学生のGHQ総得点と異常率に有意差はみられなかった。

3）複合的な影響

学科と性別の影響を検討するため、医学科男子（85名），医学科女子（89名），看護学科女子（52名）という3群を抽出し、各群のGHQ総得点と17点以上の比率を比較したが、医学科女子はGHQ総得点と異常率が有意に低値，看護学科女子はこれらが有意に高値であり、医学科男子は両者の中間に位置していた。

最後に、3群のCMI領域とYG性格類型の構成を検討した。前者の比率に関しては顕著な相違はなかった。後者の比率の有意差はなかったが、医学科男子と医学科女子はD群＞A＋C群＞B＋E群，看護学科女子はA＋C群＞D群＞B＋E群という順序であり、B＋E群は看護学科女子，D群は医学科女子に多い傾向があった。

Ⅳ. 考　察

本邦におけるGHQ-60の標準化の結果から、16／17点にCut Off Pointを設置すれば、最も良好に神経症的傾向を識別できると考えられている[2]。本研究では3種類の心理検査を併用した。GHQはストレス（State），CMIは心身の相関，YGは人格傾向（Trait）を把握する目的で採用したが、これらの諸検査の結果は良好に関連していた。

GHQ総得点が高値を示す学生の特徴を解明するために学科と性別の影響を検討したが、有意差を示したのは学科のみであり、性別の影響に関しては否定的であった。すなわち、明らかな問題性の所在を示したのは、看護学科の学生の成績であり、GHQ総得点の平均値は17点を超え、過半数の学生の数値が神経症領域に達していた。

さらに詳細に検討するために、医学科男子、医学科女子、看護学科女子という主要3群を比較したが、GHQ総得点と異常率は、看護学科女子＞医学科男子＞医学科女子の順序であった。看護学科学生がGHQ総得点を増加させる重要な要因と思われたが、性別の影響は再び否定された。

単科医科大学の約40％が、神経症的傾向を意味する高値を呈していたことは、学生の精神保健を考慮する上で重大な問題である。学科による差を説明するには、カリキュラムの相違などを考慮することも必要であるが、研究結果に2種類の制約が影響した可能性を考慮すべきである。第1は研究対象の偏りである。今回の対象は心理検査の希望者に限定されている。これらの学生が、母集団全体のどのような層から構成されているのかの検討が不可欠である。第2は性格類型の構成比が学科間の差異に影響している可能性である。有意差は観察されなかったが、看護学科女子の成績が性格類型の相違に修飾された結果である可能性も否定できない。

これらの問題点を解消するには、研究対象を拡大した追跡調査が不可欠であり、そのような意図に基づいた研究を実施している。

Ⅴ. おわりに

心理検査を希望して保健管理室を訪れた学生の約40％が、神経症的傾向が示唆されるGHQ-60の総得点を示した。このような結果に基づいて、高値の発現に関連すると思われる要因を多角的に検討するとともに、研究方法に付随する問題点を指摘した。

文　献

1) Goldberg, D. P., Blackwell, B.: Psychiatric illness in general practice: A detailed study using a new method of case identification. Brit. Med. J., 2; 439-443, 1970.
2) 福西勇夫：日本版 General Health Questionnaire (GHQ) の cut-off point. 心理臨床, 3; 228-234, 1990.

---

*香川医科大学保健管理センター
Chikako Izumi, Toshiaki Kugoh, Hiroaki Takeuchi: Heath Care Center, Kagawa Medical University.

大学生における被害観念の発生予測

The prediction of persecutory thoughts using hierarchical multiple regression analysis

森本　幸子* 　　丹野　義彦* 　　坂本　真士**

Persecutory thoughts are ideations, of less than delusional proportions, involving suspiciousness or the belief that one is being harassed, persecuted, or unfairly treated. Recent studies reported that normal people have persecutory thoughts. The purpose of the present study is to predict persecutory thoughts by using the diathesis-stress model. The diathesis-stress model predicts that people with a strong diathesis are more likely to show symptoms of psychopathology when they encounter stressors than those with a weak diathesis.

Study 1: Testing the diathesis-stress model of persecutory thoughts

Method

Questionnaires were administered to 117 college students three times at intervals of two weeks. At time 1, diatheses of persecutory thoughts were assessed with the 18 subscales that were selected from four questionnaires, such as Paranoia／Suspiciousness Questionnaire and Auditory Hallucination Experiences Scale. At time 2, the persecutory thoughts were assessed. At time 3, the persecutory thoughts and stressors experienced between time 2 and time 3 were assessed. The Persecutory Ideation Scale (Tanno, Ishigaki & Sugiura, 2000) and College Life Experience Scale were used.

Results

We found significant correlation coefficients between the 18 diatheses and persecutory thoughts. This result showed that most of the diatheses were related persecutory thoughts. A set-wise hierarchical multiple regression analysis (Cohen & Cohen, 1983) was used to predict the change in persecutory thoughts between time 2 and time 3. This prospective research design allows us to analyze the causality of persecutory thoughts, diathesis and stressors. A Hierarchical multiple regression analysis showed the significant interactions of stressors and four diatheses subscales (subscales of a) Anger, b) Resentment, c) Auditory illusion and d) Hearing negative voice). The interaction of stressors and anger is presented in Figure 1. The students who have high scores in Anger will show increase in persecutory thoughts when they experience stressors. The remaining three diatheses showed the same trend.

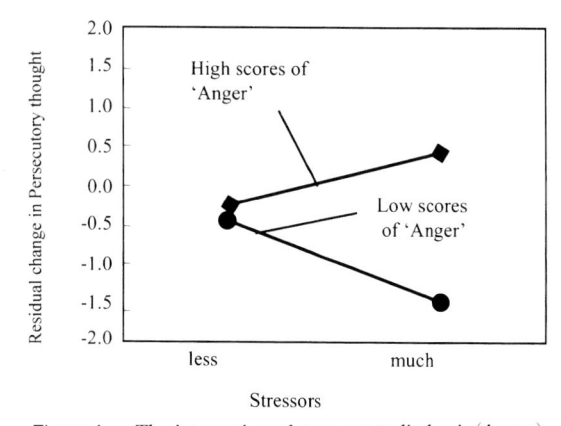

Figure 1. The interaction of stressors × diathesis (Anger)

Discussion

Most of diathesis subscales were related with persecutory thoughts. However, there were not very many interactions between each diathesis and stressors. Therefore, these subscales may not be the diathesis of persecutory thoughts. To prevent the development of persecutory thoughts, psycho-educational intervention may be effective.

Study 2: Evoluation of the diathesis-stress model of persecutory thoughts

Method

Five subjects, three male and two female, participated in the study. All of them got high scores on persecutory thoughts in study 1. The subjects were interviewed to reassess diatheses, and then questioned on stressors that they experienced and persecutory thoughts.

Results

Three of the subjects showed high diatheses scores (subscales of a) Anger, b) Resentment, c) Auditory illusion and d) Hearing negative voices). They recognised the increase of the persecutory thoughts when they encountered with stressors.

Discussion

The result of the interviews supported the diathesis-stress model of persecutory thoughts. Some subjects with high scores in persecutory thoughts had severe stressors or interpersonal problems. It may be necessary to inform them that stressors increase their persecutory thoughts, and to teach them how to cope with stressors.

Reference

1) Cohen, J., Cohen, P.: Applied multiple regression／Correlation analysis for the behavioural sciences. 2nd ed.,: Lawrence Erlbaum Associates, New Jersey, 1983.
2) Tanno, Y., Ishigaki, T., Sugiura, Y.: Construction of scales to measure thematic tendencies of paranoid ideation. The Japanese Journal of Psychology, 71; 379-386, 2000.

---

*東京大学総合文化研究科
Sachiko Morimoto, Yoshihiko Tanno: University of Tokyo.
**大妻女子大学人間関係学部
Shinji Sakamoto: Otsuma Woman's University.

精神障害（者）に対する医学生の非好意的態度を改善するための医学教育の方法についての研究
―OSCE のもたらす結果―

Studies of medical education towards reducing the unfavorable attitudes of medical students regarding psychiatry and persons with psychiatric disorders
―The effects of OSCE―

山本　和儀[*1]　　福治　康秀[*1]　　平松　兼一[*1]　　小椋　力[*1]
長崎　文恵[*2]　　比嘉　司[*3]　　大田　裕一[*4]

The effects of the OSCE (Objective Structured Clinical Examination) educational module were investigated to develop medical education for favorably changing medical students' attitudes regarding psychiatry and persons with psychiatric disorders. The following valuables were investigated through a self-rating questionnaire survey among two student groups; before the OSCE education module was adopted to medical education (pre OSCE group) and after adoption (post OSCE group). 1) Improvement of student's attitudes (C-ATDP) after the psychiatry clerkship, 2) Improvement of understanding of the object of medical interviewing (C-OBJ) and interviewing skills (C-SKILL) after the psychiatry clerkship, 3) Correlation between improvement of attitudes, understanding and skills, 4) The effects of OSCE on the improvement of attitudes, understanding and skills.

Subjects and methods

The subjects of this research were 5th year medical students during their two-week clinical clerkship from the period of September 1998 till January of 1999 (pre OSCE group) and from the period of September 1999 till January of 2000 (post OSCE group). Each group was composed of 51 students (the response rate was 100%, respectively). The scale used for investigation of attitudes was the ATDP (Attitude Toward Disabled Persons) scale form O (20 items) by Yuker (Yuker & Block, 1986). The scale is a 5-point Likert-type scale and the higher points indicate favourable attitudes. The rating scale for measuring student's understanding of objects and skills of medical interviewing was constructed originally by the first author (K.Y.). The scale is a 5-point Likert type scale and composed of 3 items for assessing understanding of objects and 20 items for assessing skills. The higher points indicate better understanding and skills.

Results

There were improvements in students' attitudes regarding psychiatry and persons with psychiatric disorders, and understanding of objects and skills of medical interviewing among the two student groups, as indicated in Table 1. However, there was no change in the attitudes, understanding, or skills, comparing the post OSCE group with the pre OSCE group. Correlations between improvement of attitudes, understanding of objects and skills of interviewing comparing the pre OSCE group and the post OSCE group were indicated in Table 2. There was strong correlation between understanding of objects and skills among both student groups. However, there was no correlation between attitudes and objects, nor attitudes and

Table 1 Comparisons of improvement in students' attitudes regarding psychiatry and persons with psychiatric disorders, understanding of objects and skills of medical interviewing, between the pre OSCE group and the post OSCE group

Items	Average score (SD)		t-value	level of significance
	pre OSCE	post OSCE		
Attitudes (C-ATDP)	2.5 (9.3)	3.8 (7.6)	0.71	0.48
Objects (C-OBJ)	2.2 (1.6)	2.2 (1.6)	−0.08	0.94
Skills (C-SKILL)	15.3 (8.6)	15.1 (7.5)	−0.10	0.92

Table 2 Correlations between improvement of attitudes, understanding of objects and skills of interviewing comparing the pre OSCE group and the post OSCE group

	Attitudes	Objects	Skills
Attitudes (pre)	1.00	−0.15	−0.08
Attitudes (post)	1.00	0.23	0.21
Objects (pre)		1.00	0.50***
Objects (post)		1.00	0.55***
Skills (pre)			1.00
Skills (post)			1.00

* $p < 0.0001$

skills, among both student groups.

Discussion

The improvement of studens' attitudes after the psychiatric clerkship regarding psychiatry and persons with psychiatric disorders was shown in both groups. However, the improvement was limited to a minimum, even among the post OSCE group. The improvements in understanding of objects and skills of medical interviewing after the psychiatric clerkship were also indicated. Furthermore, correlations between improvements in understanding of objects and improvement of skills were strong in both groups. However, there was no correlation between attitudes and understanding of objects, nor skills. This finding indicates that current psychiatric education in medical interviewing and improvement of commincation skills with persons with psychiatric disorders during clerkship is not sufficient for improvement of students' attitudes regarding psychiatry and persons with psychiatric disorders, as indicated by our previous study (Yamamoto, 1996). Adoption of the OSCE educatonal module brought no change in students' attitudes either. This study suggests the need for a specific educational program for students' attitude changes, if the development of favorable attitude changes regarding psychiatry and persons with psychiatric disorders is needed.

References

1) Yuker, H.E., Block, J.R. : Research with the Attitudes Towards Disabled Persons Scale (ATDP). Hofstra University, New York, 1986.
2) Yamamoto, K. et al. : Attitudes of medical students towards persons with mental disorders : A comparative study between Japan and Thailand. Psychiatry and Clinical Neurosciences, 50 ; 171-180, 1996.

---

[1] 琉球大学医学部精神神経講座
Kazuyoshi Yamamoto, Yoshihide Fukuji, Ken-ichi Hiramatsu, Chikara Ogura : Department of Neuropsychiatry, University of the Ryukyus.
[2] 南山病院
Fumie Nagasaki : Nanzan Hospital.
[3] 田崎病院
Tsukasa Higa : Tazaki Hospital.
[4] 平安病院
Yuich Ota : Hirayasu Hospital.

感情表出(EE)と大うつ病の再発および再燃との関連についての研究

Expressed Emotion (EE) and the relapse of major depression

植木　啓文[*1]　貝沼　諭[*1]　鈴木　泉[*1]
小川　直志[*2]　原　耕[*3]　田中　宏史[*4]

I. はじめに

家族の感情表出(EE)が精神疾患の経過に与える影響に関する研究はこれまで多くの国で行われてきた。その内，分裂病についての研究からは，EEは再発の重要な指標の一つであることがほぼ確立されている(Butzlaffら，1998)。

一方感情障害に関する研究はそれほど多くはない。Butzlaffらは6つの報告を分析し，EEは感情障害の経過に分裂病におけるよりもより重要な影響をおよぼし，さらに，低いレベルのカットオフでも影響を与える可能性があることを示唆している。

本論では，EEを測定する手段としてMagañaら(1986)が開発した5分間スピーチサンプル(FMSS)を使用し，うつ病相の寛解後の経過を前方視的に追跡し，再燃・発とEEとの関連を検討したい。

II. 対象と方法

SCID(Spitzer，1990)により大うつ病と診断され，調査に対して同意の得られた30名を対象とした。30名の平均年齢は59.0±13.6歳であり，男性10名，女性20名であった。抑うつ症状の評価にはHRSD(Hamilton，1960)を使用し，その得点が6点以下になった時点から9カ月の間，抑うつ症状の変化を追跡調査した。再発の基準は，HRSD得点15点以上が2週間以上持続した場合とした。

抑うつ症状の自己評価にはSDS(Zung，1965)も使用した。ライフイベントの評価には，SRRS(Holmes，1967)とDSM-III-R Axis IVを使用した。維持療法の薬物等価評価にはBollini(1999)を参考にした。その他の，人口統計学的な評価として，年齢，罹病期間，病相回数，うつ病の既往，家族歴，入院歴などを調査した。

EEの評価にはFMSSを使用し，以下のカテゴリー間の比較を行った；EE(1)：高いEE vs. 低いEE，EE(2)：高いEE+境界線級の高いEE vs. 純粋に低いEE，EE(3)：高いEE vs. 境界線級の高いEE vs. 純粋に低いEE，EE(4)：批判+境界線級の批判 vs. 批判なし，EE(5)：EOIあり vs. EOIなし。

III. 結　果

6名(20%)は高いEEを，残りの24名(80%)は低いEEを示した。高いEEの下位分類では，2名が「批判」，2名が「EOI(感情の過度の巻き込まれ)」，2名が「批判」と「EOI」であった。EOIの4名の内，3名は感情の現れを示した。低いEEの下位分類では，6名は境界線級の批判であり，残りの18名は純粋に低いEEであった。

再発が認められたのは12名(40%)であった。EEでは，EE(1)，EE(2)，EE(3)，EE(4)が再発と有意に関連していた。その他の変数では，ライフイベントのみが再発群に有意に多かった。

Cox比例ハザードモデルを用いた分析では，ライフイベントの数，LCUスコア(Holmes，1967)，EE(1)，EE(2)，EE(3)，EE(4)などと再発との関連が示唆された。EE(1)からEE(5)までの5つのモデルにおける，ステップワイズ法を用いたより詳細な分析では，ライフイベントは常に再発と有意に関連していた。EEでは，境界線級のEEを高いEEに含めた場合に，再発との関連がより高くなった。

IV. 考　察

1. EEの文化的特長

FMSSにおける「高いEE」の判定率には文化的な差異が認められ，アジア地域では欧米に比べ，高いEEの率は低い（Mino，1995）。感情障害の家族におけるEOIの出現はまれであると言われているが，今回の調査では30名中4名（13.3％）にEOIが認められた。しかも「感情の現れ」によってEOIと判定される傾向にあり，これは本邦のUehara（1996）の研究と一致している。この点は，EEの日本における特徴と言えるであろう。

2. EEと再発との関連

境界線級のEEを高いEEに含めること，つまり，高いEEのレベルを下げることによって，より再発を予測できる結果となった。Vaughnら（1976）は，うつ病の再発は分裂病の場合よりも低い批判のカットオフポイントで生じるとした。一方，FMSSはEE判定の原法であるCFI（Brown，1972）よりも偽陰性を多く含んでいるとされており，FMSSにおける境界線級のEEは，高いEEに含める方が妥当であろう。

EEの要素の内，EOIよりも批判の方が，感情障害の経過にとっては重要であると言われている。感情障害においてEOIは経過に負の影響を与えるという報告はこれまでなされていないが，今後も検討されるべき課題である。

3. 今後の課題

EEは家族システムの一部をとらえたものであり，しかも時とともに変化して行くものである。サポートシステムや生活の困難度との関連も言われており，「高いEE」の家族という表現はふさわしくない。従って，家族が高いEEを示していたとすると，それは家族がサポートを必要としていることをわれわれに示しているのであって，緊急の介入が必要であることのひとつの表現なのである。

そのような介入のひとつとして，心理教育的アプローチの意義がますます重要となってきている。

文　献

1) Bollin, P., Pampallona, S., Tibald, G. et al.: Effectiveness of antidepressants. Meta-anaylysis of dose-effect relationship in randomized clinical trials. Br. J. Psychiatry, 174 ; 297-303, 1999.
2) Brown, G. W., Birley, J. L. T., Wing, J. K.: Influence of family life on course of schizophrenic disorders. Br. J. Psychiatry, 121 ; 241-258, 1972.
3) Butzlaff, R. L., Hooley, J. M.: Expressed emotion and psychiatric relapse. Arch. Gen. Psychiatry, 55 ; 547-552, 1998.
4) Hamilton, M.: A rating scale for depression. J. Neurol. Neurosurg Psychiatry, 23 ; 56-62, 1960.
5) Holmes, T. H., Rahe, R. H.: Social Readjunstment Rating Scale. J. Psychosom. Res., 11 ; 213-218, 1966.
6) Magaña, A. B., Goldstein, M. J., Karno, M. et al.: A brief method for assessing expressed emotion in relatives of psychiatric patients. Psychiatr. Res., 17 ; 203-212, 1986.
7) Mino, Y., Tanaka, S., Inoue, S. et al.: Expressed emotion components in families of schizophrenic patients in Japan. Int. J. Ment. Health, 24 ; 38-49, 1995.
8) Spitzer, R., Williams, J., Gibbon, M.: Structured clinical interview for DSM-III-R（SCID）, user's guide. American Psychiatric Press, Washington, D.C., 1990.
9) Uehara, T., Yokoyama, T., Goto, M. et al.: Expressed emotion and short-term treatment outcome of outpatients with major depression. Compr. Psychiatry, 37 ; 299-304, 1996.
11) Vaughn, C. E., Leff, J.: The influence of family and social factors on the course of psychiatric illness. Br. J. Psychiatry, 129 ; 125-137, 1976.
12) Zung, W. W. K.: A self-rating depression scale. Arch. Gen. Psychiatry, 12 ; 63-70, 1965.

[*1] 岐阜大学医学部神経精神医学教室
Hirofumi Ueki, Satoshi Kainuma, Izumi Suzuki : Gifu University School of Medicine.
[*2] 社団法人　岐阜病院
Naoshi Ogawa : Gifu Psychiatric Hospital.
[*3] 岐阜市民病院
Koh Hara : Gifu City Hospital.
[*4] 高山赤十字病院
Hirofumi Tanaka : Takayama Red Cross Hospital.

うつ病の早期発見・早期治療
―琉球大学病院における総合診療科と精神科との連携をとおして―

Early detection and early treatment of depression
—Through liaison with the psychiatry department of University Hospital of the Ryukyus—

福田　吉顕[*]　　山本　和儀[*]　　平松　謙一[*]　　武田　裕子[**]

I. はじめに

　近年，抑うつ気分などの定型的症状が目立たず，身体症状を主訴として一般診療科を受診するうつ病患者が増加し，適切な時期に診断や治療を受けないまま遷延する例も少なくない。渡辺らによると，精神科を受診したうつ病患者の76.5％は，それ以前に内科外来を受診しており，そこでのうつ病診断や抗うつ薬による治療例は極めて少なかったとしている。医学・医療の高度化，専門分化が進むにつれて，包括性の不足からうつ病患者が適切に診断されず，治療開始に至るまでに長期間を要するものが少なくないものと思われる。
　琉球大学医学部附属病院では，全人的医療の実践とそれを担う医療者の育成を目的として，1999年5月，総合診療センター・総合診療科（以下総合診療科）が開設された。週2日精神科医師が直接出向し総合診療科の一員として診療を行っているが，総合診療科内での他科医師と精神科医との連携，総合診療科と精神科の連携の現状とうつ病患者の早期発見・早期治療に関して総合診療科の果たす役割という観点から若干の考察を加えて報告する。

II. 対象と方法

　2000年4月から2001年3月の1年間に琉球大学医学部附属病院総合診療科を初めて受診した患者850名のうち，総合診療科内で精神科医に紹介されるか精神神経科外来（以下精神科）へ紹介されるなど，精神科医の関与を必要とした65名について外来カルテをretrospectiveに調査した。精神科医への紹介経路，疾患分類などの他に気分障害と診断された10名については，同期間に同様に自らの意志で精神科を受診した17名の気分障害患者を対照に平均年齢，主訴，それまでの受療行動，状況因の有無，未治療期間（症状のために職業的機能ないし平常の社会的活動が障害された時点から当院受診までの期間（週数））を比較した。なお反復性の気分障害患者については今回の病相に限って調査した。

III. 結　果

　1）精神科医の関与を必要とした65名の紹介経路を見たとき，総合診療科内で精神科医に紹介されたものが18名，総合診療科から精神科へ紹介されたものが32名あり，精神科への紹介はほとんどが総合診療科初診から1週間以内であった。残りの15名は総合診療科内で精神科医が初診患者として診療した。
　2）65名のDSM-IVによる疾患分類は不安障害が最も多く26例，精神分裂病および他の精神病性障害14例，気分障害10例の順であった。
　3）総合診療科を初診した気分障害患者10名と精神科を初診した気分障害患者17名を比較したところ，平均年齢は41.9±15.5 vs 44.6±14.1（p=0.81）で有意差は認められなかった。
　4）総合診療科を初診した気分障害患者10名中6名が頭痛，めまい，倦怠感，易疲労感などの身体症状を主訴としていたが，一方精神科を初診した気分障害患者17名中身体疾患を主訴とするものは2名だけであった。
　5）総合診療科を初診した気分障害患者10名は全員がそれまでにいずれかの医療機関を受診しており，うち5名は複数の医療機関を受診してい

た。精神科を初診した17名のうちそれまでに他の医療機関を受診したことのあるものは9名であった。

6）明らかな状況因の認められるものは総合診療科を初診した10名中6名，精神科を初診した17名中10名であり2群で有意差は認められなかった。

7）総合診療科を初診した10名と精神科を初診した17名の未治療期間（週数）を比較したところ25.6±14.1 vs 6.8±4.3（Mann-WhitneyのU検定，p=0.0005）で有意差が認められた。

IV．考　察

1）精神・心理的な問題を抱えながら，精神医療への偏見や抵抗により精神科を受診する前に一般身体科を受診するものは少なくないと思われる。総合診療科においては，主訴が身体症状であっても精神面の病態が比較的明瞭な症例については，受診後の早い段階で精神科医あるいは精神科外来に紹介されていることがうかがわれた。一方総合診療科を受診した気分障害患者10名すべてが他の医療機関にかかったことがあり，複数の医療機関にかかったことのあるものも5名いたがこのことは，身体症状を主訴とした場合，過去に身体科を受診したがうつ病ないしうつ状態を見逃された結果であると思われる。

2）未治療期間を比較した場合，総合診療科を初診した気分障害患者のほうが有意に長かった。このことは，身体症状が前景に立つ気分障害患者の場合，身体症状が出現した時期のほうが精神症状が出現したときより特定しやすいこと，および精神症状によって職業的機能ないし平常の社会的活動が障害されるのは精神症状がある程度重篤となってからのことと関連があるものと思われる。また上述したこととも関係するが，身体症状が前景に立つ気分障害患者の場合，身体科を受診するが適切な診断治療が行われず症状が改善しないため，他の医療機関を受診するという悪循環がある一方，抑うつ気分，不安焦燥，希死念慮などの精神症状を持つものの方が精神医療に対し受療行動を取りやすいことによるものと思われる。

3）未治療期間を比較すると有意に長くなってしまったが，総合診療科を受診しなければ気分障害が再び見逃されている可能性があり，総合診療科での心身両面からの複合的アプローチがあればこそ的確に診断できたものと思われる。すなわち総合病院においては精神科医の参画した総合診療科はより緻密な医療サービスを提供することができるものと思われる。

4）気分障害患者に限らず身体症状を前景とする精神疾患患者は身体科を初診することが多く，精神疾患の早期発見・早期治療において身体科医は重要な役割を担っている。精神科医による身体科医への啓蒙およびコンサルテーション活動が今後一層重要なものになると思われる。

---

*琉球大学医学部精神神経学講座
Yoshiaki Fukuda, Kazuyoshi Yamamoto, Ken-ichi Hiramatsu : Department of Neuropsychiatry, University of the Ryukyus.
**琉球大学病院地域医療部
Yuko Takeda : Division for General Medicine and Community Health Care, University Hospital of the Ryukyus.

気分障害の症状・経過に与える自殺企図の影響
―自殺予防のために―

The impact of attempted suicide on the symptoms and course of mood disorder
―A contribution to the prevention of suicide―

福永　貴子*　坂元　薫**

I. はじめに

　自殺企図後にもかかわらず精神状態が不自然なほど安定していたり，むしろ軽躁的とも見える患者に出会うことも日常臨床上稀なことではない。自殺企図後の精神症状変化を検討し，その後の経過を予測することは自殺企図者の精神科的治療上重要なことであるが，その点に関する体系的な研究は意外なほど乏しいのが現状である。本研究では，自殺企図した気分障害患者の多数例を対照群と比較しながら，自殺企図前後の精神症状の変化について検討したので報告する。

II. 対象と方法

　東京女子医大精神科に入院した2800例（1986～1995年）のうち，自殺企図後に入院となった気分障害患者で，3カ月以上の治療経過が明らかな，うつ病性障害24例，双極性障害16例を自殺企図群とした。さらに，自殺企図によらない入院例（1994～1997年）のうち，うつ病性障害24例，双極性障害16例を対照群とした。
　以上80例の入院および外来病歴を遡及的に検討し，性別，発症年齢，罹病期間，自殺企図時年齢，入院までの経過型（単極性・双極性），自殺企図の手段，自殺企図時の抑うつ重症度，意識消失の有無などの背景因子と，自殺企図前後の精神症状変化ならびにその持続期間について調査した。精神症状の変化は「改善」「悪化」「病相switch」に細分して評価した。「改善」「悪化」は，DSM-IVの重症度分類に従って判定した。

III. 結果

1. 自殺企図後の精神症状変化

　自殺企図群40例のうち，自殺企図前後で精神症状の変化がみられなかったのは18例（45.0％），「改善」15例（37.5％），「病相switch」7例（17.5％）であり，悪化したものはなかった。
　自殺企図群の精神症状改善率37.5％（15/40）は対照群の改善率17.5％（7/40）に比べ有意に（Fisher's exact test，$p=0.039$）高かった。
　単極性例においては，自殺企図群の改善率50.0％（12/24）は対照群の改善率20.8％（5/24）に比べ有意に（Fisher's exact test，$p=0.034$）高かったが，双極性例においては自殺企図群の改善率18.6％（3/16）と対照群の改善率12.5％（2/16）との間には有意差は見られなかった。

2. 精神症状変化と背景因子との関連（Table 1）

　精神症状変化と背景因子との関連を調べるために，精神症状改善の有無を従属変数とし，背景因子を独立変数としたLogistic回帰分析を施行したところ，抑うつ改善には「単極性経過」が有意（$p=0.045$）に関連しており，経過型以外の背景因子と精神症状改善との間には有意な関連は認められなかった。また，病相switchの有無を従属変数とし，背景因子を独立変数としたLogistic回帰分析を施行したところ，病相switchには「意識消失」（$p=0.073$）と，「自殺企図時の重症度」（$p=0.071$）が関連する傾向が認められた。

3. 精神症状改善の持続期間（Figure 1）

　精神症状改善の持続期間は，精神症状改善例15例中，改善期間が1カ月未満の例が8例（53％），1カ月以上3カ月未満の例が3例（20％），3カ月以上持続した例が4例（27％）であった。改善期間が3カ月未満だった11例のうち，4例は退院後に

Table 1 Logistic regression model relating relevant clinical variables to improvement of depression or switching from depression to (hypo) mania

	Response Variable in Logistic Regression Analysis					
	improvement of depression			switching from depression to (hypo) mania		
Variable	b	Odds Ratio	95%CI	b	Odds Ratio	95%CI
Gender	0.70	2.01	0.41-9.94	-0.91	0.40	0.03-5.28
Age of onset (years)	-0.14	0.99	0.89-1.09	-0.083	0.92	0.76-1.12
Age of admission (years)	0.03	1.03	0.95-1.12	0.017	1.02	0.90-1.15
Monopolar course	1.69	5.41	1.04-28.29**	-1.59	0.20	0.02-2.29
Baseline severity of depression : moderate	-1.20	0.30	0.06-1.47	2.60	13.41	0.81-223.64*
Suicide attempt method : hard	-0.32	0.72	0.13-4.09	1.22	3.38	0.17-67.73
Loss of consciousness	-0.24	0.79	0.15-4.10	3.37	29.04	0.73-1149.10*

**p<0.05 *p<0.10

再燃，3例は再燃したが退院となっており，残り4例は再燃したため退院が延期となっていた。Logistic回帰分析の結果，精神症状改善期間の長短（3カ月以上，3カ月未満）と背景因子との間には，有意な関連はなかった。

IV. 考　察

1．自殺企図後の精神症状改善の要因

自殺企図後に抑うつ症状が改善する例は約1/3にみられた。その要因として，van Praagは手術やECTと同様，自殺企図による身体的侵襲が抗うつ作用を持つことを示唆している。いずれも意識消失を伴うものであり，我々の結果でも意識消失を伴う場合には病相switchが起こりやすいことを考慮すると，意識消失にいたることが「ショック療法的」に精神症状の変化に寄与する可能性が示唆された。

また van Praagは，自殺企図群の抑うつ症状が，対照群に比して有意に改善していたことから，自殺企図の「カタルシス効果」にも注目している。しかし自殺企図前の症状が実際より重く陳述され，入院後の症状が軽く申告されることによる「アーチファクト的改善」が含まれている可能性も否定できないとしている。

一方，Bronischは自殺企図群も対照群も同様に抑うつ症状が改善していたことから，症状改善は「入院効果」によるものと考えた。本研究では自殺企図群の方が対照群に比べ抑うつ症状が有意に改善していたため，抑うつ症状の改善はBronischの主張したような「入院効果」によるものではなく，van Praagらの「カタルシス効果」仮説を支持するものであった。

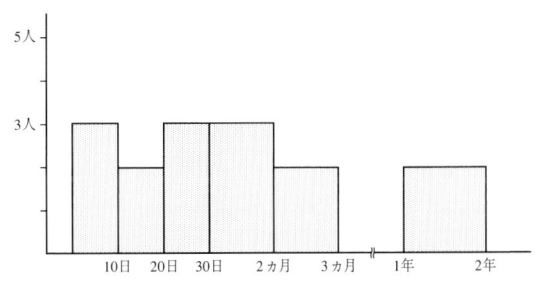

Figure 1 精神症状改善の持続期間

2．精神症状改善の持続期間

自殺企図後の改善の持続期間は3カ月未満のものが73％を占め，短期間のうちにうつ状態が再燃することが示唆された。その要因として以下の可能性が考えられた。

1）抑うつ症状改善による治療密度の希薄化
2）抑うつ症状改善により周囲の態度の好転なし（自殺企図による疾病利得の不充足）
3）抑うつ症状改善により早期社会復帰の促進
4）自殺企図の有する効果（カタルシス効果，意識消失のショック療法的効果）の減衰
5）入院効果の減衰

また精神症状改善の持続期間を予測する因子が抽出できないことからも，抑うつ状態の再燃さらには再企図の可能性に十分留意する必要があると思われた。

---

*東京女子医科大学　第二病院心の医療科
　Takako Fukunaga : Department of Psychiatry, Tokyo Women's Medical University Daini Hospital.
**東京女子医科大学　神経精神科
　Kaoru Sakamoto : Department of Psychiatry, Tokyo Women's Medical University School of Medicine.

高齢者の抑うつ症状と自殺念慮との関連について
Depressive symptoms and suicidal ideation in the elderly

田中江里子[*1,*2]　　坂本　真士[*3]　　豊川　恵子[*4]　　大野　裕[*1]

I．はじめに

　自殺には精神疾患，特に大うつ病が大きく関与していると考えられることから，自殺を予防する際には，自殺念慮だけでなく，大うつ病や抑うつ状態を早期に発見し，適切な介入を行うことが必要である。同時に，困難な状況に陥ったとき，自殺を考えたり試みたりする前に，周囲の人や専門家に相談する等の自殺以外の対処ができるようにするため，また自分や周囲の人が抑うつ状態になったとき，それに気づき適切な対応ができるようにするため，抑うつや自殺に関する心理教育も必要である。本研究では以上のような視点にたち，地域高齢者の抑うつ状態・自殺危険性を早期に発見し，保健婦や医師による早期介入・フォローアップを行うと共に，抑うつや自殺に関する心理教育を含んだ啓発活動を行う，総合的な抑うつ・自殺の予防プログラムを開発することを目的としている。そこで，まず高齢者の抑うつ症状と自殺念慮の実態を調査し，相互の関連性について検討した。

II．方　法

　手順：青森県N町の一地区に在住している65歳以上の高齢者を調査対象とした。高齢者向けの健康づくり講習会を開催し，講習会後に質問紙を実施した。その後，診断面接を含む個別面接調査を行った。講習会不参加の対象者については，後日調査員が自宅を訪問して調査を行った。なお，質問紙については原則として自己記入式としたが，視力等に問題があり独力で記入回答できない者については，調査員が質問紙を読み上げ，口頭にて回答を得，調査員が記入した。
　被検者：調査対象地区に在住する高齢者433名のうち，調査に協力し痴呆の疑いがなく，本研究で使用した変数に欠損のなかった者336名（男性121名，平均年齢73.40±5.63歳；女性215名，平均年齢73.34±6.00歳）を分析の対象とした。
　尺度：自己記入式質問紙 Self-rating Depression Scale（SDS；Zung, 1965；福田・小林, 1973；4件法20項目）を実施し，抑うつの程度を測定した。Sakamotoらの確認的因子分析の結果によると，SDSは認知症状，情動症状，身体症状の3因子に分けられることから（Sakamoto, Kijima, Tomoda, & Kambara, 1998），これらをSDSの下位尺度とみなし，各々と自殺念慮との関係を検討した。また，構造化診断面接票 Composite International Diagnostic Interview（CIDI；WHO, 1995）をDSM-IV大うつ病エピソードの現在症のみを聴取するよう改変して使用した（CIDI-MD-R）。抑うつ気分，興味喪失，易疲労性（気力低下），食欲体重の変化（増加・減少），睡眠の変化（不眠・過眠），精神運動性の障害（精神運動性遅滞・焦燥），無価値観・強い罪責感，思考の障害（集中困難・思考困難・決断困難），希死念慮（死についての反復思考・自殺念慮企図），の9種類の抑うつ症状の有無と，受診行動，機能障害の程度について聴取するものだが，この中から，希死念慮に関連する2項目（死についての反復思考「死について何度も考えたりしますか」と自殺念慮「気分がひどく落ち込んで，自殺について考えることがありますか」）を分析に用いた。この他に，Hospital Anxiety and Depression Scale，生活満足度尺度，いきいき度尺度，痴呆，ADL等について調査したが，本研究では使用しない。

III．結　果

　死についての反復思考を有している人は39名

(11.61％；男12名，女27名)，自殺念慮を有している人は8名(2.38％；男2名，女6名)おり，そのうち，死についての反復思考と自殺念慮の両方に「ある」と回答した者は4名(1.19％，男1名，女3名)であった。

SDS総合得点は31.81(SD＝7.71)であり，性差はみられなかった(t＝.18, ns)。また，SDSの認知症状得点(7項目)は13.63(SD＝4.60)，情動症状得点(5項目)は6.67(SD＝2.04)，身体症状得点(4項目)は5.26(SD＝1.79)であり，いずれも性差はみられなかった(ts＜1.08, ns)。

死についての反復思考を有している群と有していない群との間で，SDSの下位尺度得点別に平均値の差の検定を行ったところ，死についての反復思考を有している群は有していない群よりも認知症状得点が有意に高かった(t＝3.75, p＜.001)。また，自殺念慮を有している群は有していない群よりも認知症状得点(t＝2.19, p＜.05)と情動症状得点(t＝2.24, p＜.05)が有意に高かった。なお，死についての反復思考と自殺念慮のいずれか，または両方を有している者と，いずれも有していない者との間では，認知症状得点においてのみ差がみられた(t＝3.69, p＜.001)。

Ⅳ．考　察

本研究では，抑うつ・自殺の予防プログラムを作成することを最終目的として，まず地域高齢者の抑うつ症状と自殺念慮の実態を調査し，相互の関連性について検討した。面接で死についての反復思考や自殺念慮を有していると報告した者は43名(12.80％)であった。希死念慮の有無を直接的に質問して「ある」と回答した者に対しては，個別対応として医療機関への受診を勧める体制をとった。しかし自らの自殺念慮を隠す者も当然存在すると考えられ，このような場合の対処方法は今後の課題である。

また，自殺念慮は，抑うつ症状の中でも特に認知症状と関連があることが示唆された。高齢者においては身体症状を訴えることが多く，抑うつ症状との弁別が難しいと考えられているが，本研究では自殺念慮の有無によって身体症状得点に差はみられなかった。早期発見を目的とする際には，身体症状よりも情動症状や認知症状に注目すべきであろう。特に認知症状は，死についての反復思考と自殺念慮の両方に関連していることから，抑うつの認知症状を低減するのに有効と考えられる認知行動療法的な介入が，予防的介入にも適していると考えられる。

引用文献

1) 福田一彦・小林重彦：自己評価式抑うつ性尺度の研究. 精神神経学雑誌, 75；673-679, 1973.
2) Sakamoto, S., Kijima, N., Tomoda, A., & Kambara M.: Factor structure of the Zung Self-rating Depression Scale(SDS) for undergraduates. Journal of Clinical Psychology, 54；477-487, 1998.
3) World Health Organization: Composite International Diagnostic Interview(CIDI), core version 2.0., American Psychiatric Press, Washington D. C., 1995.
4) Zung, W. W. K.: A Self-rating Depression Scale. Archives of General Psychiatry, 12；63-70, 1965.

---

*[1] 慶應義塾大学
　Eriko Tanaka, Yutaka Ono : Keio University.
*[2] 日本学術振興会
　Eriko Tanaka : JSPS Research Fellow.
*[3] 大妻女子大学
　Shinji Sakamoto : Otsuma Women's University.
*[4] 青森県名川町役場保健福祉課
　Keiko Toyokawa : Division of Health and Welfare, Nagawa Town.

老年期鬱病の看護
―自殺予防や心気的訴えに対する判断や対応の難しさ―

Nursing care of patients with senile depression
—Preventing suicide and difficulties in decision or reaction to hypochondriac complaints—

兼本　恵美[*]　　上畠　茂幸[*]

I. はじめに

　福間病院は9つの病棟からなる500床の病院で，その中で私が勤務している病棟は，隔離室1床をもつ42床の急性期治療病棟(開放病棟)である。患者の病名(ICD-10による)でみると特にF3圏(気分障害)の入院が多いという特徴がある。

　H11年10月からH12年9月までの1年間の入院患者176名を見ても，F3圏(気分障害)の占める割合が77名(約44%)と高く，その中では，65歳以上の患者は19名(41%)と，高齢のうつ病患者が多く見られた。

　今回，老年期鬱病患者と関わる中での訴えに対する判断や対応の難しさ，及び自殺予防に焦点をあて，対象者10名を振り返り，クリニカルパスの視点から見直し，看護のあり方について検討した。

II. 症例の振り返り

　10症例を振り返ると，入院当初，抑うつ気分が主であり，不安も強いが何が不安なのかはなかなか話しができず，「体がきつい」「眠れない」など身体的訴えにより，自分の気持ちを表現していることがわかる。

　入院後から2週間の間は身体的訴えが多く聞かれる。高齢であることから，うつ病の症状ではなく，他科的に問題があるのではないかと判断が難しいケースが多い。看護者は戸惑いを感じながらも，医師との情報交換を行いながら援助している。

　入院1カ月から2カ月には，病棟生活にも馴染み，活動への参加や同年代の患者さんとの交流が少しずつみられ，抑うつ気分の改善にともない，意欲もでてきている。この時期に看護者は気分転換の仕方について話したり，一緒に散歩を楽しむなどの関わりをとっている。

　症状も安定し，外出・外泊ができるようになると，次第に家族関係や退院後の生活に関する不安が出現し，入院時同様，身体的訴えが主となっている。看護者は，退院後の生活について話しあい，必要時は地域サービスを紹介して退院に結び付けている。

III. 考　察

（表参照）

　10症例の振り返りをもとにクリニカル・パスの視点から看護のあり方について検討してみる。

　まずは，老年期鬱病に見られる特徴をしっかり理解することから始まる。患者が安心して休養が出来る場を提供していくことが治療の第一歩である。入院当初から2週間においては症状及び副作用の観察が重要であり，高齢者は，他の疾患により様々な薬剤を服用していることが多いので，家族より病歴を聴取し，合併症をとらえておくことも必要である。この時期は，身体的な介助を通して患者の苦悩，悲観的な発言に対して傾聴，受容し，この状態が病気であることを説明し，治療に対する意欲を持たせることが大切である。また，行動の観察を密にし，自殺予防にも努める。家族に対しては，現在の状態，症状，薬物効果について十分に説明する必要がある。

　症状が安定してくると，周囲に対しても興味を示し，動きが出てくる。看護者は機会を見て活動への参加を促しながら，関わり，適度の励まし，慰め，さらに希望を与える。この時期は，体力低下に伴う歩行障害が考えられる為，転倒などに注

表　老年期うつ病患者の看護ガイドライン（福間病院8病棟）／クリニカルパス

	入院当日～数日内	信頼関係の確立（入院～10日）	症状の改善への保証（1カ月）	体力の衰えの受容（2カ月）	退院準備～退院・外来へ（3カ月）
看護アセスメント	症状観察（行動・言動） 睡眠・食事・排泄 希死念慮の有無 家族からの情報 家族歴・病歴 医師からの情報	病像の把握 □抑うつ感, □思考・行動の制止 □身体的愁訴, □疾病恐怖 □強迫観念・強迫行為 □焦燥型 □妄想, □痴呆様症状 □意識障害, □せん妄 □社会的背景の把握	症状の改善の評価 身体的疾患の除外	退院後の生活への不安 症状再燃への不安	
検査・処置	入院時ルーチン検査 血計・生化学・検尿 ECG・EEG	ルーチン検査の異常のチェック 身体疾患合併症の有無, その検査・看護計画			
薬物療法	薬物療法の説明（医師による） 不眠時, 不穏時の指示の確認 他科からの薬との相互作用の有無	抗うつ薬の効果の評価 副作用の有無 必要なら経管栄養, ECT		服薬指導, 服薬管理	
行動範囲と安全	病棟内安静 自殺予防のための危険物を除く 窓の施錠	病棟内散歩 病院内散歩（看護者付き添い） 病棟内・院内活動の紹介 転倒の予防		院内散歩自由 外出, 外泊（同伴）	
家族相談	家族の患者への想い 退院後の患者の生活状況の予測		家族面接（医師・看護）	家族調整 外出・外泊の計画・実行	
退院計画		退院後の生活情報の収集 退院後, □家族と同居 □単身生活	介護保険, 地域サービスの紹介	外来スタッフとの連携 32条の検討	
看護・援助	身体的ケア・関わりを通して患者が自分の思いを表現できる	話を聞きながら信頼関係を築く 身体的愁訴の評価 主治医・内科医にコンサルト	（症状に対する不安） 不安の保証, 適度な励まし 患者の喪失体験への共感	体力の衰えに対する不安 体力の衰えを考慮した活動範囲の提供	退院後の生活への不安の相談に乗る 症状再燃の危険性の感知 自殺の危険性の感知

意をしながら，さらに，患者の出来ることを評価していき，孤独感，無力感の除去に努める。意欲も出てきて外出・外泊が可能になってくると，受け入れる家族のほうに不安がでてくるため，家族介入が必要となる。家族と話し合いをしていくと，特に退院後の症状再燃に対する恐れがあることがわかる。したがって，症状については主治医から説明してもらい，看護者からは日常生活に対する工夫などを助言する。また，介護保険の利用や地域サービスの紹介についてもこの時期から検討していく必要がある。

退院の話が出てくる時期には，現実的な不安から入院当初のような状態になる。これは，現実的な心配から起こるため症状ではないことを患者に伝え，安心感を与える。不安や焦りから死を考えてしまう時期でもあるので，看護者は，希死念慮に注意しながら，患者や家族と共に現実的問題について具体的に考えていくことが大切である。以上のように，それぞれの時期に合わせた看護が必要であると考えられる。

IV. 終わりに

今回，高齢鬱病患者の看護を振り返ることで，それぞれの時期にどのような看護が必要であるかを見直すことができたように思う。ここで考えたクリニカルパスを活用することでさらに検討を重ねながら，これからの看護に生かしていきたいと思う。

---

*福間病院
Emi Kanemoto, Shigeyuki Uehata : Fukuma hospital.

うつ状態や自殺念慮時の高齢者の援助希求行動
―場面想定法を用いた検討―

Help-seeking behavior for depression and suicidal ideation in the elderly—Using case vignettes method—

坂本　真士[*1]　　田中江里子[*2,*4]　　豊川　恵子[*3]　　大野　裕[*4]

I. 研究目的

　精神疾患の予防についての動きが，日本でも始まってきている。しかしいくつかの先進的な取り組みにも関わらず，我が国におけるうつ病を中心とする精神疾患の罹患率は高く，自殺者数も中高年を中心に高まっている。このような現状を見ると，高齢者を中心に地域全体を対象にした予防的な施策が必要であることは明白である。

　精神疾患の予防においては一次予防のみならず二次予防（早期発見，早期治療）も重要である。まず早期発見についてはうつ症状の認知の問題が関係する。例えばうつ症状を身体的な問題であるとか「気のせい」などと考えれば，他者への相談は望めず，早期治療には結びつかない。また変調を疑った時は，援助を求めるか，誰に求めるのかも重要である。様子が変であると思っても，専門家・非専門家を問わず誰かに相談しなければ適切な援助は受けられないだろう。したがって，地域での二次予防を考えるためには，介入対象となる地域住民のうつ症状の認知と援助希求の有無・相手について知っておく必要がある。

　そこで本研究では，調査対象となっている地区において，自分がうつ状態になったり自殺念慮を抱いたときに，それらの状態をどのように認知しているか，そしてどのような援助希求をするのか，またどのような要因が援助希求に関連するのかについて調べる。

II. 研究方法

　調査協力者：青森県の一地域の65歳以上の住民135名（男性52名，女性83名）（平均年齢74.0歳，標準偏差7.2歳）。質問は自己記入の質問紙形式で行ったが，視力等に問題があり独力で記入できない者については，調査員が質問を読み上げ，口頭にて回答を得，質問紙に記入した。

　調査項目：調査したのは，架空場面における援助希求の方法，家族構成，親戚との交流の程度，身近な友人との交流の種類，普段の外出先，家庭内の話し相手の有無，調査時点でのうつ状態の程度などである。援助希求の方法については，うつ状態および自殺念慮の状態を示し，自分がそのような状態になったときにどのように行動するかを問うた。表1に示した選択肢の中から複数選択してもらった。家族構成については，「独居，一世代，二世代，三世代，その他」の中から単一選択してもらった。親戚との交流の程度については，「よく会う，盆・正月のみ，電話で話す程度，ほとんどつきあいはない」の中から単一選択してもらった。身近な友人との交流の種類については，「お茶を飲みお喋り，共通の趣味，電話で話す，ほとんどつきあいはない，その他の交流」の中から複数選択してもらった。普段の外出先については，「仕事，通院，買い物（以上義務的な外出）；趣味，運動，デイサービス，町内会や老人クラブ，友人宅や知人宅のところ，子供や親戚のところ，散歩（以上娯楽の外出），外出はほとんどない」の中から複数選択してもらった。家庭内の話し相手の有無については，「ある，ない」のどちらかを選択してもらった。うつ状態の程度については，Zung Self-rating Depression Scale（SDS）の短縮版5項目で測定した。オリジナルのSDSとは異なり，「はい，いいえ」のどちらかを選択してもらった。得点化に際しては，症状なしには0点，症状ありには1点を与えた。

表1　提示したケースごとの援助希求の仕方（人数）[1,2]

援助希求の方法	うつ状態(%)	自殺念慮(%)
普通のことなので何もしない	13(9.6)	8(5.9)
普通ではないと思うが特に何もしない	15(11.1)	18(13.3)
家族や友人，知人に相談する	77(57.0)	74(54.8)
保健婦・医者などの専門家に相談する	14(10.4)	21(15.6)
その他	20(14.8)	15(11.1)

1) 重複選択を許している
2) N=135

Ⅲ．結果・考察

ケース別の援助希求行動は表1のようになった。大まかにいって，「何もしない」人が2割，「誰かに相談する」人が7割近くいた。このことは二次予防の可能性を示唆している。非専門家については，地域において精神保健に関する正しい知識を普及させれば，相談を受けた場合にうつ状態や自殺念慮を看過することなく，保健婦や医者などの専門家へ連絡する態勢をとることができるかもしれない。専門家への相談では，自由記載を調べたところ現在かかっている病院の医師や保健婦に話すという回答がほとんどであり，精神科へ相談するという回答はほとんどなかった。地方農村部では開業する精神科も少なく，また偏見のためもあって精神科への受診はためらわれ，かかりつけの医師や保健婦へ相談することが多いだろう。今後は，非精神科の医師や保健婦にも精神科についての知識を普及させ，早期発見・早期治療につとめる必要があろう。

調査した諸変数との関連であるが，家族構成や家庭内の話し相手の有無と援助希求の方法との間には有意な関係は見いだされなかった。また「普段の外出先」のうち，「義務的な外出」の有無と援助希求の方法との間にも有意な関係は見いだされなかった。

親戚との交流との関係では，「盆・正月のみ」「電話で話す程度」を「ほとんどつきあいはない」と併せて「ほとんどもしくはあまり会わない」というカテゴリーにまとめ，「よく会う」と比較した。その結果，親戚とよく会う人はそうでない人と比べて，うつ状態や自殺念慮を抱いたときに「普通でないと思うが特に何もしない」ということは少なく，非専門家に相談することが多いことが見いだされた。同様の結果は，身近な友人との交流との関係，娯楽外出の有無，現在のうつ状態の高低でも見られた。すなわち，身近な友人との交流がある人，娯楽のための外出先がある人，現在のうつ状態が低い人では，うつ状態や自殺念慮を抱いたときに「普通でないと思うが特に何もしない」ことが少なかったり，非専門家に相談することが多かったりした。親戚や友人との交流がなく地域で孤立している高齢者は，うつ症状や自殺念慮を経験しても援助希求をしにくいと思われる。このような人々に保健婦などによる訪問を手厚くする必要が示唆された。

[*1] 大妻女子大学
　Shinji Sakamoto : Otsuma Women's University.
[*2] 日本学術振興会
　Eriko Tanaka : JSPS Research Fellow.
[*3] 青森県名川町役場保健福祉課
　Keiko Toyokawa : Division of Health and Welfare, Nagawa Town.
[*4] 慶應義塾大学
　Eriko Tanaka, Yutaka Ono : Keio University.

郷土文化を媒介とした回想法
Reminiscent therapy by local folk culture

赤嶺　政信*　　与那覇康博*

Ⅰ. 郷土文化の導入

　痴呆高齢者は，言葉による意思伝達がとりにくく，会話を中心とした回想法が難しい。従って，非言語的な媒介物として，地元で古くから歌われてきた民謡，わらべうた，琉歌（和歌に対して）を介して回想法を行った。民謡，わらべうた，琉歌は民衆のうちがわから自然発生するかのようにわき起こり，滅びることがなかった。それらには，論理を越えて情動にうったえる力をそなえている。言葉での自己表現が困難な痴呆高齢者には，若い頃に親しんだ民謡をくちずさんだり，琉歌を難なく口にする場面が見うけられる。郷土文化を介した回想法において，どのような側面に効果があったか，検討する。

Ⅱ. 対象と方法

　対象は当院痴呆療養病棟に入院中の患者さんで，痴呆の重症度に関係なく，身体的に安定していて，重度な難聴を有さない8人（男性4人，女性4人）で，年齢は67〜97歳（平均年齢81.7歳）とした（表1）。

　方法は週1回1時間，平成12年4月〜平成13年3月の1年間，グループ療法室で行った。室内には観葉植物や水槽，郷土の民芸品を配置し，和らいだ雰囲気にした。参加メンバーは円卓を囲んでイスに座る。スタッフは精神科医1人，心理士1人，看護職1人であった。テーマは前もって決めておくが，特に限定せず当時の想い出を語る体験を重視する。

Ⅲ. 結　果

　評価にあたっては，実施の前後に改訂長谷川式簡易知能評価スケール（HDS-R）とN式老年者用精神状態評価尺度（NMスケール）を測定した。また，毎回ごとに東大式観察評価スケールを用いて，各メンバーの状態変化を見た。統計学的検討はt検定にて行った。

　HDS-R，NMスケールの結果を表2，東大式観察評価スケールの結果を表3にそれぞれ示す。HDS-R，NMスケール，東大式観察スケールとも，試行前後において得点変化に有意差は認められなかった。

表1

氏名	年令	性別	疾患名
O・Y	97	男	アルツハイマー型痴呆
Y・T	93	男	アルツハイマー型痴呆
M・S	86	男	アルツハイマー型痴呆
A・T	67	男	血管性痴呆
U・M	79	女	血管性痴呆
G・H	78	女	アルツハイマー型痴呆
T・Y	78	女	血管性痴呆
S・S	78	女	血管性痴呆

表2

氏名	HDS-R		NMスケール	
	施行前	試行後	施行前	試行後
O・Y	3	1	29	27
Y・T	4	4	33	33
M・S	1	6	25	29
A・T	12	12	27	27
U・M	6	6	31	31
G・H	7	4	29	27
T・Y	3	3	35	35
S・S	20	20	27	29
平均	7	7	29.5	29.8
標準偏差	6.23	6.16	3.34	3.01

表3

氏名	言語的コミュニケーション		非言語的コミュニケーション		注意・関心		感情	
	施行前	試行後	施行前	試行後	施行前	試行後	施行前	試行後
O・Y	1	2	3	4	1	1	4	5
Y・T	4	5	5	5	4	5	5	5
M・S	1	3	3	3	3	4	5	5
A・T	4	3	4	5	5	5	5	5
U・M	4	3	5	5	4	4	5	5
G・H	4	4	5	5	4	3	5	5
T・Y	4	3	4	5	5	4	5	5
S・S	5	4	4	4	5	5	5	5
平均	3.4	3.4	4.1	4.5	3.9	3.9	4.9	5.0
標準偏差	1.51	0.92	0.83	0.76	1.36	1.36	0.35	0.35

Ⅳ. 事 例（わらべ歌）

沖縄のわらべ歌「赤田首里殿内 黄金燈篭サギィテ ウリガ アカリバ 弥勒ウンケ」（赤田の首里殿内に黄金の燈篭を下げて，それに火がともったら弥勒様をお迎えしょう）をメンバー全員で歌う。「そうとう，小さい頃の歌だ」と90才を越えたYさんは覚えていた事に感嘆しながら発言する。Uさんは歌が終わると続けて同じ曲で「東明ガリバ 墨ナレガ イチュン 髪結テ タボレ 我親ガナシ」（東の空が明るくなると，学問を習いに行きます。髪を結ってくださいお母さん）と歌い，他のメンバーも想い出したかのように歌う。さらにUさんは「こういう歌もあるよ」と同じメロディーで「月ヤ昔カラ 変ワル事 ネサミ 変ワティ イクムヌャ 人ヌ心」（月は昔から変わることはあるまい。変わっていくものは人の心だ）わらべ歌をきっかけに，学校の話となり，弁当の中身や当時の服装の話題が次々と出てくる。

Ⅴ. 考 察

今回の結果から，有意差は統計学的にも認められなかったが，得点の変化から回想法が痴呆患者さんに良い効果を与える可能性が示唆された。特に，東大式観察評価スケールにおいて非言語的コミュニケーションと感情の側面でスコアの維持，上昇がみられる。記憶を呼び戻すきっかけとして，古くから郷土文化を用いたことが回想法の効果をあげた要因だと考えられる。琉歌を手がかりに，出身地の風景を思い浮かべたり，わらべ歌を聞いたり，歌ったりすることで子供の頃を懐かしむことがあって，記憶の想起が容易に促されたといえる。痴呆患者さんに対して過去の記憶にはたらきかけることは容易ではないが，今後，一人一人の高齢者のレベルに応じた導入方法を工夫する必要があると考えられる。

文 献

1) 黒川由紀子：痴呆老人に対する回想法グループ. 老年精医誌, 5; 73-81, 1994.
2) 黒川由紀子, 斎藤正彦, 松田修：老年期における精神療法の効果評価―回想法をめぐって. 老年精医誌, 6; 315-329, 1995.
3) 須貝佑一, 竹中星郎：痴呆性精神疾患の非薬物的アプローチの臨床的意義と適応. 老年精医誌, 6; 1471-1475, 1995.

*医療法人アガペ会北中城若松病院
Masanobu Akamine, Yasuhiro Yonaha : Kitanakagusuku Wakamatsu Hospital, Okinawa.

老人性痴呆疾患治療病棟でのヒヤリハット
―インシデントに学ぶ医療事故防止―

Characteristics of advers events in the psychiaric hospital with wards for senile dementia

阿河　礼子* 　井田　能成* 　御手洗裕子* 　増田貴美子*

Ⅰ．はじめに

当院は254床の単科の精神科神経科病院で平成4年に老人性痴呆疾患治療病棟を併設した。適応能力の低下した痴呆老人においては痴呆という疾患の特徴的要因や環境の変化から，情緒的混乱を招き易く，医療事故へつながる事も多いと言える。今回，医療事故防止対策委員会の行った「医療事故防止に関する調査」のアンケート結果・意識調査の結果・事故報告書の提出結果を基に，痴呆病棟で起こる事故について分析を行った。

Ⅱ．目　的

1) 患者に起こりやすい事故の内容を明らかにする。
2) 予防可能な事故へのアプローチ内容を明らかにする。
3) 事故防止の為の対策を明らかにし医療の質を保証する。

Ⅲ．方　法

当院看護職を対象に，厚生省の「医療リスクマネージメント・システム構築に関する研究班の，看護のヒヤリハット事例，領域別収集事例」より，精神科に関連した項目を選出して当院の医療事故防止対策委員会が実施した調査結果を基に，事故の危険因子について分類・分析を行った。

Ⅳ．結果・考察

厚生省が一般病院を中心として218病院を調査した結果では，診察の補助業務の事例が62%，療養上の世話業務の事例が31%を占めていた。当院では，診察の補助業務の事例が22%，療養上の世話業務の事例が56%を示し結果が反転していた。更に当院では，精神科系・老人系にわけ分類分析をした結果，老人系での療養上の世話業務は72%となった。この事に注目し，療養上の世話業務における事故内容を分類した結果，転倒転落・誤食異食・誤飲誤嚥の報告が多く確認できた。その中で上位を占める転倒転落について着目した。医療事故防止に関するアンケート調査では転倒転落の体験事例は全体の82%に見られた。事故やインシデント体験後には，その予防に対する注意や観察をする意識が高まってくるようになったという意見や所属部署での取り組みでは予防の為の統一したマニュアルを作るといったリスクの頻度・結果の重大性に伴った発展的な取り組みと予防意識の向上が伺えた。しかし，インシデントレポートをどのレベルで判断してよいのか分かりにくいという意見が33%あり，インシデントを体験しても書かなかった事があるに対しては，62.7%と高値であり報告基準を定めるようにした。

表1は，厚生省研究班・川村治子氏のヒヤリハットが教える，医療における危険要因とその分類を使用し，痴呆病棟での療養上の世話における危険要因とその分類へ評価し直したものである。厚生省施設基準に基づき，自力歩行が可能な痴呆老人が入院の対象となっているが，実際には歩行障害の為杖伝い，伝い歩きなど歩行不安定な状態で入院してくるケースも多いのが現状である。精神症状や行動障害・睡眠障害の為，薬物治療として向精神病薬を投与した場合，過鎮静となり車椅子使用や床上安静の為ベット抑制が必要となるケースも多々ある。そうした場合にはADLも低下し，排泄・食事・入浴・着脱衣・洗面・整容・安全についてのケアが増大する事で事故に対する患

表1 痴呆病棟での療養上の世話における危険要因と分類

		内　　容
患者側要因	患者の特性	★痴呆(記憶障害, 認知障害)(せん妄, 妄想, 徘徊, 異食) ★高齢に伴う身体特徴 ・視力障害(白内障, 老視) ・聴力障害(難聴) ・歩行障害(脳血管性痴呆に伴う下肢筋力低下, 片麻痺, 変形性関節症) ・筋, 神経障害(嚥下, 咀嚼障害, 運動能力の低下) ・コミュニケーション障害(失語)
	服用の薬剤	★トランキライザー, 降圧剤, 睡眠導入剤, 血糖降下剤の使用 ・睡眠, ふらつき, せん妄, アカシジア, ジスキネジア, 低血糖症状, パーキンソン症状, 脱力, 過鎮静作用
状況的要因	状況(患者)	★日常生活動作(排泄, 食事, 入浴, 着脱衣, 洗面, 整容) ・車椅子, 杖の使用による移動 ★療養環境上の要因 ・病棟という閉鎖的な環境 ・住み慣れた環境との違い(トイレ, 風呂, 洗面所の場所, ベット)
	状況(医療者)	★勤務体制の変わり目, 他の業務の遂行, 多忙 　注意を促す特定患者への対応 ・申し送り, カンファ, 休憩中 ・夜間勤務といった手薄な状況 ・急変者, 要観察者への関わり 　多忙による緊張状況
医療側要因	医療従事者	★ヒューマンエラー(認知―判断, 動作エラーを誘発しやすい条件) ・過労, 睡眠不足, 体調不良など ★知識, 経験, 技術上の要因 ・新人の(知識, 経験, 技術)不足による要因 ・慣れによる確認不足 ★医療従事者間のコミュニケーション 　(情報伝達ミス, 確認, 情報漏れ)

者側要因, 状況的要因が拡大する。更に医療側要因として, 定められた人数で業務内容の質・量が共に増し, 多忙となり, 事故の起こりやすい状況を作るという悪循環ともなり得る。現在, 痴呆の特徴的要因や精神症状により予測のつかぬ事故への完全な予防対策・方法は難しく, リスク回避の為, 医療部門での情報共有する事を重要と認識し対応へ努めてきた。昨年10月より提出された報告書は医療事故防止対策委員会の定例会にて事故分析され, 議事録として各部署へ配布している。今後は更に病棟独自の評価を加え, 事故防止のポイント, 体制整備, 対応の改善策を打ち出し, 予防可能な事故内容を明らかにアプローチする事を質の評価, 指標とし我々の医療の質を保持して行きたいと考える。

V. 結　　論

1) 患者側要因によって起こる転倒転落・誤飲誤嚥・誤食異食が療養上の世話において60％を占めていた。

2) 医療側要因の備品, 設備環境の不備による事故は17％を占めるが, これは予防が可能である。

3) 状況要因においてはADLの拡大, QOLの向上に対する積極的アプローチと医療者の業務意識の改善が必要である。

VI. 終わりに

医療事故についての社会の関心度が高まり患者の権利が尊重される中, 痴呆患者の医療現場においては「痴呆患者だから仕方がない」という医療者側の事故防衛的な説明に患者家族も仕方なく同意している状況にあるのではないだろうか。私達医療者側の問題を「痴呆だから」にすりかえるのではなく, 患者家族から信頼・安心・満足を受ける為にはどうすればよいのかの観点を定め「身内を看るこころ」で事故防止に努めたいと思う。

*小倉蒲生病院
Ayako Agawa, Yoshishige Ida, Hiroko Mitarai, Kimiko Masuda : Kokura Gamoh Hospital.

二次予防のうえで重要な精神科急性期治療棟と分裂病の様態

The importance of the psychiatric acute-care ward in secondary prevention and the pathophysiology of schizophrenia

佐々木勇之進*

'96年，保険診療に精神科急性期治療病棟の制度が導入された。そこで，早々に隔離室1床を含む定床42床の開放病棟である8病棟，またさらに，'99年1月から隔離室8床を含む定床40床の閉鎖病棟である西2病棟を精神科急性期治療病棟として発足させた。それから丸々2年を経過した。

筆者は，精神科急性期治療病棟の運営に関しては，基本的にはF2（精神分裂病）を中心に検討すべきであると考えているので，当然のことながらF2を中心に述べることにする。

福間病院の年間の入退院件数は，併発疾患による帰院を除くと概して1日1件の入院と退院である。

年間入院件数1日1件
新入院 55% ┌ 20% 分裂病
             └ 35% その他
再入院 45% ┌ 25% 分裂病
             └ 20% その他

図1

入院	新	再	計	新／計	再／計
'99	52	55	107	49%	51%
'00	54	61	115	47%	53%
計	106	116	222	48%	52%

※退院に関しては西2病棟から退院するとは限らないので省く。
図2　西2病棟の'99と'00年のF2入院の動向について

入院	新	再	計	新／計	再／計
'99	23	39	62	37%	63%
'00	30	40	70	42%	58%
計	53	79	132	40%	60%

※退院に関しては8病棟から退院するとは限らないので省く。
図3　8病棟の'99と'00年のF2入院の動向について

西2病棟と8病棟のF2の要約

1）西2病棟と8病棟の入院件数を併せると，'99年が169件，'00年が185件である。多少，微増の傾向か？

2）入院患者のうち新入院患者は，'99年が75件と'00年が84件。再入院患者は，94件と101件でいずれも微増。新入院と再入院の比率は44％対56％，45％対55％である。概して，45％対55％である。

期　間	8病棟	西2病棟	計
《退院患者》	62 (100%)	92 (88%)	154 (93%)
1年以内	54 (87%)	87 (84%)	141 (85%)
1カ月以内	13　40	5　48	18　88
1～3カ月以内	27　(65%)	43　(46%)	70　(53%)
3～6カ月以内	9	25	34 (20%)
6カ月～1年以内	5	14	19 (11%)
1年～1年6カ月以内	3	5	8　13
1年6カ月～2年以内	4	0	4　(8%)
2年以上	1	0	1
《在院患者》	0 (0%)	12 (12%)	12 (7%)
1年～1年6カ月以内	0	2	2
1年6カ月～2年以内	0	5	5
2年以上	0	5	5 (3%)
合計（退院＋在院）	62	104	166

（'01年6月1日現在）
図4　'99年に入院したF2患者の退院・在院の状況

図4解説

1）3カ月以内の退院患者は開放棟が65％。閉鎖棟が46％計では53％。3カ月以内の退院に限ると開放棟の退院率が高い。

2）1年以内の退院患者は開放棟が87％，閉鎖棟が84％，計では85％。1年以内の退院に限ると開放棟，閉鎖棟ではほとんど差がない。

3）長期在院患者の退院（1年以上）は，開放棟

評価	期間	'96年		'97年		'98年		'99年		'00年	
×	90日以内	10 11.6%	25.6%	10 9.7%	23.3%	9 10.8%	19.2%	5 5.3%	18.1%	8 7.5%	14.0%
−	91日を超えて 180日以内	12 14.0%		14 13.6%		7 8.4%		12 12.8%		7 6.5%	
±	6カ月を超えて 1年以内	13 15.1%		8 7.8%		12 14.5%		12 12.8%		16 15.0%	
＋	1年を超えて 3年以内	23 26.7%	59.3%	27 26.2%	68.9%	21 25.3%	66.3%	28 29.8%	69.2%	29 27.1%	71.0%
＋＋	3年を超える	28 32.6%		44 42.7%		34 41.0%		37 39.4%		47 43.9%	
合　計		86		103		83		94		107	

('96年～'00年)

図5　F2再入院患者の前回退院より入院迄の期間

では13％あるが現在の在院患者は0である。一方，閉鎖棟では5％が長期在院患者として退院しているが，現在，入院している長期在院患者は12％である。開放・閉鎖棟を併せて考えると，1年以上の長期在院患者数の退院は8％。7％は入院していることになっている。しかしながら，2年以上の長期在院患者は3％で，いずれも閉鎖棟である。

要は，1年を越える長期入院患者15％に注目するべきである。ただし，その3分の2は2年以内に退院し，3分の1が2年以上に及ぶようである。

図5の解説
1) 90日以内の継続入院は，10％標準から6％標準へ減少している。
2) 180日以内の再入院は，20％前半標準から15％標準に減少している。
3) 6カ月を越えて1年以内の再入院は概して15％といえそうだ。
4) 1年を越えての再入院は70％標準と考えられる。
   ただし，3年を越えるものは40％強である。

＊福間病院
　Yunoshin Sasaki, M. D., Ph. D. : Fukuma Hospital.

大学保健管理センターにおける「精神障害の早期発見・早期対応プロジェクト」についての7年間の経験

Experience over the first seven years of the "project for early detection and intervention in psychiatric disorders" in the University Health Administration Center

福治　康秀[*1]　小椋　力[*1]　仲本　晴男[*2]　新垣　元[*3]　古謝　淳[*4]
大田　裕一[*5]　平松　謙一[*1]　山本　和儀[*1]　外間　宏人[*1]　宮里　洋[*1]　古川　卓[*6]

精神分裂病を中心とした精神障害の早期発見・早期介入に関するプロジェクトを1994年4月から実施し，その概略は，シンポジウムでも報告した。本講演では，いくつかの症例を提示した。

琉球大学保健管理センターが実施する新入生を対象とした一般健康診断のさい，Chapman らが開発した Psychosis Proneness Scale（一部 GHQ）を配布し，高得点者で同意が得られた者を介入プロジェクトの対象者とした。方法についての詳細は，シンポジウムで述べたのでここでは省略した。

症例1　20歳　女子

入学時の GHQ は13点で，「自殺しようと考えたことが」の項目に対し「一瞬あった」と答えていた。手紙による面接への案内で来所した。自殺に関しては，生きていてもしょうがないと思うことはよくあるが，実際に死のうという程ではない。また，リストカットを何度かしたことがあり，最初は浅い傷だったが次第に深くなってきていると話した。初回は，上記のことも含めいくつかの問題を抱えて来ていたので，十分に傾聴し，SCID-Ⅱは後日行うこととした。その後の面接継続については，本人から希望があり，定期的に週1回で継続した。2回目に SCID-Ⅱを施行し，どの診断基準にも該当しなかったが，急激に生ずる希死念慮やリストカットに対して急いで対処する必要があると思われ，本人とともに検討した。その結果，希死念慮の急な増悪やリストカットへの衝動が出現した時に向精神薬を内服してみることとし，その後リストカットは減少した。また，対人関係における不安定さに対し実際的なアドバイスを行い，比較的安定して学生生活を送れるようになった。1年次の終了とともに継続の面接は終了し，現在は必要時に相談に訪れている。

症例2　23歳　女子

入学時の GHQ は11点で，手紙による案内で来所した。健康診断時には不眠と抑うつ感があったが，依然それが残存し自己不全感が強く対人関係の困難さを述べ，過度の緊張が認められた。SCID-Ⅱはどの診断基準にも該当しなかったが，回避性と依存性のポイントが高かった。精神医学的な診断は下せなかったが，面接を継続した方が良いと判断し，本センターの利用を促したところ，自ら必要な時に来所して相談を受けた。相談の内容は，主に家族関係や友人関係そして学業面であり，それぞれに対し具体的なアドバイスを行った。特に，友人関係で疎外感を強く自覚しており，その背景には家族，特に母親や姉との関係の問題があると述べた。家族関係について十分傾聴すると同時に，友人関係や学業面の問題に対して，その都度一つ一つ具体的にアドバイスをした。次第に，家族の中での関係の問題，特に母親や姉に対する敵意は和らいでゆき，現実面に対して目を向けられるようになった。面接は，おおむね月に1回であった。その後，2年次，3年次と無事に進級し，比較的順調にやれていることや本センター校医の変更などで相談の回数は減少し，3年次の来所は2回であった。4年次になり，卒業論文や将来への不安，学業および対人関係における軽度の不適応が生じ，再び相談の継続を希望して来所した。以後，ほぼ毎週面接を継続している。対人関係の問題，特に同級生に対する不信と逆に認められたいという欲求，関係念慮的傾向，

自己評価の揺れ，受動的でなかなか自分の意志が出せないことやその背景にある家族との関係の問題などが，卒業論文に対する不適応に伴い再び出現している。これらの問題に対し，まず優先順位をつけ具体的なアドバイスを行いながら，家族関係，人への不信感，自己評価の揺れなどについても少しずつ触れるようにしている。徐々に適応は改善しており，来春には無事に卒業する見込みである。

症例3　21歳　男子
　入学時のGHQは8点で，カットオフポイントよりも低い評点であったが，面接を希望していたため，案内を発送した。主訴は，忘れ物がないか気になるため確認行為を繰り返してしまうことや，テストやレポートの計算を繰り返して止まらなくなること，入浴時の洗浄強迫などの強迫症状であった。その持続は数時間に及び，深夜まで床につけない日もたびたびあった。強迫神経症と診断し，まずは保健管理センターで数ヶ月の間面接を継続して，主に精神療法的なアプローチを行ったが，症状は改善しなかった。そのため，薬物療法の目的で大学病院に紹介し，同医が担当となって，Fluvoxamineの内服を開始し，症状は軽減した。現在も大学病院で通院を継続している。

症例4　24歳　男子
　入学時のChapman's Scalesは受けていない。3年次の12月，つきあっていた女性との別れ話で，暴力などの問題行動があった。結局別れたが，その後も浮気を疑っていた友人宅に忍び込んで殴ったり，夜中からアパートを一軒一軒回って彼女を捜したりと落ち着き無い行動が出現していた。1月，指導教官の勧めで，保健管理センターのカウンセラーへの相談を開始した。2月頃にはカウンセラーからの紹介で，2回校医へ相談に訪れた。そのときの症状は，不眠や意欲の低下，集中力の低下などであった。3月，指導教官との相談で休学し，実家へ帰省した。帰省後，不眠や，雨の中を歩き続けたり夜中中ホットケーキを作り続けるなどの奇妙な行動が著しくなった。5月，家族で相談して，実家近くの精神科病院を受診し，精神分裂病の診断にて医療保護入院となった。約3ヶ月で症状は改善し退院した。その後は実家で過ごし，通院を続けていた。10月に復学し，しばらくは問題なく過ごしていたが，紹介されたクリニックへの通院は中断し，内服も中断した。12月頃より，不眠がちとなり疎通性が悪くなった。指導教官が会いに行ったところ，疎通がとれず食事の摂取もほとんどしていなかった。12月下旬，他人の車に乗ろうとしているところを警察に保護され，翌日，指導教官と伴に当大学病院の救急部を受診し，当科へ入院となった。当初は，疎通困難で食事もほとんど摂れない状態であったが，薬物療法にて，改善した。翌1月上旬に退院となったが，その後も休学を続けており，実家にて治療を継続している。復学のめどは立っていない。

　以上のことより，以下のことが考察された。
1．症例1と2は，本プロジェクトを通じて，本センターに継続して来所するようになった例である。症例1は定期的に，症例2は本人の必要に応じて相談に訪れた。本プロジェクトの立ち上げにより相談がよりしやすくなったと考えられた。
2．症例3は，本センターにしばらく相談に訪れた後，薬物療法を目的に大学病院精神科に紹介し治療を継続している例である。本プロジェクトが早期の治療導入に役立っていると考えられた。
3．症例4は，本プロジェクトに参加せず，後に精神分裂病を発症した例である。このような症例をできるだけ少なくすることが大事であろう。そのためには，スクリーニングの回収率を上げることが重要ではないかと考えられた。

---

[1]琉球大学医学部精神神経科学講座　Yasuhide Fukuji, Chikara Ogura, Ken-ichi Hiramatsu, Kazuyoshi Yamamoto, Hiroto Hokama, Hiroshi Miyazato : Department of Neuropsychiatry University of the Ryukyus.
[2]沖縄県立精和病院　Haruo Nakamoto : Okinawa Prefectural Seiwa Hospital.
[3]新垣病院　Hajime Arakaki : Arakaki Hospital.
[4]宮里病院　Sunao Koja : Miyazato Hospital.
[5]平安病院　Hirokazu Ohta : Hirayasu Hospital.
[6]琉球大学保健管理センター　Takashi Furukawa : Health Administration Center University of the Ryukyus.

前駆期が5年間継続した後に発症した精神分裂病の一女性例
―二次予防の観点から6年間の継続した対応の経験―

A case report of a female diagnored with schizophrenia following a five-year prodromal period

備瀬 哲弘* 仲本 晴男** 大田 裕一*** 福治 康秀*
平松 謙一* 外間 宏人* 小椋 力*

I. はじめに

演者らは1994年4月から，当大学保健管理センターにおいて，新入生を対象に精神分裂病の早期発見・早期介入を目的とした試みを，実施している。これは，Chapman's Scales, GHQ (General Health Questionnaire) などを用いたスクリーニングにより，新入生から精神分裂病の高危険者を推定した後，二次面接を行い，要介入と診断された学生には，ひきつづき精神分裂病の顕在発症の予防を目的とした継続的介入を行うというプロジェクトである（図1）。当大学の早期介入プロジェクトで，精神分裂病の前駆状態と診断され，大学在学中4年間の治療的介入を行い，その後も，引き続き大学病院で介入を続けている女性例の経過について報告する。

II. 症　例

症例は23才の女性。伯母とその娘，および伯父が自殺している。母方祖母が，診断は不明だが，東京の精神病院に入院歴がある。家族構成は，感情的になりやすい父親と厳格で教育熱心な母親，弟の4人暮らし。生活歴としては，4才頃夜になると「家がまわる」と言って泣くといったエピソードがあった。小学校は成績は優秀だが，友人は少なく，虫を殺して土に埋め，墓を作って遊んだりウサギを餓死させたりしたという。高校では，受験勉強に打ち込み，現役で当大学に入学。厳格な両親から離れての一人暮らしがはじまった。

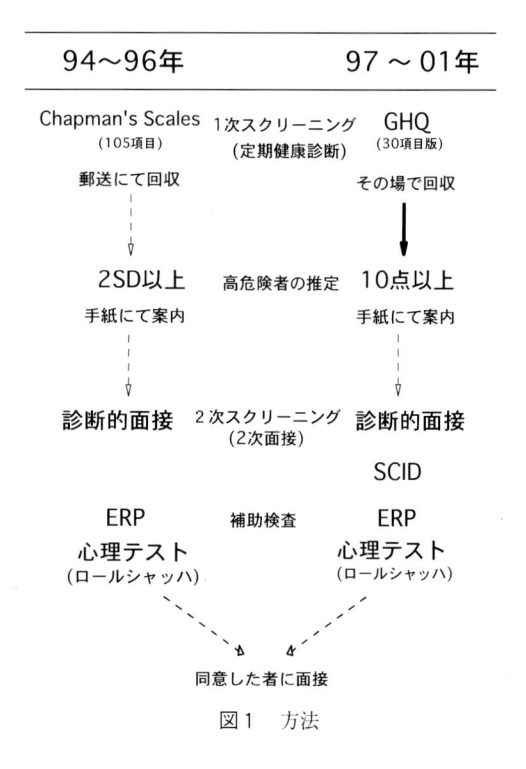

図1　方法

III. 入学時スクリーニングと大学4年間の介入の経過

入学時スクリーニングとして実施したChapman's Scalesが高得点（図2）で精神分裂病のハイリスク者として同意を得て，精神科医の診察。その結果，精神分裂病の前駆期を疑い，図3のような精神分裂病の発症予防を念頭においた介入を行った。BPRS得点の経過は，図4に示すとおりであった。

Chapman's Scales 55点(105項目中)にて high risk
初回面接所見
精神症状：感覚過敏，自生思考
検査所見：ERP 波形：健常者平均波形型
　　　　　BPRS：6点
　　　　　Rorshach Test：
　　　　　R＝31, R＋％＝51.6
　　　　　空想的傾向
診　　断：分裂病型人格障害(DSM Ⅲ-R)
　　　　　要介入

図2　94年入学時スクリーニング

94年　4月：早期発見・早期介入プロジェクトにて要介入
　　　　　　大学保健管理センターで年数回の面接
　　　　　　学業や生活習慣に対する具体的指導
95年　6月：「指が虫に見える」，「体に虫が這っている」
　　　11月：「身の回りの物から猫の尿臭がする」
96年　1月：「人の声が聞こえて目がさめる」，「家にいたくない」
　　　10月：不安感増強，diazepam 開始，
　　　　　　「家族へは知られたくない」
97年　11月：叔父の焼身自殺
98年　1月：「駐車場に人の首が見える」thioridazine 開始
　　　3月：大学卒業，マスコミ関係へ就職
　　　4月：保健管理センターから精神病院へ紹介したが不穏
　　　　　　大学病院外来で初診
　　　6月：「虫が見えて怖い，体が溶ける，色が怖い」
　　　　　　家族へ連絡，当科入院

図3　介入の経過

Ⅳ．まとめ

1) 早期発見・早期介入プロジェクトで精神分裂病前駆期を疑われ，精神分裂病に対する予防的介入を行ってきた一女性例について報告した。

2) 大学4年間の介入により，在学中に関しては精神病期への進展を防ぎえたと考えられた。大学卒業後，就職，家族の問題，治療環境の変化などの諸要因が関係し精神病期に至ったと考えられた。

3) 今後も，陰性症状の悪化と急性増悪を防ぐため，家族指導や精神科リハビリテーションの導入を行いたいと考える。

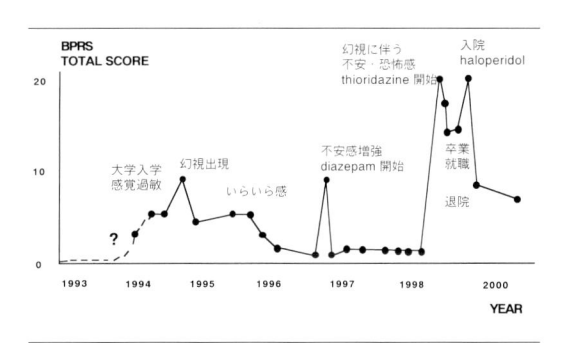

図4　本症例の経過とBPRS得点の変化

＊琉球大学医学部精神神経科学講座
　Tetsuhiro Bise, Yasuhide Fukuji, ken-ichi Hiramatsu, Hiroto Hokama, Chikara Ogura : Department of Neuropsychiatry University of the Ryukyus.
＊＊沖縄県立精和病院
　Haruo Nakamoto : Okinawa Prefectural Seiwa Hospital.
＊＊＊平安病院
　Hirokazu Ota : Hirayasu Hospital.

分裂病の1次・2次予防への寄与を目指す
疾患教育プログラムの実施経験

A new psychoeducational approach to the primary and secondary prevention of schizophrenia

原田　誠一* 　岡崎　祐士*

I. はじめに

筆者らは，分裂病の1次・2次予防への寄与を目指す疾患教育プログラムを作成し，予防のための心理教育を開始した。その経緯は本学会のシンポジウム（1A-10）で発表したので，本論では「予防教育での幻聴の悪影響の説明法」を紹介する。

II. 予防教育での「幻聴体験の悪影響」の説明法

筆者らの「予防教育での幻聴の悪影響の説明法」は，筆者らが考案した認知療法[1-4]をもとに作成した。

「幻聴体験の悪影響」の説明方法を，1）幻聴の直接的な悪影響，2）幻聴から考想伝播が生じる過程の説明，3）幻聴から個人情報漏洩体験が生じる過程の説明，4）幻聴から二次妄想形成に至る過程の説明に分けて説明する。

1）幻聴の直接的な悪影響

幻聴では，しばしば「悪口」「中傷」「荒唐無稽な内容」が聞こえてくるので，様々な誤解，不快，混乱が生じがちであると説明する。さらに，幻聴で指示や命令が聞こえて，圧倒的な影響力のもとで危険な行動をとってしまう場合があると解説する。加えて，幻聴ではその場にいない知らない人の声が聞こえるため無気味であるし，謎めいた未知性がついてまわり，超自然的な出来事と受け止めて，「お告げ」「テレパシー」「電波」などと勘違いしやすい事情を理解してもらう。

2）幻聴から考想伝播が生じる過程の説明

次に，幻聴から考想伝播体験が生じる場合がある理由を，次のように説明する。

幻聴のルーツは本人の考えなので，「どこかで自分に関する事実，自分の心の動きに正確に符合し対応している」「声が聞こえてくる間合いが良く，ピッタリ合ったタイミングで聞こえる」「どこにいても聞こえる」「相手と対話できるように感じられる」「自分しか知らないはずの内容が聞こえる」場合があると理解してもらう。

幻聴体験がこうした特徴を持つのは，自分自身の考えが幻聴のルーツなので，ある意味で当然であるが，体験している本人はこの事情を知らないため理由を考えて，「隠しマイクで盗聴されているのではないか？」「組織的に監視されているのでは？」「テレパシーや超能力で心を読まれているのでは？」「心を見通せる新しい機械で人体実験されているのでは？」などと誤解しがちである。すると，心の自由，内界のプライバシーを保ちにくい苦しい状況に陥り，「自分の気持が誰かに時々刻々つつぬけになる」と感じがち，と説明する。

3）幻聴から個人情報漏洩体験が生じる過程の説明

同じように，「幻聴自体の性質」から「自分に関する情報が周りに知れ渡り，噂になっている」という体験（=個人情報漏洩体験[4]）が生じうる理由を，次のように説明する。幻聴で，「街中の面識のない人が，自分に関する噂話をしている」体験がある場合，それを率直に受け止めると自分の個人情報が広く漏れ伝わっているとの確信につながる。また，「テレビやラジオの音声と一緒に声が聞こえる。自分のことが放送されている」という幻聴体験から，やはり自然に「自分の個人情報が不特定多数の人に伝わる」という信念が生まれがちな事情を理解してもらう。

表　幻聴の悪影響の説明
―幻聴から二次妄想形成に至るプロセスの説明―

（1）　幻聴の出現
（2）　自我障害（つつぬけ体験）の出現
・考想伝播
・個人情報漏洩体験
（3）　関係妄想，注察妄想，説明妄想の出現
（＊）　以上は「説明の手順」であり，必ずしも「実際に症状が出現する順番」ではない。

4）幻聴から二次妄想形成に至る過程の説明（表）

　幻聴から二次妄想形成にいたる過程を，次のように説明する。先ず，幻聴から考想伝播や個人情報漏洩体験などのつつぬけ体験が生じる経緯を再確認する。そして，これらのつつぬけ体験を前提として疑心暗鬼の目で周囲を見ると，色々な偶然が自分と関係あるように感じられ，関係妄想，注察妄想，説明妄想が生じがち，と説明する。

Ⅲ．おわりに

　筆者らが考案した「分裂病予防のための心理教育プログラム」での「幻聴体験の悪影響の説明法」を紹介させていただいた。分裂病の予防教育や幻覚妄想体験への精神療法的接近法を工夫する際に，筆者らの方法に参考になる点が少しでもあれば幸いである。

文　献

1) 原田誠一：幻声に対する精神療法の試み―患者の幻声体験のとらえ方に変化を与え，幻声への対処力を増すための認知療法の接近法．中安信夫編：分裂病の精神病理と治療8―治療をめぐって．星和書店，東京，1997.
2) 原田誠一，吉川武彦，岡崎祐士ほか：幻聴に対する認知療法的接近法（第1報）―患者・家族向けの幻聴の治療のためのパンフレットの作成．精神医学，39；363-370, 1997.
3) 原田誠一：幻覚の認知療法．臨床精神医学，27；953-958, 1998.
4) 原田誠一：幻覚妄想体験への認知療法．精神医学，43；1135-1140, 2001.

---

*三重大学医学部精神神経科学教室
Seiichi Harada, Yuji Okazaki: Department of Neuropsychiatry, Mie University School of Medicine.

学校交流会に対する長期入院患者の意識調査
Attitude of long-term inpatients concerning interaction with school

赤崎恵理子*　千綿　雅彦*　宮川　由香*　出口　昭典*　長岡　興樹*

I. はじめに

　出口病院は昭和41年の開設以来，精神科の病院として地域との接点は少なく，閉鎖処遇の歴史も長かった。医療，福祉の現場において，社会復帰が謳われるようになり，次第に病院も地域とのつながりを模索するようになってきた。学校との交流は，そうした試みの一つであり，作業療法士宮川らの報告にもあるように平成9年より積極的に続けている。一方で，病院に入院している患者は，このような時代の流れや，病院の試みをどう受け止めているのか，患者自身に社会に対するニーズは存在するのかを知っておく必要を感じた。そこで，出口病院に入院する患者を対象に，学校との交流会という具体的エピソードを題材として，アンケート調査を行った。その結果を若干の考察を加えて報告する。

II. 対象と方法

　1）平成12年9月現在，出口病院に入院している患者を対象に，学校交流会に対する意識調査をアンケート方式で行った。2）9問からなるアンケート調査を，PSWが病棟にて個別に聞き取り調査で行った。3）対象患者として，アンケート方式という質問事項理解度等の問題により痴呆疾患，知的障害のケースは除外した。4）上記の方法で，147名中72名の患者が対象となったが，そのうちアンケートに対する拒否または疎通困難の例が12名あり，60名を対象とした。対象者の平均年齢は53歳，男女比は男性35人対女性25人であった。

III. アンケート内容

　問1．学校との交流会に参加したことがありますか。問2．参加した理由を教えてください。問3．参加したときの感じを教えてください。問4．交流会を行った病棟の雰囲気をどう感じましたか。問5．今後の交流会にも参加したいと思いますか。問6．OTでの創作物を学校に送っています。それについてはどう思われますか。問7．学校からの手紙が時々届きますが，それについてはどう思いますか。問8．最近では，病院と地域との交流が次第に盛んになってきていますが，そのことについてどう思われますか。問9．前回の夏祭りで報道されたことについては，どう思われますか。

IV. アンケート結果

　問1（参加）．参加したことがある78%，参加したことがない22%。問2（理由）．興味があったから32%，職員(OT)に誘われたから26%，なんとなく23%，子供が好きだから11%，患者仲間に誘われて4%，わからない4%。問3（感じ）．楽しい・うれしい60%，別に感じない28%，わからない9%，つまらない・退屈2%，その他2%。問4（雰囲気）．明るく楽しい28%，活気があり生き生きした17%，いつも通り13%，緊張した・張り詰めた13%，わからない8%，回答なし20%。問5（今後）．ぜひ参加したい12%，参加したい30%，参加してもよい28%，参加したくない13%，その他12%，回答なし3%。問6（創作物を送ること）．喜んでもらえるのならうれしい43%，よいことだ37%，どうでもいい7%，わからない7%，余計なことだ無駄なことだ2%，その他2%，回答なし3%。問7（学校からの手紙）．かわいい45%，うれしい35%，喜んでもらえるのならうれしい5%，関心ない7%，余計なことだ2%，その他3%，回答なし3%。問8

（地域との交流）．大切なことだと思う37％，積極的に行うべきだ22％，大切なことかもしれないがあまり賛成できない17％，できればそっとしておいてほしい7％，わからない13％，その他2％，回答なし3％。問9（報道）．大変よいことだ45％，報道されても別にかまわない25％，関心ない7％，迷惑だ7％，わからない13％，回答なし3％。

V．結果のまとめ

1）学校交流会に対する入院患者の回答に，拒否的な姿勢はみられず，むしろ積極的な意見が多かった。（問3，問4，問5，問8の結果）　2）交流会参加の理由が，患者の主体的な動機でなくとも（職員からの働きかけ，なんとなく参加），交流を楽しめたという回答が多かった。（問2，問3の結果）　3）長期入院の患者が，社会に対する関心を失っていない様子が窺えた。（問8，問9の結果）　4）新聞やテレビ報道に関しては，寛容な反応が多く否定的な意見は少数であった。（問9の結果）

VI．考　察

交流会が，入院患者に積極的に受け入れられる傾向にある理由として，参加患者の年齢層が高く，交流の相手が小中学生（子供）であったことが考えられる。また，病院という閉鎖的な空間の中で長期に入院してきた患者にとって，院外の「人」との出会いは，新鮮であったためとも考えられる。長期入院患者の場合，二次的障害として，社会に対する関心が低下したり，出会いを喜んだり楽しむといった感情が動きにくい等といわれるが，アンケートの結果からはそういう傾向は見られなかった。特に報道に関しては，積極的な意見も多く，患者自体の障害に対する負い目（偏見を恐れる気持ち）が，交流を経験していくことで，いくらか薄らいできたのではないかと考えられる。

先日の大阪児童殺傷事件については，当初精神科分野への偏見につながりかねない報道もあったが，当院の患者側の不安や動揺はほとんど見られなかった。偏見を恐れる気持ちよりも，事件に対する怒りや，そうした人物に対する恐れ（もし自分たちの病院に入院してきたら…という心配）を感じているようであった。自分たちとは次元の違う話であるという様子であった。事件後すぐに行われた交流会では，従来と変わらず，病棟は小学生の明るい屈託のない笑顔や声に包まれた。意思疎通困難な患者の中には，子供たちとのふれあいの中でスタッフには見せた事のない豊かな反応を見せたケースもある。こうしたケースにとっても子供たちとの交流の過程は，精神科リハビリテーションの意義があると思われる。

VII．終わりに

今回の調査によって，長期の入院患者であっても，意識の中に社会に向かうニーズが存在することがわかった。しかし，病状は安定していても退院に結びつくケースはまだ少なく，患者が主体的に社会に向かっていくことは困難である。私たちは，社会と病院，社会と患者をつなげる役割を担っていると考えている。小学生を対象に行った病院へのアンケート調査の結果では地域からの手ごたえを感じた。また患者自身に社会に向かうニーズが存在する事もわかった。そうした現状をふまえて，今後も病院が，地域の受け入れを整えながら，患者にも働きかけていかなければならないと考えている。

---

*長崎県医療法人昌生会出口病院
Eriko Akasaki, PSW., Masahiko Chiwata, PSW., Yuka Miyagawa, OT., Akinori Deguti, MD, Koki Nagaoka, MD : Deguch Hospital, Nagasaki.

精神科の病院に対する地域の小学生の意識調査
Attitude of elementary school pupils toward psychiatric institutions

宮川　由香*　　田中　悟郎**　　出口　昭典*　　長岡　興樹*

I. はじめに

出口病院では、平成9年より、地域の学校との活発な交流を続けている。しかし一方で、入院患者が、地域の中の生活場面に関わっていくまでには至っていないというのが現状である。病院としては、入院中であっても、患者が抵抗なく、街に繰り出していけるような地域との関係作りのひとつとして、学校との交流に積極的に取り組んできた。

今回報告するアンケート調査は、地域のK中学校区にある3つの小学校の6年生に対して行った当院に対する意識調査である。各学校において、病院との間に直接、間接的な交流等の接点を持つ地域の小学生が、病院に対してどのような認識を持ち、また、交流がどの程度子供たちの意識の中で受け入れられているのかをモニタリングする目的で調査を行った。

調査の過程や結果に加え、その後の交流の展開についても報告したいと思う。

II. 対象・方法

1）K中学校区の小学校（S小学校，K小学校，T小学校）を対象に病院に対する意識調査をアンケート方式で行った。

2）各学校とは平成9年度より直接的、間接的な交流を続けている。

3）対象学年を小学校6年生とした。S小学校の6年生とは、平成10年度、病院内や地域の施設で直接交流した経験があった。また、K小学校の6年生とは、平成10年度から11年度にかけて、手紙等の文章での交流の経験があった。T小学校6年生とは、平成11年度現在、病院から作品を送るのみで、具体的な交流の経験はなかった。

4）全15問からなるアンケート調査を、各学校の担任教諭の協力を得て、それぞれのクラス単位で行った。アンケートの開始から回収までの期間は平成11年11月から平成12年1月までであった。

5）このアンケート内容は、児童の主観的な回答によるものであり、特別な統計処理は行わず、単純集計とした。そのなかで、特にポイントと思われる質問事項については以下にまとめた。

III. アンケートの内容

Q1．あなたは出口病院を知っていますか。Q2．出口病院がどういった病院か知っていますか。Q3．あなたは出口病院をなぜ知っていますか。Q4．出口病院に何のために行きましたか。Q5．出口病院の建物やバス、そこにいる人たちを見たことがありますか。Q6．見たときどう感じましたか。Q7．病院からの展示物を見かけたことはありますか。Q8．展示物からどんな感じを受けましたか。Q9．病院から展示物等が送られてくることをどう思いますか。Q10．交流会に参加したことがありますか。Q11．交流会で患者さんと触れ合いはありましたか。Q12．交流会時、どんな気持ちがしましたか。Q13．病院を知るようになって、以前と比べ、病院に対する考え方等が変わりましたか。Q14．病院へ行って患者さんと触れ合ってみたいと思いますか。Q15．性別を教えてください。

IV. 結果のまとめ

1）病院と何らかの関わりを持つ地域の小学6年生の病院に対するマイナスイメージは少ない傾向にある。

Q6の病院の印象についての回答は、「明るく楽しそう」32％、「別に何も感じない」29％の順

に多かった。Q8の展示物に対する印象については「明るくきれい」が61.4％，次いで「上手」が60.1％で多かった。

2）接点の多い学校の生徒がより正しい認識を持った上で，好印象を持ち，反応も積極的な傾向がある。

Q2で病院が精神科の病院であると答えた率は，直接交流したS小学校が68.5％と最も多かった。また，Q6の病院の印象については，S小学校が「明るく楽しそう」に最も多い41％の回答があり，K小学校は8.1％，T小学校は1％であった。Q13の病院に対する考え方の変化について，「変わった」という回答は，S小学校が49.2％，K小学校39.7％，T小学校1％であった。Q14の患者さんと触れ合ってみたいかという質問に関して，「行きたい」という回答が，S小学校52.3％，K小学校41.7％，T小学校30.9％であった。

3）交流に関しては，どの学校も積極的な意見が多い。

Q14の患者さんと触れ合ってみたいかという問いに対しては，「行ってもよい」という回答まで含めると，全体で75.1％であった。

4）交流会における生徒の反応は，好印象の回答が多い。

Q12の交流会した時の気持ちについて，「やさしい」45.3％，次いで「楽しい」43.4％の順に回答が多かった。

V．その後の展開

アンケートの実現にあたり，各小学校の校長をはじめとした教諭の皆さんに多くの協力を得ることができた。アンケート実施から報告に至るまでのプロセスの中で学校側の病院に対する関心の高まりが見られた。アンケート後，直接交流のなかった学校が積極的に病院に関わってくるようになり，平成12年度からは，S小学校，K小学校，T小学校との直接交流は頻度も増え，学校間の格差なく年間3～4回行われるようになった。交流の場も病院から学校，地域の中（子供会，地域のお祭りなど）へと広がってきた。平成12年8月に病院で行われた夏祭りには，各学校から教師の付き添いなしで任意に，約120名の児童の参加があった。集計の結果以上に，アンケート調査ということが手段となり，地域の学校と一つの具体的な事柄について取り組めたことが，今回の最も大きな収穫であったように思う。

VI．平成13年6月8日（金）大阪児童殺傷事件の影響

あまりに悲惨で衝撃的な事件であり，当初の報道は精神科疾患を前面に押し出すような内容であったため，今後の交流に関しては相当慎重に行わなければならないと考えた。あるいは，しばらく自重せざるを得ないのではないかとも考えた。しかし，学校の反応は意外にも事件に大きく影響されることはなかった。事件の動揺収まらない6月11日（月）には，職員会議を経て，予定通りK小学校との交流会が行われた。事件後，1カ月もたたないうちに，新たに交流の依頼を受け，S小学校，T小学校，K中学校とも交流を行った。学校側から，安全面についてのコメントを求められることもなく，以前と変わらない関係を続けている。K小学校の担当の教諭が「学校は，何度も出口病院に来て患者さんたちと会って，彼らをよく知っている。病院のことも信頼しているから，何の心配もしていない。事件と病院は次元の違う話だ。」と言われた事が印象的だった。継続してきた交流の成果であると確信できたように思う。

---

*長崎県医療法人昌生会出口病院
Yuka Miyagawa, Akinori Deguchi, Kouki Nagaoka : Deguchi Hospital, Nagasaki.

**長崎県長崎医療技術短期大学部
Goro Tanaka : School of Allied Medical Science, Nagasaki University.

児童青年期発症精神分裂病患者の保護者の意識調査
Attitude survey of guardians of schizophrenic patients with onset in childhood and adolescence

柳下　杏子* 　棟居　俊夫* 　中谷　英夫* 　武藤　宏平* 　下田　和紀* 　越野　好文*

I. はじめに

　児童青年期発症の精神分裂病は前駆症状が多彩であるばかりでなく，患者が症状を表現する能力が未熟なため，周囲の者は患者の変化を児童青年期特有の心性として解釈する傾向が強い。そのため専門医への受診に時間を要し，疾患が進行し，明らかな幻覚妄想状態が出現してはじめて治療へ導入されることが多い。また，治療が開始されても治療抵抗性であり，入院期間も長期を要する場合が多い。このため患者や家族の社会的損失がたいへん大きい。今回われわれは，入院治療が必要であった児童思春期発症の精神分裂病患者とその保護者に面接法により後ろ向きの意識調査を行い，前駆症状出現から発症，専門科への受診に至るまでの経過を調べ，効率的な治療を阻害する問題点を明らかにすることを試みた。

II. 対象と方法

　対象は1998年1月から2001年3月までの3年3カ月に金沢大学医学部附属病院神経科精神科に医療保護入院し，DSM-IVにより精神分裂病と診断された18歳以下発症の患者とその保護者15例（男性9例，女性6例）である。診療録から家族歴，発達歴，初診時年齢，初診時症状，入院期間患を調査し，これらの症例の保護者に対して，面接法により後ろ向きに患者の変化に気付いた時期，初診までに要した期間，精神科受診までの相談者の有無，受診を決意した理由，病名の告知の有無，退院時と現在の心配点について聞き取り調査を行った。

III. 結　　果

　初診時平均年齢は14.9歳（11～18歳）であった。精神分裂病あるいはうつ病の家族歴のあるものがそれぞれ2例あり，発達歴では言語発達の遅れが2例，精神遅滞を1例認めた。
　保護者が患者の変化に気付いた年齢は平均13.4歳（10～17歳）であり，変化に気付いてから精神科専門医を受診するまでに要した期間は平均13.5カ月（2～27カ月）で，入院までの期間は平均5.1カ月（0～12カ月）であった。図1に示すように周囲が気がついた変化（前駆症状）は，強迫症状，成績低下，あるいは不登校などであり，精神分裂病に特異的症状ではなかった。初診時症状としては幻覚，妄想が多かった。専門医受診までに保護者が担任教師や患者の同級生の父兄に相談した例は9例で，相談者のいないものは6例であった。図2に示すように専門医受診を決意した理由としては，幻聴など精神病症状の出現が最も多く，以下患者の希望，前駆症状の増悪が挙げられた。保護者がこれらの理由が出現する前に専門医受診を考えていたが，躊躇していたケースが多く，受診を躊躇して専門医受診を決意できずに1年以上の期間を要した理由として，保護者や相談を受けた人の知識不足と患者の病識の乏しさが多かった。病名の告知は保護者全員になされていたのに対して，患者へは1例もなされていなかった。入院期間は平均5.1カ月（2.0～9.5カ月）であった。退院後は，完全に復学している者が6例，不定期ながら保健室登校も含めて復学しているものが5例であり，半数以上が何らかの形で社会復帰を果たしていた。他の4例は復学せずに家で過ごしていた。保護者の退院時と調査時の心配点を図3に示した。退院時の保護者の心配としては，どのような状態を症状再燃と考えるかが分からないというのが12例と多く，次いで復学の可能性やその時期についてであった。特に心配点はないという保護

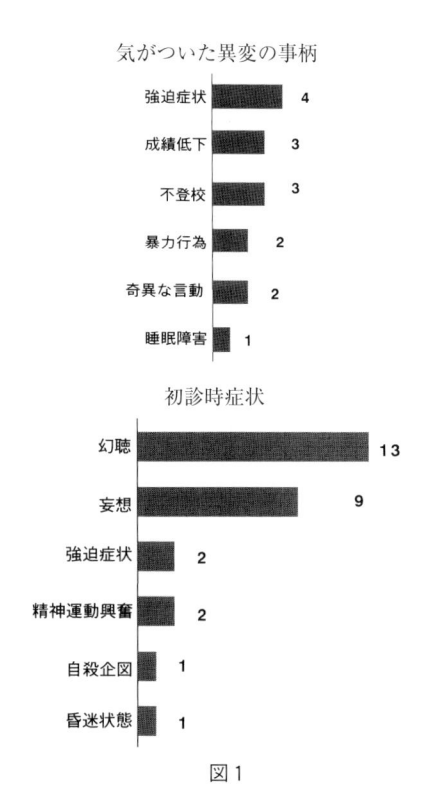

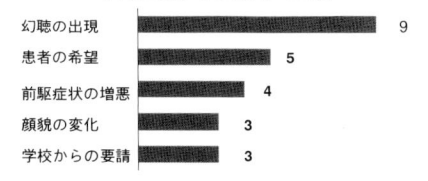

気がついた異変の事柄
- 強迫症状 4
- 成績低下 3
- 不登校 3
- 暴力行為 2
- 奇異な言動 2
- 睡眠障害 1

初診時症状
- 幻聴 13
- 妄想 9
- 強迫症状 2
- 精神運動興奮 2
- 自殺企図 1
- 昏迷状態 1

図1

専門医受診を決意した理由
- 幻聴の出現 9
- 患者の希望 5
- 前駆症状の増悪 4
- 顔貌の変化 3
- 学校からの要請 3

専門医受診までに期間を要した理由
- 患者の拒絶 9
- 学校で病気ではないと言われた 6
- 病気ではないと思っていた 5
- 保護者の精神科への偏見 3

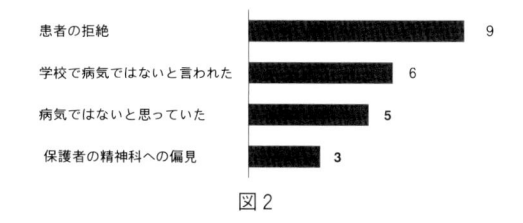

図2

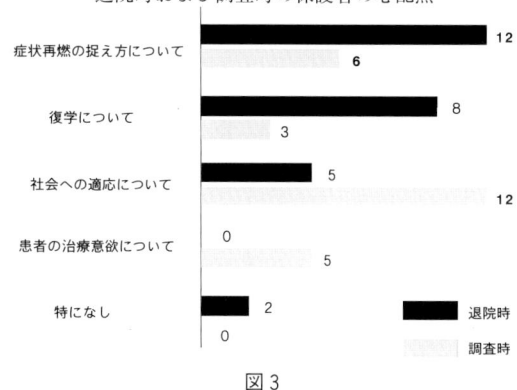

退院時および調査時の保護者の心配点
- 症状再燃の捉え方について 12 / 6
- 復学について 8 / 3
- 社会への適応について 5 / 12
- 患者の治療意欲について 0 / 5
- 特になし 2 / 0

■ 退院時　■ 調査時

図3

者も2例あった。これに対して調査時の心配点としては，意識調査を行った症例の半数以上が社会復帰していることもあり，復学よりもさらに先の将来の社会適応についてが12例であった。また，患者自身の病気に対する理解の乏しさから治療意欲に乏しい症例が多く，治療継続，服薬遵守についての心配が挙げられた。症状が軽快して退院し，さらに病状が好転したことで復学が可能になっているにもかかわらず，保護者の心配点は解消されておらず，患者の治療意欲の乏しさに対する心配が加わっていた。

IV. 考　察

入院を要した児童青年期発症の精神分裂病15例の保護者に対して調査を行った。保護者が患者の前駆症状としての変化に気付いても専門医受診には1年以上の期間を要し，その理由としては，保護者や保護者から相談を受けた学校関係者の知識不足や患者自身の病識の乏しさが窺えた。そのため，症状が出現してから受診までの未治療期間を短縮するには保護者や学校関係者に前駆症状について啓発することが必要と考えられた。また，症状が好転しても保護者の心配は解消されておらず，むしろ患者の治療意欲の乏しさに対する心配が加わっていた。これは保護者に対しては病名告知がなされ，精神分裂病に対する知識，理解も得られていくのに対して，患者自身への病名告知はされておらず，患者自身の知識，理解が得られていないことが原因と思われた。それに対しては児童青年期発症の患者に対しても，成人発症例にならって，極めて慎重に患者教育を行っていくことが必要であろうと思われる。

---

*金沢大学医学部附属病院神経科精神科
Kyoko Yagishita, Toshio Munesue, Manabu Kaneda, Kouhei Mutou, Kazuki Shimoda, Yoshifumi Koshino : Neurochiatory, Kanazawa University School of Medicine.

症状改善の観点から見たデイケアの有効性
—当院の事例を通して—

Analysis of the efficacy of day care services from the point of symptom improvement
—Through our own cases—

志喜屋　昇*　　金城　修*　　名城　真治*　　松本　庄司*　　宮平　裕江*　　久場　兼功*

I. はじめに

精神科デイケアの地域生活支援の有効性は、すでに報告されているが当院においても、デイケア通所前と通所後の入院回数の比較調査を実施し、支援効果の有無の検証を試みた。当初の調査目的を症状改善の有効性としたが、調査方法の設定に矛盾があり、その点を踏まえて精神障害者への生活支援の有効性に関する報告をする。

II. 調査方法と結果

1. 方法

1) 調査症例

定期的な利用があり、スタッフの状態把握のあるケース

2) 期間

平成元年初〜平成13年2月末

3) 内容

症例のデイケア入所日を基準に以前2年間と以後2年間の入院回数を群別比較する。尚、期間中は初入所日から4年以降の再入所は事例を2と数える。

2. 結果（図1：全体例、図2〜4：疾患別、図5〜6：種目別）

図1　全体例（症例156・サンプル172）：以前群145・以後群106⇒27%の減少率

図2　精神分裂症（症例133・サンプル146）：以前群121・以後群94⇒22%の減少率

図3　躁うつ（症例7・サンプル9）：以前群12・以後群1⇒92%の減少率

図4　非定型精神病（症例3・サンプル4）：以前群2・以後群2⇒増減なし

図5　プログラム：SST（サンプル23）：以前群14・以後群1⇒93%の減少率

図6　プログラム：手芸（サンプル64）：以前群60・以後群32⇒47%の減少率

表1

運営方針と支援内容
1. 安心して過ごせる場所であること。 ＊職員は障害者自身の自由な意志を尊重し、過度の干渉を控える。受け入れに当たっては緊張しないインテークを行う。 【障害者の不安な心境】 …（嫌なことをさせられないかなぁ。他の障害者とうまく付き合っていけるかなぁ。入院させられないかなぁ。）
2. 自分の為になると思える場所であること。 ＊支援プログラムは、目的として、暇つぶし・友人作り・趣味活動・心身のトレーニング・栄養管理・相談（悩み・福祉・健康）・仕事復帰などに対応できるようにする。 【障害者の不安な心境】 …（自分のためになるかなぁ。やりたいものは何もないんじゃないかなぁ。無意味じゃないかなぁ。）
3. 容易に通える場所であること。 ＊デイケアの職員が無料送迎バスを運行する。 【障害者の不安な心境】 …（バスは何時のバスで行けばいいのかなぁ。また、変な目で見られないかなぁ。往復だとお金がいくら必要かなぁ。バス停はどこで乗り降りすればいいのかなぁ。）
4. 障害の回復に答えられる場所であること。 ＊職員は、主治医の情報・デイケアでの観察・面接・プログラムでの実際の行動・家族からの情報などで障害の評価をまとめ、共通の認識を持つ、可能な場合はインフォームド・コンセントする。これらの対応により、症状改善・技能改善・生活維持の支援を行う。 【障害者の前向きな心境】 …（やればできるかもしれないなぁ。少し肥っているからスポーツでもしようかなぁ。あの人と友人になりたいなぁ。本当のことを言っても馬鹿にされないかもしれないなぁ。）

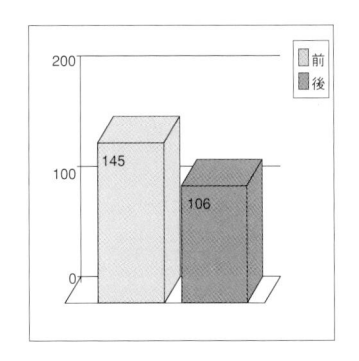

図1 全体（症例156・サンプル172） 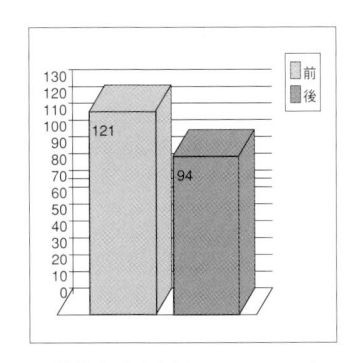　　図2 精神分裂症（症例133・サンプル146） 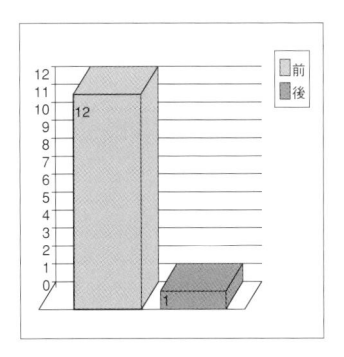　　図3 躁うつ（症例7・サンプル9）

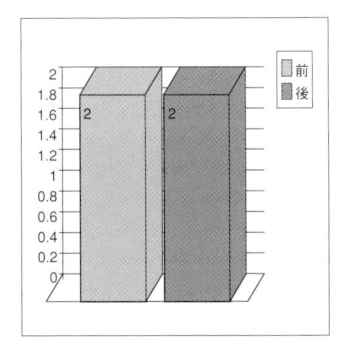

図4 非定型精神病（症例3・サンプル4） 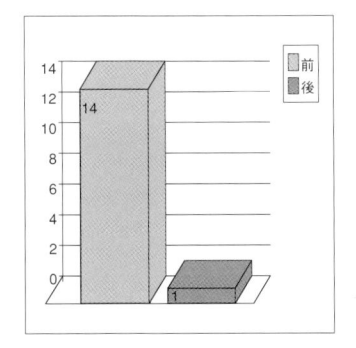　　図5 プログラム：SST（サンプル23） 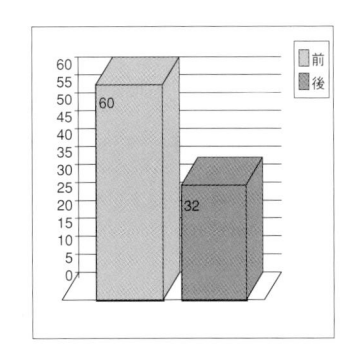　　図6 プログラム：手芸（サンプル64）

Ⅲ．調査結果の検討と課題

入院回数の増減を目安に，症状改善の有効性の検討を試みたが，社会的入院の存在，症状改善の評価の仕方，早期治療のための入院。又，慢性アルコール依存症例の内科治療の入院などの問題点が挙がり，統計処理に至らなかった。減少率が極端に高い，躁うつはサンプル数が少なく，入院期間の比較でも明らかな特徴はなかった。クローズに訓練するSSTは，入院歴のない方や適応水準の高い参加者が多いので減少率は高い。

Ⅳ．まとめと施設紹介

今回は調査設定に問題があり検証に至らなかったが，全体事例で約25％の入院回数減少率や，デイケア利用者の増加に比例し，入院患者が減少している現状から，デイケアは精神障害者の地域生活支援に大きな役割を果たしていると思われる。

最後に調査施設となった当院デイケアの「運営方針と支援内容」を表1に示した。開設当初は利用する精神障害者が少なく，継続した参加が20名前後という状態が3～4年程続いた。10年が経過した現在は，1日平均80名前後の利用者がありその半数以上は継続利用者である。専門職員と精神障害者の継続した関わりは信頼関係や状態把握に必要な事である。それによって症状改善，能力改善，生活維持というデイケア機能は発揮される。

なお，訓練プログラムは，SST，集団心理療法，室内レク・手芸・園芸などの作業療法，調理実習，前職業訓練など平均的な活動種目である。今後も，効果的な支援を模索したい。

---

*沖縄中央病院
Noboru Shikiya, Osamu Kinjo, Shinji Nashiro, Shoji Matsumoto, Hiroe Miyahira, Kenko Kubo : Okinawa Chuoh Hospital.

精神科デイケアを切り口とした再発予防の取り組み
―地域精神医療の限界を考察する―

Approach to relapse prevention from the perspective of psychiatric day care
− Considering the limits of psychiatric treatment in the local community −

市来　真彦*　　川口　宏一*　　執行すみ子**　　市川　貴子**　　宮本めぐみ***

　筆者らは「再発予防すなわち2次予防の推進」という視点から「デイケア(以下DC)を切り口として休息入院の増加や外来中断防止を中心とし，様々な社会資源のフル活用による地域精神医療の展開」を実践してきた。今回は長期入院者と措置入院頻回者という地域支援がかなり困難と思われる患者さんの代表2例に対する取り組みを提示し，地域精神医療の限界を考察した。

症例1　精神分裂病の48歳女性
　治療歴：高卒後会社に就職するが1週間で自室閉居。約1年後に2カ月間精神病院に入院。精神分裂病の診断を受ける。退院後再び自室閉居，母や物への暴力行為にて3カ月間入院。退院後，怠薬により計8年にわたる入退院を繰り返し医療中断。平成6年から2年半入院後，当院に転院。大量の抗精神病薬投与下で，無為に閉鎖病棟に暮らしていた。本人からの強い退院希望により主治医が交代となった。
　治療経過1（入院後期）
　1）段階的に薬剤を整理し，1日70錠以上の薬剤が20錠程度になる。症状がとれている実感を確認し，今出来ることを共に考えてsupportiveに接し，Positive Feedbackし続けた結果，不安の訴えは減少した。
　2）Key Personの弟に対し濃厚な心理教育後，課題の明確化を行った外出・外泊を依頼，定期的な面接時に家族の苦労を受け止め，共に考える姿勢を継続した。
　3）作業療法を導入し退院への意識を高め，早期よりDC見学参加とし，早期介入による休息入院を保証し，退院となった。

　治療経過2（退院直後―再入院）
　4）予想通り初日からDCには来られず，2日目に往診。仕切治しの早期介入・休息入院（1カ月間）とし，1週間後から送迎付き外泊訓練を行い，high EEである母親への心理家族教育と共に高齢の母親自身の福祉サービス利用の調整を行った。
　治療経過3（再退院直後）
　5）週3回，送迎付きのDC参加開始。本人のDCへの帰属意識を高める一方，Positive Feedbackを与え，送迎時に引き続き家族への心理教育を行った（この後主治医は転勤となる）。
　治療経過4（再退院後中期）
　6）本人が毎回の送迎を遠慮し，単独通所を試みたが1週間で破綻。毎回の送迎を復活し，通所日以外もDCスタッフによる電話カウンセリングを行い，SOSを出すことが出来る本人にPositive Feedbackを与えた。
　その結果家族のEEも低下し，現在は週1回迎えのみ（帰りは自分で帰る）のDC利用で，残りの日は家事手伝いをし，DCのみの利用にて家庭生活を送っている。

症例2　精神分裂病の32歳男性
　背景：生後5歳で両親離婚し父と二人暮し。中卒後暴走族に所属し有機溶剤を乱用し少年院に入所。23歳時結婚するが精神変調にて離婚。以後父と二人暮し。その後何度も精神変調をきたしては警察に保護される。
　治療歴：幻聴，被害妄想，支離滅裂にて，平成3年9月から精神分裂病の診断で約3年間医療保護入院。退院4カ月後より症状再燃，平成6年10

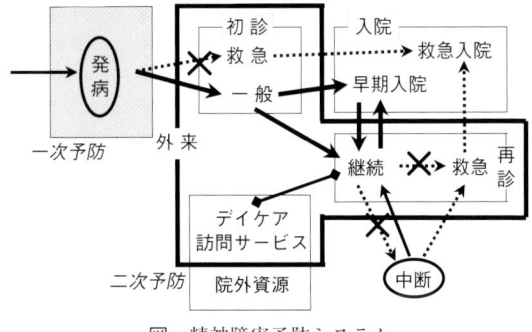

図 精神障害予防システム

月措置入院となり10カ月間入院。2年9カ月後より異常行動が増加し，近隣の住民自治会から市長，市議会，保健所，民生委員宛に「早期入院願」が提出され，半年間措置入院。退院後怠薬し，他害行為が増加。1カ月後に当院に措置入院となる。

「精神症状の鎮静と，自己中心的な態度や思考，反社会的な言動や態度を自覚させ，問題を認識し，上手な人間関係や社会性を確立する」治療課題を通し，医療中断防止を目標とした。

治療経過1（入院中期）

1) 濃厚な薬物療法を行い，陽性症状はほぼ鎮静した。

2) 病識不完全ながら内服・デポ剤使用に協力的になったため，Positive Feedback を用いた評価表の刷り合わせ（平易な目標を本人と治療チームで共有し，2週間毎にそれぞれがつけた4段階の評価表を刷り合わせ，修正していった）により，病棟スタッフが信頼感を獲得し，Key Person である父親に対し濃厚な心理教育後に定期的な面会を依頼した。主治医や特定スタッフとの関係作りも強化された。

治療経過2（入院後期）

3) 他者への攻撃性が減少した事を褒め，併せて作業療法を導入，早期よりDC見学参加を利用し，人間関係や社会性の訓練を行った。

4) 父親はもとより，保健所，福祉事務所など治療段階に合わせて医療チームの人数を増やし，院外資源を加えた医療チームカンファレンスを施行。本人及び父に「多くの人がSupportしている」という意識を与え退院への焦りを軽減した。

治療経過3（退院後前期）

5) 仲間を得た喜びからDC通所も定期的で服薬良好であった。

6) 父に対し，担当医やDCスタッフとの定期的なミーティングへの参加を依頼した（ここで主治医は転勤となる）。

治療経過4（退院後中期）

7) 退院後3カ月目からDCメンバーに対するSexualな問題勃発し，エスカレート。8カ月目に止む無くDC中止となる。その後Y病院に4回目の措置入院となった。

病棟，外来といった枠組みを越えたチーム医療の視点から，DC，訪問サービス，本人および家族への心理教育を含めた手厚い外来サポートが成されれば，超長期入院患者さんであっても外来サポートが出来，外来サポート充実，急性期医療減少のためには「早期介入→早期休息入院→早期退院」という二次予防の意識が大切と思われた。しかし社会資源をフル活用して手厚いサポートシステムをもってしても支えきれない患者さんの特徴として①性衝動が強い，②金銭的に破綻を来しやすい，③家族サポートが弱い等の悪条件を「複数」持っている場合が挙げられ，これらのハイリスク群が二次予防の限界と思われた。

---

*横浜相原病院社会復帰支援部
　Masahiko Ichiki, Kouichi Kawaguchi : Yokohama Aihara Hospital.
**相模病院リハビリテーション課
　Sumiko Shigyo, Takako Ichikawa : Sagami Hospital.
***東京医科歯科大学附属病院精神神経科
　Megumi Miyamoto : Tokyo Medical and Dental University Hospital.

SSTが慢性分裂病者に及ぼす影響
―閉鎖と開放を比較して―

Influence of SST on chronic schizophrenic patients—Comparing closed and open wards—

大野　宏明* 　村上　泰子* 　浅田　恵子*

I. はじめに

今回，過去2年間に，慢性の閉鎖病棟と開放病棟で実施されたSSTグループの経験者と未経験者を対象として，LASMIを用いた断面的調査を行い，SSTが慢性分裂病患者の社会生活技能面に及ぼす効果の比較検討を行った。

II. 目　的

SSTが，開放（慢性安定群）と閉鎖（慢性増悪群）病棟の患者に与える効果の違いを，生活障害の視点から捉え，対象患者に見合ったSSTの方針を再検討することを目的とした。

III. 対象と方法

対象は，慢性の閉鎖病棟と開放病棟に入院中の精神分裂病患者の内，過去2年間にSSTを経験した患者（対象群）各10名と未経験者（コントロール群）各10名を選出した。

対象患者のSST参加期間は，閉鎖病棟が0.98年，開放病棟が1.68年であった。

訓練の構成は，各病棟で週1回2時間のセッションを，6カ月を1クールとして，2年間に4クール実施した。リーダーは，積極的にHTA技法を活用しながら行った。

実施したモジュールの内容は，閉鎖病棟では，会話（2クール）・身だしなみ（1クール）・問題解決（1クール）を，開放病棟では，会話（1クール）・身だしなみ（1クール）・問題解決（2クール）を実施した。

調査方法は，慢性の閉鎖病棟と開放病棟の対象群各10名，コントロール群各10名に，2年間SSTを実施した後にLASMIの評価を行い，Wilcoxon検定により有意差（$P<0.05$）を求め，病棟ごとに対象患者の生活技能の比較を行った。

表1

閉鎖病棟患者の背景因子　　（N=20）

項　目	対象群		コントロール群	
年齢	42.6歳	(SD=11.8)	42歳	(SD=8.7)
性	男7：女3		男8：女2	
初発年齢	21.8歳	(SD=5.9)	22.1歳	(SD=4.7)
平均就学年数	11.9年	(SD=2.1)	13.3年	(SD=1.9)
就労経験	有7：無3		有6：無4	
入院期間	11.8年	(SD=9.8)	11.8年	(SD=6.7)
婚姻状況	有1：無9		有2：無8	

開放病棟患者の背景因子　　（N=20）

項　目	対象群		コントロール群	
年齢	50.2歳	(SD=8.9)	50.9歳	(SD=11.1)
性	男7：女3		男6：女4	
初発年齢	25.3歳	(SD=5.7)	26.1歳	(SD=4.7)
平均就学年数	11.2年	(SD=2.7)	13.1年	(SD=2.1)
就労経験	有8：無2		有6：無4	
入院期間	17.7年	(SD=10.7)	18.3年	(SD=6.8)
婚姻状況	有2：無8		有2：無8	

IV. 結　果

表2，3は，閉鎖・開放病棟のLASMI評価項目ごとに平均値と標準偏差を比較したものである。表が示すように，閉鎖病棟においては，「D12：自由時間の過ごし方」の項目において有意差が認められたものの，他の領域において，差は認められなかった。開放病棟においては，『D：日常生活』，『I：対人関係』の領域において，多くの項目で有意差がみられた。

V. 考　察

今回の調査の結果を，①調査対象患者の背景因子，②有意差のみられた項目の2点から考察してみた。①について，表1，2に示すように，開放病棟の患者は閉鎖病棟の患者と比べ，初発年齢が高く，SST参加期間も長い。このことは，病前の社会体験の有無及び，訓練への参加期間が，SSTによる生活技能の獲得に影響があると考えられる。精神症状も軽症期に移行しつつある50代の患者には，SSTにおける生活技能面への刺激を与えると変化する可能性があることが示唆された。閉

表2　閉鎖病棟

LASMI評価項目	対象群	コントロール群
1. D日常生活　　　　(D合計)	2.0±0.43	2.1±0.74
D1. 生活リズム	1.4±0.97	1.7±1.83
D2. 身だしなみ(整容)	1.8±1.14	2.2±1.40
D3. 身だしなみ(服装)	1.8±0.92	2.2±1.14
D4. 居室の掃除・整理	1.6±0.97	2.0±1.49
D5. バランスのよい食事	1.1±1.10	0.9±1.10
D6. 交通機関	4.0±0.0	3.5±1.08
D7. 金融機関	4.0±0.0	3.8±0.63
D8. 買い物	1.6±0.97	1.4±1.07
D9. 大切な物の管理	1.8±1.03	1.1±0.74
D10. 金銭管理	1.6±0.70	2.1±1.29
D11. 服薬管理	1.4±0.52	1.0±0.0*
D12. 自由時間の過ごし方	2.4±0.84*	3.5±0.97
2. I対人関係　　　　(I合計)	1.9±0.63	2.2±0.97
I1. 発言の明瞭さ	1.6±1.35	1.5±1.08
I2. 自発性	1.6±0.84	2.1±1.20
I3. 状況判断	2.3±0.95	2.3±1.34
I4. 理解力	2.6±0.70	2.1±1.37
I5. 主張	1.3±0.95	1.7±1.06
I6. 断る	1.2±0.92	1.7±0.95
I7. 応答	1.7±0.67	1.8±1.03
I8. 協調性	2.3±0.95	2.7±1.25
I9. マナー	1.4±0.84	1.0±1.15
I10. 自主的な付き合い	1.9±0.88	2.8±1.14
I11. 援助者との付き合い	1.6±0.70	1.9±1.20
I12. 友人との付き合い	1.7±1.06	2.5±1.18
I13. 異性との付き合い	1.9±2.31	4.7±3.77
3. W労働・課題の遂行(W合計)	2.8±0.90	2.7±1.16
W1. 役割の自覚	2.1±1.37	2.6±1.65
W2. 課題への挑戦	3.0±1.05	2.9±1.10
W3. 課題達成の見通し	3.2±0.79	3.1±1.45
W4. 手順の理解	2.6±1.17	1.9±1.52
W5. 手順の変更	2.9±0.99	2.4±1.17
W6. 課題遂行の自主性	2.9±0.99	2.6±1.35
W7. 持続性・安定性	2.6±1.07	2.6±1.17
W8. ペースの変更	2.6±0.97	2.9±1.10
W9. あいまいさに対する対処	2.8±0.63	3.2±1.03
W10. ストレス耐性	3.0±0.82	2.6±1.07
4. E持続性・安定性　(E合計)	5.5±0.0	5.5±0.0
E1. 現在の社会適応度	5.0±0.0	5.0±0.0
E2. 持続性・安定性の傾向	6.0±0.0	6.0±0.0
5. R自己認識　　　　(R合計)	2.9±0.86	2.6±0.77
R1. 障害の理解	3.0±0.94	2.8±1.14
R2. 過大(小)の自己評価	2.9±0.88	2.8±0.92
R3. 現実離れ	2.7±0.95	2.2±1.03

Wilcoxon Signed Rank Test　*P＜0.05

表3　開放病棟

LASMI評価項目	対象群	コントロール群
1. D日常生活　　　　(D合計)	1.2±0.49*	2.0±0.34
D1. 生活リズム	0.1±0.32	0.9±1.29
D2. 身だしなみ(整容)	0.6±0.97*	1.7±0.82
D3. 身だしなみ(服装)	1.0±0.82	2.0±1.05
D4. 居室の掃除・整理	1.3±0.82	2.4±1.58
D5. バランスのよい食事	1.1±0.88	1.6±1.43
D6. 交通機関	2.2±1.23*	3.5±0.71
D7. 金融機関	2.9±0.32*	3.7±0.67
D8. 買い物	1.2±0.92*	2.2±0.63
D9. 大切な物の管理	0.5±0.71	0.6±0.52
D10. 金銭管理	1.8±1.14	2.0±1.25
D11. 服薬管理	1.3±1.16	1.6±0.97
D12. 自由時間の過ごし方	0.8±0.63*	2.2±1.23
2. I対人関係　　　　(I合計)	1.2±0.58	2.3±0.50
I1. 発言の明瞭さ	1.0±1.15	1.7±0.82
I2. 自発性	0.8±0.63*	2.0±0.94
I3. 状況判断	1.2±1.14*	2.0±0.67
I4. 理解力	1.4±1.35	2.2±1.03
I5. 主張	1.4±0.84	2.0±0.82
I6. 断る	1.2±0.92	1.7±0.67
I7. 応答	0.8±0.79*	1.8±0.63
I8. 協調性	1.2±1.32	2.3±0.82
I9. マナー	0.9±0.74*	1.7±0.67
I10. 自主的な付き合い	1.4±1.07	2.4±0.70
I11. 援助者との付き合い	0.8±0.79*	1.9±0.74
I12. 友人との付き合い	1.5±0.97*	2.7±0.95
I13. 異性との付き合い	1.4±0.70*	5.1±3.41
3. W労働・課題の遂行(W合計)	2.5±0.30	2.5±0.66
W1. 役割の自覚	2.6±0.70	2.6±1.26
W2. 課題への挑戦	2.9±0.57	3.2±0.79
W3. 課題達成の見通し	2.8±0.42	3.0±1.63
W4. 手順の理解	1.6±0.97	1.7±0.82
W5. 手順の変更	2.7±0.67	2.8±1.03
W6. 課題遂行の自主性	2.6±0.70	2.6±1.07
W7. 持続性・安定性	1.7±0.48	1.9±0.74
W8. ペースの変更	2.5±0.97	2.7±0.82
W9. あいまいさに対する対処	2.4±0.70	2.1±0.99
W10. ストレス耐性	2.7±1.06	2.7±0.95
4. E持続性・安定性　(E合計)	5.5±0.0	5.5±0.0
E1. 現在の社会適応度	5.0±0.0	5.0±0.0
E2. 持続性・安定性の傾向	6.0±0.0	6.0±0.0
5. R自己認識　　　　(R合計)	1.6±0.55*	2.4±0.99
R1. 障害の理解	1.4±0.70*	2.7±0.95
R2. 過大(小)の自己評価	1.9±0.57	2.5±0.85
R3. 現実離れ	1.6±0.97	2.1±1.60

Wilcoxon Signed Rank Test　*P＜0.05

鎖病棟の患者は，それだけ精神状態が重症であり，般化に至りにくいと考えられる。

次に，②について考察する。開放の対象群において，対人関係の付き合いの項目で差がみられたのは，病棟スタッフのサポーティブな関わりが，患者の学んだ技能を引き出すきっかけとなり，また，SSTを経験した患者同士の交流が，相互に技能を実生活で使おうとする意欲を高める結果につながったと考える。このことから，SSTを経験した患者は，スタッフとのコミュニケーションで安心感が生まれ，それが他患者との関係へと広がったと考える。また，外出などの自由度が高い開放病棟では，訓練の成果を発揮する機会が多いため，身だしなみや交通機関，自由時間の過ごし方など，日常生活を豊かにするための生活技能を獲得できる効果があると思われる。

今回調査した閉鎖病棟は，精神症状の不安定な患者も対象とした。しかし，対人関係の項目において僅かながらも有意差がみられたことから，SSTを，コミュニケーション能力を少しでも高める事に焦点をあてることで，日常生活における不安やストレスを軽減させ，生活の安定化(再燃の予防)につなげていけるのではないかと考える。

VI. 終わりに

今回の調査は，訓練前後の評価との比較がなかったため，十分な結果を得ることはできなかった。しかし，以下のように開放・閉鎖病棟におけるSSTの方針について確認することができた。

1) 慢性閉鎖病棟患者へのSSTの方針
   - 技能獲得よりコミュニケーションに焦点付けたアプローチ
   - 日常生活における不安・ストレスの軽減(再燃の予防)
2) 慢性開放病棟患者へのSSTの方針
   - 療養生活におけるQOLを高めることで安定を図る
   - 個々人の生活技能の獲得

---

*福間病院
Hiroaki Ohno, Yasuko Murakami, Keiko Asada : Fukuma Hospital.

関連施設連絡協議会の試み

A liaison council trial among related facilities—As preliminary training for care manager—

大月　紀子*　　増冨　信子*　　秀島　幸子*　　杉田　育子**　　堤　真理**

I．はじめに

福間病院は開設以来，分裂病のリハビリテーションに強い関心を寄せてきた。精神科医療改革の中で，ケアマネジメントシステムの必要性を痛感するようになり，平成10年4月，地域生活支援センター「みどり」を開設した。福岡県では，最初の認可と聞く。

これまで，当事者への支援は，病院関係者は医学モデル，社会復帰施設等関係者は生活モデルでのアプローチを試みていた。しかし，精神障害者は，疾病と障害を併せ持ち，立場の異なる医学モデルと生活モデルとの協同により，支援することが求められる。そこで，精神障害者ケアマネジメント従事者の予備訓練として，事例を中心に各関連施設のスタッフが勉強する場，「関連施設連絡協議会」(以後，「関連協」とする)を開始した。

今回は，「関連協」の平成12年度までの2年半の経過を報告する。

1) 規約(表1)
2) 構成メンバー

部署，資格，職種別に分類。15部署，7つの職種からなり，看護とソーシャルワーカーの人数がほぼ同数。経験年数も3年から30年と幅広い。

3) 開催状況(表2)
4) 議題分類(図1)

提出された議題を「医療継続支援，退院援助等」7つに分類。開催当初と比較し，平成12年度は，「退院援助」「社会復帰施設利用支援」に分類される議題が増加。

5) 議題傾向(図2)

議題を提出した部署を「社会復帰施設・GH，DC・DNC等」6つに分類。部署別に議題内容の傾向を分類。

表1
関連施設連絡協議会規約
略称「関連協」
H10.10. 1
H10.10.28改正
H11.11. 1改正
H12. 5. 1改正
H12. 9. 1改正
H12.12. 1改正

1．「関連施設連絡協議会」は，地域生活支援センター「みどり」主催のもとに行なう。
2．「関連施設連絡協議会」は，関連施設のスタッフがあいより，事例検討会や情報交換などを通して，チームワークの重要性を認識し，ケースマネジメントシステムの推進，明確化を期し，適切なケアの実践を目的とする。
3．関連施設とは，地域生活支援センター「みどり」，生活訓練施設「緑の里」，通所授産施設「緑の里」，グループホームガーデンサンシャイン，ガーデンサンシャイン2号，共同住居「ふじ」，緑陰クラブ，陽光クラブ，悠々クラブ，悠々2科，外来，デイホスピタル，訪問看護，もろもろの特性をもつ病棟などをいう。
4．各施設から，代表幹事1名が参加．但し，欠席の場合は代表幹事が出席のこと。代表幹事は，その都度代理幹事の他，事例担当者などを指名すること。
5．開催日　毎週月曜日　15：30〜
　場　所　　研修医　研修センター
6．事務局は，地域生活支援センター「みどり」におく。
　常任顧問　理事長　　　　　　　佐々木勇之進
　議　　長　地域生活支援センター所長　増冨　信子
　副議長　看護センター看護部長　　　原田智恵子
　※書記以下は，省略。

6) 議題の経過(図3，4)

議題分類の中で「退院援助」「社会復帰施設利用支援」として分類したケースにおいて，議題提出時とその後の経過で，当事者の状況がどう変化したか。入院の割合が減り，社会復帰施設やその他へ移行したケースの割合が増加。

II．まとめ

2年半を振り返り，開催当時と現在を比較してみると，出席者の意識，姿勢と共に「関連協」自体のあり様も大きく変化してきた。今回，これまでを振り返ると共に，今後の「関連協」の方向性について検討するため，出席者へのアンケートを試みた。

一部紹介すると，「議題提出の難しさ，他部署のケース内容の理解の難しさを感じていた」「緊張した雰囲気であった」という意見が多かったが，現在では「当事者の所属に関係なく，出席者

全員で当事者中心に協議できるようになった」「ほぼ固定の参加者であることと，感情的な発言が減ってきたためか，参加者自身の緊張感が和らいできた」といった意見が聞かれた。結果，他出席者もこの変化を感じ取っていることを，アンケートを通して知ることができた。

開催当初は，出席者が所属する部署によっての視点の違いや自分たちの依拠するモデル（医学モデルと生活モデル）を絶対とする立場での，意見のぶつかり合いや感情的な摩擦もあった。しかしながら，回を重ねるごとに，お互いの機能や役割，立場が理解し合えるようになり，アプローチの違いによる距離も縮めることができてきているように思う。

それにより，特に具体的な支援を要するケースにおいて，報告者への批判や言い合いに終わることなく，当事者を中心とした協議ができ，共に学ぶ姿勢が感じられるようになった。

これまでの「関連協」の経過の中で，入院から施設への移行がスムーズとなったいくつかの事例を踏まえ，この会が再発・再燃防止の視点からも。改めて当事者への適切なサービス，支援につながってきつつあることも認識した。

なお，当法人内では，医療機関と社会復帰施設が合同で，定期的な事例検討等の場をもつことは，「関連協」が初めての試みである。この会の運営によって，依拠するモデルによって生じるアプローチの間隙が定かになり，またその間隙を埋めるべく，当事者を中心としたチームアプローチを形成できるということを経験できた。「関連協」の目指すケースワークやケアマネジメントの重要性についても，各自認識が深まったように思う。

これからも，当事者を中心としたアプローチを実践できるよう，「関連協」を運営していきたいと思う。

＊（医・財）恵愛会　社会復帰施設「緑の里」
  Noriko Otsuki, Nobuko Masutomi, Sachiko Hideshima :
  Rehabilitation Facility, "Midori no Sato"
＊＊（医・財）恵愛会　福間病院
  Ikuko Sugita, Mari Tsutsumi : Fukuma Hospital.

表2　「関連施設連絡協議会」開催状況

	平成10年度	平成11年度	平成12年度	計
開催回数	17	28	19	64（回）
出席者数	312	561	401	1,274（名）

◆ 第1回開催日　平成10年10月5日
◆ 開催回数　　年度平均　　21,3回
　　　　　　　月平均　　　2,1回
◆ 出席者　　　年度平均　　424,6名
　　　　　　　1回平均　　19,9名

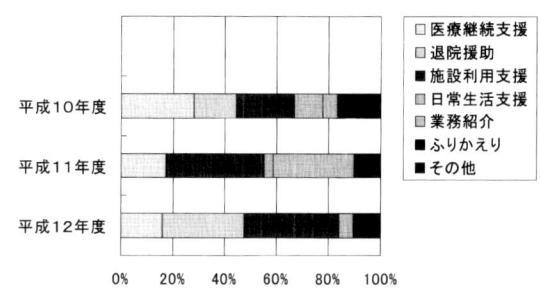

図1　「関連施設連絡協議会」議題分類

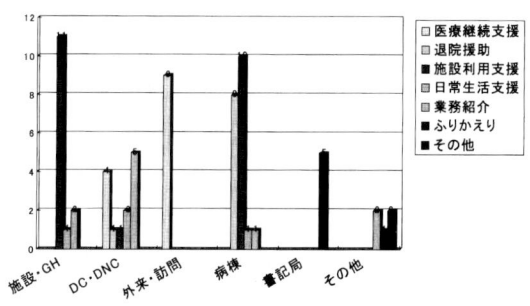

図2　「関連施設連絡協議会」議題傾向―諸題提出部署別―

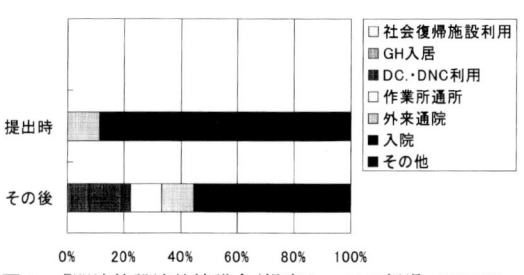

図3　「関連施設連絡協議会」提出ケースの経過―退院援助―

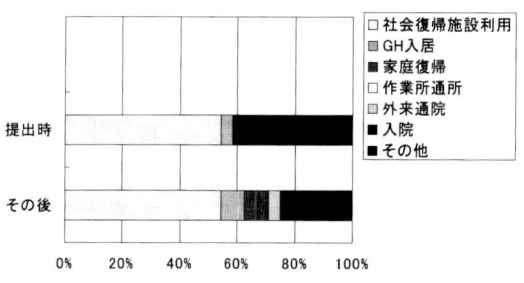

図4　「関連施設連絡協議会」提出ケースの経過―社会復帰施設利用支援―

強固な妄想体系で全生活史を置き換えていたケースが
地域で自らの人生を再発見するまで
―地域での20年間のサポート―

Psycho-social treatment and community support for a schizophrenic patient
with severe systematic delusion which led to fabrication of his life history
―20 years community support and rediscovery of his real life―

金子　忍* 　藤田　一隆* 　清水さつき* 　石川英五郎* 　平松　謙一*, **

I. はじめに

　グループ・オアシスでは単に利用者に作業を提供するだけではなく，作業所での集団を最大限に利用し，利用者が自らの人生を再発見する場としての機能を重視してきた。

　本報告の事例は，人生の中で繰り返された挫折体験のすべてを妄想に置き換え，「40歳になれば世界の支配者になれる」という強固な妄想を構築した。そのような事例に対して地域の作業所を中心に支援を行ってきたものである。

　本事例を通して，分裂病治療において自らの人生の再発見とその実現がいかに重要であるかを検討する。

　事例は現在52歳の男性。3歳の頃父親の入院を機に母親の実家に預けられた。のちに父親は退院するが，仕事と住居を転々とし，事例も転校を繰り返すこととなる。この頃の一家の生活は困窮を極め，面倒を見てくれたのは父親の兄である事例の伯父であった。伯父はエリートで自ら仕事を興し，事例から見れば人生の成功者で父とは正反対の存在であった。母親は事例への期待を示したが，事例は中学を卒業し，単身で上京する。両親ものちに上京するが，事例は職を転々とし，19歳頃から仕事もせずに引きこもりがちとなった。

　21歳の時に幻覚妄想が出現し，精神科へ入院となる。惨めな現実世界を経験した事例は，不幸な環境のもとでいつかは父親と同じ人生の落後者となっていくことを受け入れられず発病している。そして，入退院を繰り返す中で妄想体系が構築されていった。

　事例の妄想はすべて，惨めで悲惨である自らの受け止めがたい現実生活を置き換えたものであった。そして，これまで世話になった人生の成功者である伯父のようでありたい，または伯父を超えたいという思いによって「40歳になると人生の成功者である伯父を超え，世界の支配者になる」といった妄想体系が形成された。

　このような事例の強固な妄想は，一日あたり最高ハロペリドール60mg以上の投与によっても改善されなかった。

　事例は33歳で地域の保健所デイケア，そして35歳になると「40歳までの暇つぶし」として作業所の利用を開始した。それ以降，作業所と保健所保健婦は情報交換を密に行い，具体的な支援の方針を共有しながら，事例に対する支援を継続して行ってきた。

　当初事例は，集団内でリーダー的な立場を取れるようになりながらも，見通しが持てない場合などは，妄想に逃避しようとすることが度々あった。しかし，徐々に自信のない課題に対しても，自ら周りに助けを求めながら取り組めるようになった。そして事例は他の利用者から頼りにされる存在になってきた。実際の生活場面で充足感が得られることが多くなってくると，現実世界と妄想世界の間で揺れ動くようになった。また，この頃から妄想で置き換えていた過去の惨めな自分を語り始め，「40歳になっても世界の支配者になれなかったら死ぬしかない」という不安も表出され

た。

　このような事例に対して，妄想を否定せず，事例にとって「仮の生活」である現実生活を充実させ，事例の中の妄想世界と現実世界の比重を逆転させていくことを支援の方針とした。そして「伯父のような他人に頼られる存在」になりたかったという気持ちを受け止めながら，事例に対しては支配者になる40歳までを単なる暇つぶしではなく「他人に役立つように過ごそう」と現実生活の目標を設定した。

　作業所では，様々な活動でリーダーの役割を期待し，それが達成できるように支援をした。40歳の誕生日は作業所の改装主任として迎え，その時の事例の責任感は集団から高く評価され，事例自身も充実感を得ることができた。

　そして，妄想については「世界の支配者になるのは1年延ばす」と語り，その後は「5年延びた」「50歳になったら」などと語るようになってきた。

　その後，事例の就労希望を受け止めT木工所への就労が実現した。事例の実生活がさらに充足してくると，妄想は激減した。就労2年10ヶ月後，雇用主への被害的な反応や後輩との関係を上手に作れず，職場を離職し，1年後に作業所通所を再開する。通所再開後も事例は作業所の様々な場面で周りから頼りにされる中心的な存在となる。また，事例自身が表立ってリーダー的な役割を担うのではなく，次のリーダーを育てる役割を期待した。するとそのような立場であっても「みんなの役に立っている」という充足感が得られるようになった。

　事例は「息子はくるだろうか」と不安になるが，その妄想の内容も「不況でみんなが大変だから，息子が帰ってきたらそれをなんとかいしたい」と，単に「世界の支配者になる」という当初の妄想とは変わってきている。

　事例は50歳の誕生日も無事に過ごし，作業所の利用を継続している。「5年後も作業所にいるんだよなぁ」と語り，妄想表出は時折あっても弱いものとなった。最近では，近い将来の自分の姿を具体的に見つめ始めるようになってきた。

II．まとめ

- この事例が世界の支配者になる40歳をただ待って過ごした場合は，強固な妄想を一生持ち続けるか，絶望寛解して死にいたる事が容易に予測できた。
- 事例が構築した妄想は決して根拠のないものではなく，事例の幼い頃からの惨めな経験をもとに形成されたものであった。そのため支援者は妄想を否定せず事例の気持ちに寄り添い，現実と妄想の間の揺れを受け止めながら，具体的な課題を設定し支援を行ってきた。
- 「他人の役に立つように」という目標設定の中で20年間支援を続けてきた結果，事例は他の利用者から頼られる存在となり，実際の生活場面で充足感が得られるようになった。「世界の支配者」にはならなかったものの，現実世界の中に自らの存在意義を見いだせるようになった。

III．考　　察

　精神分裂病患者の再発予防には，社会の中で彼らが自らの人生を再発見し，実現していくことが重要となる。これは単なる再発予防にとどまらず，急性期の薬物療法を中心とした症状軽減後の社会心理的治療の中心課題である。その際の薬物治療は，それを効果的に行うための補助的なものにすぎない。

　本事例に対する作業所の支援は，再発予防にとどまらず，事例の人間性の回復を目指すものである。

---

*東京都江東区グループ・オアシス
　Shinobu Kaneko, Kazutaka Fujita, Satsuki Shimizu, Eigoro Ishikawa, Ken-ichi Hiramatsu : Group Oasis Koto Ward Tokyo Metropolitan.

**琉球大学医学部精神神経科学講座
　Ken-ichi Hiramatsu : Department of Neuropsychiatry, University of the Ryukyus.

精神障害者の就労支援と地域ネットワークの試み

Employment support to the patients with psychiatric disorders and a local networking trial

一杉　光男＊　　譜久原朝和＊

I. はじめに

沖縄県における障害者別の就職率は1998年度では，求職者が身体障害者514名，知的障害者245名，精神障害者92名に対し，就職者が身体障害者457名，知的障害者281名，精神障害者16名などとなっており，沖縄における全障害者就職者数の中に占める精神障害者の割合は全体の約2.1%であった。（表1・2参照）

精神障害者と他の障害者とを比較した時，非常に低い就職率は，単に労働市場や障害自体の問題にとどまらず，病院から地域にいたるトータルリハビリテーションの課題がそこにあることを暗に示しているとも言える。

南山病院を基点とした，この5年間の沖縄県南部地区での就労支援と地域ネットワーキングの試みについて報告する。

II. 沖縄県内の雇用状況

沖縄県の雇用状況は失業率7.9%（2000年度）と，全国平均の約2倍。企業規模も30人以下の零細企業が全体の9割を占めており，新卒者でも就職が決まりにくい状況が当然となっている。このような状況の中で，就労を前提とした職場訓練適応制度や職業訓練を受け入れてくれる事業所を開拓すること自体が容易ではない。（表3参照）

III. 周辺資源の開拓と連携

このような厳しい雇用状況の中，南山病院では，長期入院療養者の社会復帰を進めるために1996年10月から，地域生活援助事業（グループホーム）に着手。女性療養者3名が入所。

これと並行して社会復帰を強力に推し進めるために，地域の中で働く場の確保をしていかねばな

表1　県内障害者求職／就職状況1991年

1991	身体障害	知的障害	精神障害
求職者	556	240	18
就職者	198	187	4

表2　県内障害者求職／就職状況1998年

1998	身体障害	知的障害	精神障害
求職者	514	245	92
就職者	457	281	16

表3　那覇職安管内の事業所構成1999年

人　数	事業所数	(%)
0～4人	5,980社	56.9
5～29人	3,535社	33.7
30～99人	738社	7.0
100～299人	187社	1.8
300～499人	31社	0.3
500～999人	16社	0.2
1,000人～	6社	0.1
合　計	10,493社	100%

（表1・2・3ともに那覇職安調べ）

らなかった。糸満市近辺のGS，養鶏場，大学，幼稚園など計10カ所をあたったが，軒並み断られ，結局，飛び込みで持ち込んだ流通関係の組合の支所にグループホームの2名を受け入れてもらうことになった。これと並行してデイケア療養者を那覇市内の作業所「アトリエ種子」や「ふれあいセンター」へと送り始めた。翌1997年には，糸満市PHNの紹介で糸満市内にある身体障害者の作業所が労働力として受け入れてくれるようになり，デイケア療養者や福祉ホーム利用者などがハ

ーブ管理に通うようになった。糸満市保健予防課では，この年，家族教室を定期的に開催。南山病院からもデイケアスタッフ等が参加。翌年，1998年4月，糸満市精神療養者家族会を結成。同月，糸満市保健予防課からの南山病院への要請があり，家族会作業所設立に向けて，南山病院外来療養者を組織。南山病院 PSW，デイケアスタッフが全面支援して活動を開始。赤十字奉仕団による高校生ボランティアにも協力してもらい，糸満市役所玄関前でのパンと野菜の販売を中心に3カ月間行い，同年7月に作業所「ひかり」は正式開所に至った。これと並行して，作業所やグループホームの当事者を職業訓練として受け入れてくれる地域事業所を南山病院 PSW が開拓。糸満市内のハーブ農園や豊見城村の地場産業の染め物工房と契約。翌，1999年春より，職親制度を活用し，工房の仕事の下請けをひかり作業所で行う一方，ひかり作業所の他院の療養者をハーブ農園にて職親として受け入れてもらうとともに，福祉ホームの療養者もハーブ農園にてアルバイトができるようにもっていった。同年春，市役所玄関前でのパンの販売を禁じられたため，作業所指導員と PSW とで販売先を一緒に開拓。2つの大学の生協と新聞社労組販売店にて了解を取り付けたが，最終的には，マスコミで売り場探しを知った糸満市内の結婚式場から，ランチタイムでの販売をしてもよいとの申し出があり，2001年5月まで毎週火曜日と木曜日に販売を行ってきた。

Ⅳ．ネットワーキングの試み

現在，ひかり作業所を利用している南山病院外来療養者は作業所登録者数全体の約8割にあたる19名。このうち，福祉ホーム「やすらぎの里」入所者が6名。グループホーム「やすらぎ荘」入所者が2名となっている。

この他，「ふれあいセンター」に3名，「アトリエ種子」に1名，「ひまわりハウス」に1名が通所している。流通関係組合の豊見城支所での職親には，この4年間で南山病院外来療養者が延べ10人。また，他院の外来療養者が1名通所してきた。こうした，福祉的就労支援と並行して，職安と障害者職業センターとの連携を徐々に深める中で，障害者緊急雇用安定プロジェクトでの訓練生や職域開発援助事業などでの業務上の関わりの中から，障害者職業センターのカウンセラー，総合精神保健福祉センター OTR，地域生活支援センター職員，地域 PHN，作業所関係者たちと2000年8月から「精神障害者の就労支援を考える会」というインフォーマルな集まりを月1回のペースで開くようになった。各現場での活動報告を行う中，翌，2001年2月，作業所関係者と医療機関関係者たちとの連携が深まり，那覇北地区での民間のタコ焼き屋さんに職親を導入するため，近隣の3つの作業所からメンバーを派遣。制度活用のための県への要請活動も3つの作業所と「就労支援を考える会」が連携し，病院 PSW もこれに加わり支援。南山病院デイケアにて前職業訓練を行っているケースと，障害者緊急雇用プロジェクトを終了した「アトリエ種子」に通所しているケースの2人が，アルバイトと職親を行っている。

また，「就労支援を考える会」に集った1つの作業所が支持母体の市民組織の NPO 法人の認証申請を行い，この団体を通じて，職親の期限が切れた南山病院外来療養者を在日米軍基地で就労してもらうべく障害者枠雇用の要請を団体として行うなどネットワーキングは確実に地域へと広がりを深めつつある。

---

*医療法人陽和会　南山病院
Mitsuo Hitsugi, Tomokazu Fukuhara : Nanzan Hospital, Okinawa.

精神分裂病圏障害者の人生形成と地域リハビリテーション機能
The formation of life on schizophrenias and the community rehabilitation function

加藤　欣子*　　加藤　春樹**

Ⅰ．研究目的

1998年10月現在のわが国の精神障害者社会復帰施設利用者数は6,236人であるが[3]，補助金の支給があるとはいえ国の施策外である小規模作業所は，その4倍の障害者が利用しているといわれている。筆者らは1992年，保健婦らの作業所設立活動の高まりの中で，次は早急に作業所の中身づくりに取りかかる必要性があることを説き，その中で「かつて患者の滞留を担保した精神病院に代わって作業所がその任を負う。作業所内滞留，作業所内適応に甘んじるということも生じている」ことを予見した[2]。それから8年後の2000年に，菱山[1]は「かつてのホスピタリズムに代わって，社会参加とは似て否なる『地域内施設症』や『地域内逼塞』を助長することにもなりかねない，極論すれば，社会の受け入れ条件の悪さを理由に社会的入院を安易に容認することと同次元の，リハビリ関係者の責任放棄にも通じよう」と述べており，私達の予見は，不幸にも現実になったといえる。いま，そのサービス内容の改善と高次化が課題になっていると考える。本報では作業所のリハビリテーション機能を提示することを目的とする。

Ⅱ．研究方法

対象は，作業所で5年以上安定してリハビリテーションを受けている精神分裂病圏障害者とした。事前に事例研究，並びに発表の了解を得た上で，本人へのインタビューの記録と本人が大学生を対象に講演した時の原稿を分析した。インタビューは2回行い，内容は録音し，テープ起こしをして逐語記録にしたものを分析した。

Ⅲ．結　果

事例：40歳，女性，生活保護受給，都営住宅で単身自立生活。家族は，長兄夫婦が東京近郊都市に，次姉夫婦が東京都内に在住し，交流も有る。

1．生育歴および病歴

幼少時両親に死別し，兄妹3人別々に里親に預けられた。学童期に理由もなく気分が全然休まらない，何もしないのにすぐ疲れた感じがし，自分でも変じゃないかと感じるという病的体験があった。小学校の教師は，通知表に「やや神経質」と書いていた。高校卒業後就職したが，人間関係のトラブルで解雇され，以来，求職と就労の失敗を繰り返した。

養母の世話で，精神科を受診するが，効果なしと自己判断し中断した。23歳の時，自殺を企図したため，里親は養育放棄し，東京の兄に引き取られた。新しい生活環境で緊張し，無為自閉状態に陥った。兄が保健所に相談に来所し，保健婦の紹介で精神科を受診したが，何度も治療を中断し，自己判断による就労にも失敗した。数度の失敗の後，義姉と保健婦の説得により作業所利用を開始した。作業所でも，保健婦や指導員のサポートを得て求職に数度挑戦するが，先方から婉曲に拒否され，現在は，作業所に落ち着くことを決めた。

2．本人が語る自己像

1）時々追い詰められた感じで苦しくなる。頭の中がプツンと切れそうになる。一生病気の生活は嫌だ。緊張しているときの自分の顔は怒ったようにきつい表情で別人のようだ。これではどこの会社も勤まらない。恥ずかしい。自分が嫌になる。

2）普通の人より疲れやすい。何もしなくても疲れる。他の人は買い物篭をもってレジの順番を待てるのに，自分は疲れて篭が持てない。無理しなければ生きてゆけない。休むと工賃がもらえない。生きている以上トラブルは避けられない。生きることは辛いことが多い。

3．本人が語る作業所の人間関係

作業所を利用してからも何度も就職に失敗し，辛かった。それがショックで作業所にずっと居ることにした。作業所には自分を理解してくれる人もいるが，嫌な人もいる。指導員も住いに電気器具をつけたりしてくれるので有難いが，精神障害者の気持ちを解っていない。指導員の言葉に傷つく。自分の欠点ばかり指摘されるようで落ち込む。泣きながら帰ることもある。

Ⅲ．考　察

精神分裂病圏障害者の障害像は，障害と慢性の疾病の共存，すなわち，生活のしづらさ，それに伴う緊張感や不安，易再発などの併行を特徴とする。従って，自己の人生をストーリーテーリングすることはリハビリテーション効果の明確な指標となる。

小児期からの精神疾患体験をもつ事例は，過去のつらいリクルート体験から，共同作業所の枠組内に自己の人生を留めようとしている。生活保護と公営住宅が得られ，生活の基本的枠組みは確保されているようでありながら，常時緊張感が続き均衡が崩れると自己否定感にさいなまれ，生活的自己価値は定立されない。それがストーリーテーリングを整序することが十分出来ないことに表現されている。

臺は，精神障害リハビリテーションは，何よりも当事者への直接個人サービスに基づくと述べている[4]。このような事例には，強化モデルに典型的な本人の「強さ」に着目した個別的持続的な支援が必要であろう。わが国の地域リハビリテーションの中核となっている共同作業所に，この種の専門的といえる支援方略の必要性が顕在化しつつある。

文　献

1）菱山珠夫：リハビリテーション実践上の原則と課題．村田信男，川関和俊，伊勢田堯編：精神障害リハビリテーション．医学書院，東京，p.13-14，2000．
2）加藤欣子，加藤春樹：今，中身づくりのとき―保健婦として作業所に関わることを問い直す．生活教育，Vol. 36, No 3, p.16-26, 1992．
3）国民福祉の動向．厚生統計協会，p.334, 2000．
4）臺弘：精神障害者リハビリテーションの現場と実学．村田信男，川関和俊，伊勢田堯編：精神障害リハビリテーション．医学書院，東京，p.1-12，2000．

---

*札幌医科大学保健医療学部
Kinko Kato : School of Health Science, Sapporo Medical University.
**北海道浅井学園大学人間福祉学部
Haruki Kato : School of Human Welfare, Hokkaido Asai University.

お互いの語り合いの場が再発予防に
―『つどい』の効果を考察する―

The effectiveness of mutual conversation among patients in relapse prevention
―Consideration of the effect of "Meeting"―

金城　和代[*]

『ふれあいセンター』の正式名称は『障害を持ちながらも自立と納得のいく社会参加を目指すふれあいセンター』といいます。

『ふれあいセンター』では，障害を持ちながらも，働きがいの持てるような，職場作りに努力していますが，それと平行して，働き続けるために必要な，生きる力，苦手な対人関係の改善を目指して，週1回の『つどい』を行っています。

6年前にスタートした『那覇のつどい』では，すでに第300回を越えるようになりました。

『つどい』は，テーマを決めての意見交流と，『2分間の自己アピール』の2つの柱で運営されています。

『つどい』は，学習の場でも，討論の場でもなく，それぞれが，自分の思いを語り，意見の交流を図ることを目的とした場です。

設定されるテーマにも，一貫性や継続性が無く，その都度の参加者の思いにゆだねられています。その時点，その時点での興味を優先させているのです。

しかし，主に取り上げられるテーマとしては，お互いに共通して切実な話題でもある，「病気や医療に関する話題」「経済的・精神的自立に関する話題」「対人関係に関する話題」が多くなっています。

『つどい』の場では，意見の交流を大切にし，議論にはならないように気を配っています。なかには，必ず激論になる会場もあるようです。その会場では参加者が減る一方で，停滞気味だとのことです。

意見の一致や結論を求めないので，気軽に自分の意見が出せるようなホットな雰囲気がありま
す。気軽ゆえに，いろんな意見が飛び出すので，人間理解の場となっています。

はじめて参加した人や口下手な人でも，発言を強制されることが無いので，気軽に参加できます。私自身もそうでした。

口下手な人でも，身近な話題なので，いつの間にか，意見交流のなかに加わり，ポツリポツリと意見を述べるようになってきます。

『2分間の自己アピール』も，表現力を豊かにし，対人関係での自信を回復させるものとなっています。

『2分間の自己アピール』では，単なる自己紹介ではなく，テーマに関連した内容や，過去の出来事，これからの希望など，ありとあらゆる話題を2分以内で述べてもらうものです。

『2分間の自己アピール』の時は前もってタイマーが4人選ばれます。その4人のタイマーが向かい側の自己アピール者のタイムをカウントし，1分30秒経過したときに手を上げつづけて合図し，1分55秒からは2分までの残りの秒数について声を出してカウントします。2分を経過したら，たとえ発言の途中でも直ちに終らなければなりません。

名前だけ述べて終えることも，自己アピールをパスすることも出来ますが，可能な限り1分30秒はアピールできるようにすることが努力目標として強調されています。

『2分間の自己アピール』の時は隣り同士の私語は禁止されます。原則として席を立つのも禁止です。自己アピール者の発言中に質問したり発言することも禁止です。

ひたすら自己アピール者が自分の思いを語り，

その他の参加者がそれを真剣に聞くということが『2分間の自己アピール』の特徴です。

最初の頃はとても緊張し，自分の名前さえも蚊の鳴くような声でしか語れなかった人でも，回を重ねることで，しだいに2分近く喋れるようになり，表現力が向上してくるので不思議です。

表現力の向上は，対人関係での自信にもつながってきました。多くの仲間たちが，講演会活動などでも，対外的に自己を語れるようになってきました。

自信の回復と社会的存在感，支え合う仲間の存在が再発の予防に大きな効果を発揮しているものと確信しています。

毎週同じ時刻に，身近な場所で『つどい』が開かれることで，社会や仲間から孤立することなく，自信回復へのきっかけとなることから，県内各地での『つどい』の開催も呼びかけてきました。

現在では，県内16箇所で開催されるようになりました。これからも，県内各地で数多くの『つどい』の輪が広がるように目的意識的に取り組んで行きたいと思います。

私が，この『つどい』に参加するようになったのは10カ月前のことです。初めて参加した当時は，自分からあまり意見を言えず，心を開いていない自分がいました。

子どもの頃から両親ともあまり会話がなく，喋る内容もありませんでした。

最近では，少し自分が調子のいいときは，今日の『つどい』はどういうテーマが上がって，誰々がこういうことをいっていたとか，を自分から母に語り，会話のきっかけになっています。

この10カ月の積み重ねで，少し自信がついてきたように思いますが，第1回日本国際精神障害予防会議の場で，私が意見発表を述べるとは，思いませんでした。

まだまだ未熟で対人関係の苦手な私ではありますが，これからも欠かさず『つどい』に参加して，自分自身をみがいていきたいと思います。

---

*ふれあいセンター，沖縄
Kinjou Kazuyo : Fureai Center, Okinawa

人格目録における自己制御の減退と補足運動野の体積減少との関係

Lack of self-control in personality inventory and reduced volume of supplementary motor area

松井　三枝* 　　米山　英一** 　　住吉　太幹** 　　野口　京***
野原　茂** 　　瀬戸　光*** 　　倉知　正佳**

Introduction

According to the dimensional personality-based continuity models, the trends toward psychopathological personality in healthy people predisposes to mental illness. Some studies reported that schizophrenia-related personality may be linked to a neural substrate (Farde et al., 1997 ; Matsui et al., 2000). The purpose of this study was to investigate the relationship between schizophrenia-related personality and brain morphometry. We applied voxel-based analysis of the magnetic resonance imaging (MRI) using statistical parametric mapping (SPM) techniques (Wright et al., 1995), and related the data with results of the Minnesota Multiphasic Personality Inventory (MMPI).

Methods

Subjects

We administered the MMPI to all freshmen who entered our university in 1998 to check their mental health. Forty-two students (21 males and 21 females) were selected from 267 freshmen (115 males and 152 females) entering Toyama Medical and Pharmaceutical University who had taken the new Japanese version of MMPI (New Japanese MMPI Committee, 1997), and the MRI scan was administered to each subject. The mean age of these subjects was 20.3 (SD = .61) years. All subjects were right-handed. Written informed consent was obtained after the purpose of the study had been explained to all participants.

Schizophrenia-related measure

The Harris-Lingoes subscales for the Schizophrenia (Sc) score provide more detailed information on this domain, and allow more subtle analysis of an individual's clinical scale elevations than the basic score alone (Greene, 1991). The Sc subscale includes Social Alienation (Sc1), Emotional Alienation (Sc2), Lack of Ego Mastery, Cognitive (Sc3), Lack of Ego Mastery, Conative (Sc4), Lack of Ego mastery, Defective Inhibition (Sc5), and Bizarre Sensory Experiences (Sc6). We focused on these schizophrenia subscales to examine the relationship between schizophrenia-related personality and MRI data.

MRI Scan Acquisition and Analysis of structural MRI data in SPM

The subjects underwent brain MRI scans with a Simens 1.5-T Magnetom Vision system using a three-dimensional gradient-echo sequence (fast low-angle shot, FLASH) yielding high-resolution T1-weighted images with good contrast between gray and white matter. Image analysis was performed on a Unix workstation using ANALYZE and SPM96 software running in MATLAB. Imaging processing was based upon the method reported previously by Shah et al (1998). Briefly, images were first spatially normalized into the standard space of Talairach and Tournoux (1988), and then segmented into gray matter, white matter, cerebrospinal fluid, and skull／scalp compartments. The spatially normalized segments of gray matter were smoothed with a 12-mm full-width at half-maximum isotropic Gaussian kernel to accommodate individual variability in gyral anatomy. Correlational analyses were performed using SPM 96. Each schizophrenia-related MMPI subscale (Sc1-Sc6) was treated as the covariate of interest, and global gray matter and age as confounding covariates.

Results

The Sc3 score was negatively correlated to gray matter volume of the supplementary motor area (SMA), while the Sc3 score was positively related to gray matter volume of the cerebellar vermis. The Sc5 was also negatively correlated to gray matter volume in region adjacent to the precuneous. There was no significant correlation between other scores including Sc1, Sc2, Sc4 and Sc6 and gray matter volumes.

Discussion

This study obtained results indicating that self-control in the MMPI subscales is related to the morphological changes in the SMA, the precuneus and the cerebellar vermis that govern voluntary movements and motor imagery. This finding provides important clues for understanding the neural basis responsible for the disturbance of the self associated with such schizophrenia-related disorders as schizotypal personality and schizophrenia.

Acknowledgements : This study was supported by Grant-in-Aid for Exploratory Research, 12871016 from the Ministry of Education, Science, Sports and Culture of Japan.

References

1) Farde, L., Gusiavsson, J. P., Jonsson, E. : D2 dopamine receptors and personality traits. Nature, 38 ; 590, 1997.
2) Greene, R. L. : The MMPI-2／MMPI : An interpretive manual. Allyn & Bacon, Boston, 1991.
3) Matsui, M., Gur, R. C., Turetsky, B. I., Yan, M., Gur, R. E. : The relation between tendency for psychopathology and reduced frontal brain volume in healthy people. Neuropsychiatry, Neuropsychology & Behavioral Neurology, 13 ; 155-162, 2000.
4) New Japanese MMPI Committee : Study of standardization for the New Japanese MMPI. San-Kyo-Bo, Kyoto, 1997.
5) Shah, R. J., Ebmeier, K. P., Glabus, M. F., Goodwn, G. M. : Cortical grey matter reductions associated with treatment-resistant chronic unipolar depression : controlled magnetic resonance imaging study. Br. J. Psychiatry, 172 ; 527-532, 1998.
6) Talairach, J., Tournoux, P. : A co-planar stereotactic atlas of the human brain. Thieme, Stuttgart, 1988.
7) Wright, I. C., McGuire, P. K., Poline, J. B., Travere, J. M., Murray, R. M., Frith, C. D., Frackowiak, R. S. J., Friston, K. J. : A voxel-based method for statistical analysis of gray and white matter density applied to schizophrenia. Neuroimage, 2 ; 244-252, 1995.

---

*富山医科薬科大学医学部心理学教室
Mie Matsui : Department of Psychology, School of Medicine, Toyama Medical and Pharmaceutical University.
**富山医科薬科大学医学部精神神経医学教室
Eiichi Yoneyama, Tomiki Sumiyoshi, Shigeru Nohara, Masayoshi Kurachi : Department of Neuropsychiatry, School of Medicine, Toyama Medical and Pharmaceutical University.
***富山医科薬科大学医学部放射線医学教室
Kyo Noguchi , Hikaru Seto : Department of Radiology, School of Medicine, Toyama Medical and Pharmaceutical University.

精神分裂病の発症年齢と N200異常
―患者の発症年齢が若いほど異常は高度か？―

Abnormality of N200 and onset age in schizophrenia
―Does increased N200 amplitude reflect early onset?―

王　継軍* 　外間　宏人* 　平松　謙一*

Auditory ERPs were recorded from 58 drug free or drug naive patients with schizophrenia. Twenty-five normal healthy subjects were included as the control group. N200 measurements were measured from ERPs at Fz. The significant group difference was detected only for the N200 latency. However, the N200 amplitude correlated with the age factor in the schizophrenic patients ($r = 0.393$, $P = 0.002$), but not in the normal controls ($r = 0.363$, $P > 0.05$). Furthermore, the N200 amplitude showed a more significant correlation with the onset age factor ($r = 0.4609$, $P < 0.001$). Increased N200 amplitude in schizophrenic patients might reflect an early onset in schizophrenia. It is suggested that the N200 amplitude could play some role in the early intervention and prevention of schizophrenia.

Introduction

The N200 component of event-related potentials (ERPs) is an endogenous components as well as P300, indexing cognitive processes involved into the categorization of deviant stimuli. The developmental process of cognitive function among normal subjects, is also reflected in the correspondingly age-related ERP changes. For instance, the N200 amplitude showed a linear decrease with age from childhood to adulthood.[1] Schizophrenia has been regarded as one kind of psychodevelpomental disorder. It is well recognized that for the patients, the earlier the onset age, the poorer the prognosis, and the more important the early intervention. This study was made to investigate the possibility of using the N200 component of event-related potentials (ERPs) as an indicator of early onset in the intervention and prevention of schizophrenia.

Subjects and methodology

Subjects

There were 58 patients (male: 31; female: 27) and 25 healthy controls (male: 13; female: 12) included into the ERP test. All patients met the diagnostic criteria of schizophrenia according to DSM-Ⅲ-R, and were drug naive or drug free for above 4 weeks (25: drug naive; 33: drug free) when they undertook the ERP test. Among the patients, 26 were classified as the paranoid subtype, and the other 32 as the non-paranoid subtype. The mean age was 28.1 ± 8.6 years for the patient group, and 26.2 ± 8.7 years for the control group. All the subjects, including the patients, were free of neurological disease, mental retardation, and physical illness that might affect cognitive function or produce hearing loss. All subjects except one normal control were right handed as determined by the handedness questionnaire of Rackowski and Kalat (1974). Informed consent to the experiment was obtained from every subject.

Procedure

Auditory ERPs were obtained using an oddball paradigm. The procedure of ERP test used in this study was the same as in our previously reported studies. ERPs were recorded from Fp1, Fp2, F7, F3, Fz, F4, F8, C3, C4, T5, P3, Pz, P4, T6, O1 and O2, but only the data obtained from Fz were reported in this pilot study.

Results

The significant group difference was found only with the N200 latency ($F = 16.64$, $P < 0.001$), not with the N200 amplitude ($F = 0.14$, $P > 0.05$). The patients showed a prolonged N200 latency as compared to the control subjects (238.5 ± 27.3 ms Vs 213.4 ± 21.3 ms). However, the N200 amplitude correlated with the age factor in the patient group ($r = 0.393$, $P = 0.002$), and this correlation was insignificant for the control group ($r = 0.363$, $P > 0.05$). More important, for the patient group, the partial correlation analysis revealed that the N200 amplitude correlated with the onset age more significantly when controlling for the illness duration factor ($r = 0.4609$, $P < 0.001$). The N200 latency showed no correlation with the age or onset age factor. The N200 amplitude of the non-paranoid patients was higher than that of the paranoid patients (-5.4 ± 3.9 μV Vs -2.5 ± 3.1 μV, F = 9.02, $P = 0.004$). However, this difference disappeared when the onset age was included into ANOVA as a covariate ($F = 2.05$, $P > 0.05$). The onset age was significantly earlier in the non-paranoid than in the paranoid patients (21.0 ± 4.8 years Vs 28.0 ± 8.0 years, $F = 17.60$, $P < 0.001$). In addition, no change was observed with the N200 amplitude after the antipsychotic treatment (paired t = -0.009, $P > 0.05$).

Conclusion

The prolonged N200 latency in schizophrenic patients was a finding consistent with the previous reports. Our unique finding was that, the significant correlation of N200 amplitude with age, which had been reported among normal children, had also been observed in drug free patients with schizophrenia. More importantly, schizophrenic patients showed the N200 amplitude correlating more remarkably with their onset age. Within the patient group, it was the non-paranoid patients that had the increased N200 amplitude and the earlier onset age as compared to the paranoid patients. The N200 component of ERPs is maximal over the frontal area, indicating the cortical activity over this area, which is closely related to the mental development. Schizophrenic patients, especially the non-paranoid subtype, not only had the remarkable frontal dysfunction, but also suffered from this abnormality more enduringly. The N200 amplitude might be developed into an indicator of the early onset in schizophrenia, suggesting the necessity of early intervention in schizophrenia.

References

1) Johnstone, S. J., Barry, R. J., Anderson, J. W. et al. : Age-related changes in child and adolescent event-related potential component morphology, amplitude and latency to standard and target stimuli in an auditory oddball task. Int. J. Psychophysiol., 24(3) ; 223-238, 1996.

---

*琉球大学医学部精神神経科学

Wang Jijun, Hokama Hiroto, Hiramatsu Ken-ichi : Department of Neuropsychiatry, Faculty of Medicine, University of the Ryukyus.

沖縄県名護市における脳検診4年間の報告
—痴呆関連疾患の予防と早期発見，早期治療の試み—

A report on four-year brain medical checkups in Nago City, Okinawa : A trial study for the prevention of dementia as well as early intervention and treatment

城間　清剛* 　古謝　淳* 　玉城　直** 　岩田　正一* 　宮里　好一*

I．はじめに

当院では沖縄県名護市の委託を受け，平成8年度から，痴呆関連疾患の1次，2次予防を目的とした，一般住民が対象の「すこやか脳検診」を実施している．地方自治体による痴呆関連疾患の住民検診は全国的に見てもほとんど例がなく，痴呆性疾患の予防と治療の試みとして意義が深いと考えられたので，今回，平成12年度までの4年間の結果を報告した．

II．方　法

対象は60歳以上75歳未満の名護市在住者で，受検時に痴呆性疾患治療中でないもの．しかし，市民の希望があり，実際には53歳から86歳までの市民が受検した．

1次検診は，脳血管障害の危険因子や痴呆性疾患にみられる症状を項目に取り入れた調査票を作成し，スクリーニングとして本人と家族もしくは民生委員など，本人のことを比較的よく知っている者に記入を依頼した．その結果，痴呆が疑われたり，脳循環不全症状のある者，脳血管障害の危険因子を有する者を抽出し，2次検診を施行した．

2次検診では，頭部MRI検査，血液尿一般検査，心電図，簡易知能判定，精神科医による診察を行った．簡易知能判定として，改訂長谷川式簡易知能評価スケール（以下，HDS-R）および空間失行を簡易的に判断する目的で五角形模写を，さらに実際の生活状況を勘案して検討するため柄澤式「老人知能の臨床判定基準」（以下，柄澤式）を実施した．費用は，1次検診は無料．2次検診は自己負担が1万円で，2万円を市が負担した．

表1　痴呆が疑われた症例一覧

症例（歳,性）	柄澤式基準	HDS-R	五角形模写	基礎疾患・嗜好	MRI所見	診断
66 男	+	11	正常	—	多発梗塞	VD
67 男	±	20	正常	高脂血症・高血圧喫煙・飲酒	小梗塞萎縮	SDAT
68 男	±	18	異常	高血圧・喫煙・飲酒	多発梗塞	VD
69 男	+	20	正常	高脂血症	梗塞・萎縮	VD
83 男	+	23	異常	高血圧・心電図異常高脂血症・喫煙・飲酒	多発梗塞萎縮	SDAT or MIX
68 女	+	26	異常	高脂血症・心電図異常	出血・梗塞	VD
69 女	+	18	正常	高血圧・心電図異常	多発梗塞	VD
72 女	+	26	異常	高脂血症・心電図異常	小梗塞	VD
73 女	+	25	異常	—	多発梗塞	VD

（VD；脳血管性痴呆，SDAT；アルツハイマー型痴呆，MIX；混合型痴呆）

III．結　果

1次検診受検者は，4年間合計で男性136人，女性204人，計340人であった．年齢構成は，60歳未満の受検者が9人，60歳から64歳が67人，65歳から69歳が143人，70歳から74歳が90人，75歳から79歳が23人，80歳以上が8人であった．2次検診受検対象は340人中，212人，62.4％であった．このうち2次検診を受検した者は男性55人，女性103人の計158人であった．

2次検診の結果では，頭部MRI検査で小梗塞5個以上などの異常を認めた者は158人中，101人（63.9％）．HDS-Rで，痴呆の疑いとされる20点以下の者が6人（3.8％），五角形模写の異常が19人（12.0％），柄澤式の軽度以上の異常が6人（3.8％）に認められた．

医師の最終判定で，痴呆が疑われた者，すなわちHDS-Rで20点以下，もしくは五角形模写の異

表2 痴呆疑群と非痴呆群の背景

	痴呆(疑)	非痴呆 人(%)
平均年齢	71歳	69歳
高脂血症	5 (56)	91 (61)
高血圧	4 (44)	75 (51)
糖尿病	0 (0)	33 (22)
心電図異常・心疾患	4 (44)	49 (33)
喫煙	3 (33)	30 (20)
飲酒	3 (33)	20 (13)
頭部MRI異常	9 (100)	92 (62)

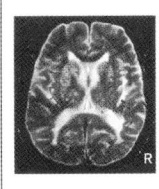

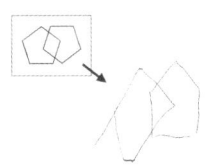

図1 症例1の頭部MRI所見と五角形模写
両側大脳基底核に多発性小梗塞を認め脳室周囲高信号を認める。五角形模写は変形が著しい。

常があり，かつ柄澤式で異常のある者があわせて9人(5.7%)であった。そのほか頭部MRIで比較的大きな脳梗塞，もしくは5個異常の小梗塞があり，脳循環改善薬の服用や定期的受診が必要と判断された者が15人(9.5%)であった。

表1に痴呆が疑われた症例9人の一覧を示した。脳血管性痴呆の疑いが7人，アルツハイマー型痴呆の疑いが1人，アルツハイマー型痴呆もしくは混合型痴呆の疑いが1人であった。

痴呆が疑われた群と非痴呆群の背景を表2に示した。痴呆が疑われた群で心電図異常，喫煙，飲酒，頭部MRIの異常が比較的多く認められた。

IV. 症　例

症例1は68歳男性，団体役員で地域の世話役をしている。既往にアルコール過剰摂取や喫煙歴がある。高血圧症を指摘され，近医にて降圧剤の投薬を受けている。

受検前の状況では，物忘れを自覚し，物の置き場所を思い出せない，スケジュール等メモ書きしてやっと仕事をこなすことなどがみられた。

症例1の2次検診の結果(図1)，頭部MRIで，大脳基底核を中心に多発性の脳梗塞や，脳室周囲高信号を認めた。HDS-Rは18点で軽度痴呆が疑われ，五角形模写は図形の変形が著しく正確に描けなかった。検診の後，本例に対して外来受診を勧め，精密知能検査を行い，その結果脳血管性痴呆の極初期として脳循環改善薬による治療を開始した。日常生活指導を行い，脳活性化訓練として本人の趣味である三味線の継続を奨励した。

V. 今後の課題とまとめ

今回のわれわれの結果では，2次検診受検者158人中，最終的に痴呆が疑われた者が9人，5.7%で，65歳以上の4.0～6.7%に痴呆が認められるとの報告[1,3]に一致している。今後の課題として，痴呆の診断基準や痴呆と他の検査結果との関連性について，さらに継続した予防的介入のあり方について検討する必要性があると考えられた。

自治体の委託による痴呆性疾患を対象とした住民検診は，国立琉球大学精神神経科が中心となって実施した渡嘉敷村での例があるものの，全国的にみてもほとんど例がない。

脳血管性痴呆の予防には，無症候性脳梗塞例を早期発見して，危険因子の管理とライフスタイルの改善を徹底し，脳卒中リスクを減少させることが重要であるとの報告があり[2]，一般住民を対象とした脳検診は脳血管性痴呆の予防や早期発見，早期治療に有意義であると考える。

文　献

1) Chikara O., Haruo N., Takeshi U. et al. : Prevalence of senile dementia in Okinawa, Japan. Int. J. Epidemiol., 24 ; 373-380, 1995.
2) 小林祥泰：痴呆の予防は可能か―成人期からの対策は？　脳血管性痴呆は予防できるか．臨床成人病，27 ; 647-652, 1997.
3) 大塚俊男，柄澤昭秀，松下正明ほか：わが国の痴呆性老人の出現率．老精医誌，3 ; 435-439, 1992.

*医療法人タピック　宮里病院
Seigo Shiroma, Sunao Koja, Syoichi Iwata, Yoshikazu Miyazato : Miyazato Hospital.
**国立療養所琉球病院
Naoshi Tamaki : National Ryukyu Hospital.

長寿県沖縄における健常高齢者の頭部MRIによる形態学的検討
―定量的MRIによる痴呆の早期診断の試み―

A brain MRI study in healthy aging in Okinawa, known as the longevity :
For the early diagnosis of dementia using a quantitative MRI

宮平　良尚* 　Yu Jin* 　田中　晋* 　外間　宏人* 　平松　謙一*
小椋　力* 　島崎　順之** 　宇都宮　尚** 　村山　貞之** 　武田　祐子***

I. 目 的

頭部MRIによる痴呆高齢者脳の病的萎縮は数多く検討されているが健常高齢者脳の生理的萎縮を定量的に検討した報告は少ない。今回，我々は健常高齢者の頭蓋内容積，全脳容積，そしてアルツハイマー型老年痴呆の初期病変とされている海馬，内嗅領皮質の各容積を定量的MRIによって計測し，画像処理・解析ソフトを用いた形態学的検討を行ったので報告する。

II. 対象と方法

対象は長寿県沖縄に在住の健常高齢者で男性15名，女性16名の計31名。全員右利き。年齢は61歳から91歳で平均年齢は74.8±8.62歳。全員にMini-Mental State Examination (MMSE) を施行し24点以上(平均28.2±1.56点)であった。頭部MRI上，明らかな脳梗塞その他異常所見は認めなかった。撮像装置はSiemens Vision 1.5T MRI, Flash法によるT1強調撮像を行い，撮像条件はTR 35 ms, TE 5 ms, Flip angle 45deg, Field of View 240mm, matrix 256×256, Voxel size 0.9375×0.9375×1.5mmとした。頭部MRIにより得られた画像データをMEDx (Sensor Systems Inc.) を用いて画像処理を行い頭蓋，全脳，海馬，内嗅領皮質の各容積を自動および手動により計測した。

III. 結 果

MEDxによる画像処理を示す (Figure 1)。頭蓋内容積で補正した全脳，海馬および内嗅領皮質の各容積は年齢と有意な相関を認めた (Table 1, Figure 2)。海馬と内嗅領皮質の容積比は年齢との相関を認めなかった (Figure 3)。また海馬では左右差を認め右側が有意に大きかった。各補正容積では性差を認めなかった。

IV. 考 察

今回得られた結果は生理的萎縮を反映するものと推測でき，病的萎縮の客観的評価に有用と思われる。アルツハイマー型老年痴呆では，海馬，内嗅領皮質に初期病変が認められることが神経病理学的に確認されており，病的萎縮では両者の萎縮の割合や左右差などが生理的萎縮と異なることが推測される。

V. まとめ

1) 定量的MRIによって，全脳，海馬，内嗅領皮質は加齢により萎縮することが推測された。
2) 海馬と内嗅領皮質の萎縮の割合は同程度であった。
3) 海馬は右側が大きく，各補正容積では性差を認めなかった。
4) 今後は対象を増やして縦断的にfollow-upし，痴呆に至る対象群において検討を行うことにより，定量的MRIを用いた痴呆の早期診断を試

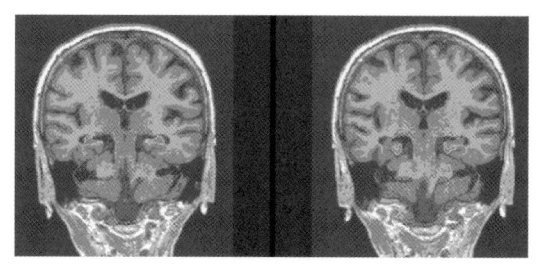

Figure 1　Manual segmentation of the Hippocampus (left side), and the Entorhinal cortex (right side).

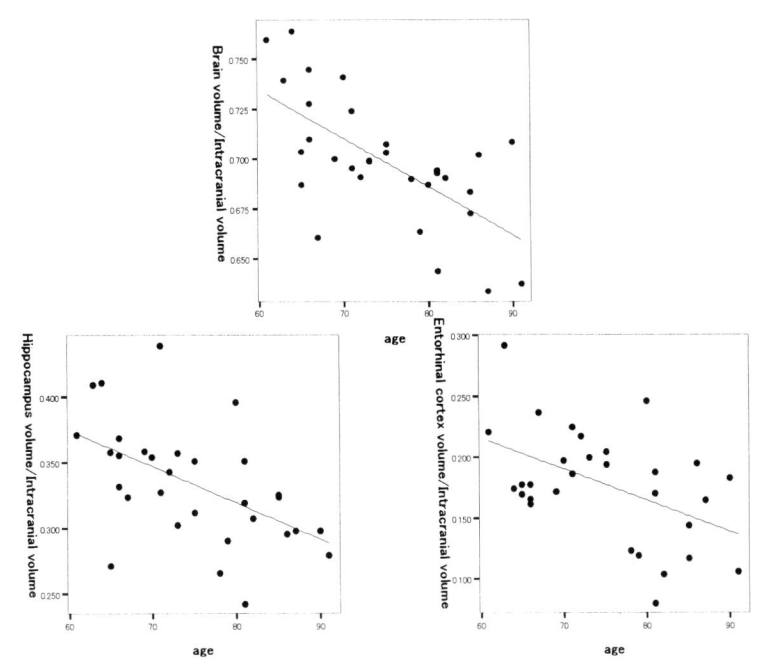

Figure 2 Age-related changes in volumes of interest.

Table 1 Quantitive MR measures

	mean±SD (mm³)	min - max	adjusted for ICV (mean±SD)	r (age)	
Intracranial volume (ICV)	1460800.61 ± 115.71	1231437 - 1690013	-	-	
Brain volume	1020418.32 ± 85.78	828878 - 1196355	0.699 ± 0.032	-0.656	**
Hippocampal volume	4862.28 ± 662.47	3642.62 - 5953.71	0.334 ± 0.045	-0.530	**
Right	2485.40 ± 346.27	1716.50 - 3050.68	0.171 ± 0.024	-0.560	**
Left	2376.88 ± 345.02	1825.93 - 2996.63	0.163 ± 0.027	-0.449	*
Entorhinal cortex volume	2603.29 ± 677.87	1294.63 - 4221.38	0.178 ± 0.045	-0.485	**
Right	1272.05 ± 326.43	632.8 - 1998.40	0.087 ± 0.022	-0.482	**
Left	1331.25 ± 382.36	585.35 - 2231.98	0.091 ± 0.026	-0.447	*

Associations between the adjusted brain volumes and age (Pearson product-moment correlations). *$P<0.05$; **$P<0.01$

みる。

*琉球大学医学部精神神経科学講座
Yoshinao Miyahara, Yu Jin, Shin Tanaka, Hiroto Hokama, Ken-ichi Hiramatsu, Chikara Ogura : Department of Neuro psychiatry, Faculty of Medicine, University of the Ryukyus.

**琉球大学附属病院放射線部
Yoriyuki Shimazaki, Nao Utsunomiya, Sadayuki Murayama : Division for Radiology, University hospital of the Ryukyus.

***琉球大学附属病院地域医療部
Yuko Takeda : Division for General Hedicine and Community Health Care, University hospital of the Ryukyus.

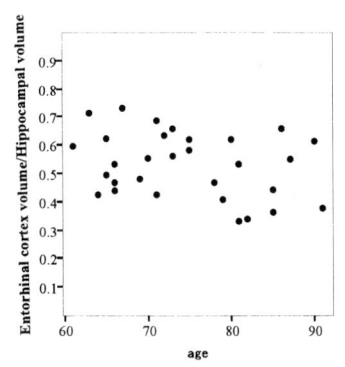

Figure 3 Age-related changes in The Hippocampus-Entorhinal cortex ratio.

事象関連電位P300は痴呆の予測,早期発見に役立つか
Is event-related potentials helpful for prevention and early detection of dementia?

Yu Jin*　平松　謙一*　小椋　力*　外間　宏人*　田中　晋*　宮平　良尚*
武田　裕子**　島崎　順之***　村山　貞之***　宇都宮　尚***

I. Introduction

事象関連電位(event-related potentials, ERPs)の変化は,注意,認知,判断などの情報処理機能の客観的指標とされている。事象関連電位(ERPs)のP300潜時が加齢により延長することは多くの報告で認められている。加齢によるP300潜時の延長は知的機能の低下とおおまかに相関するとされている。しかしながら,加齢による,脳の形態学的な変化,P300成分を指標とする脳内情報処理機能の変化,知的機能の変化が相互にどのような関連を持つかは,詳細には検討されていない。すなわち,それぞれが独立の事象なのか,関連があるとすればどの程度寄与しているのか,またこれらの指標で痴呆の早期発見にどの程度有用であるか,などを明らかにすることが求められている。

II. Methods

Subjects:沖縄県内の60歳以上の健常な高齢者で,精神神経疾患の既往がなく,Mini-Mental State(MMS)の高得点(24点以上),並びに脳のMRI(1.5T)検査で明らかな脳梗塞のない48人を分析対象者として選択した。

比較に使用した60歳以下の若年者のデータは本講座でERPの測定を実行した健常者の中から年齢,性の偏りのないように男女それぞれ36名計76名を選んだ。

MRI:頭部MRI 1.5T

ERP:ERPsの測定は音刺激を用い,目標刺激を数えるodd-ball課題を遂行中のERPsを記録する。

Scale:MMSE, Benton, GDS, QOL,他

Data analysis

P300成分の頂点潜時と振幅を測定し,年齢の差や性差の有無と程度について検討を行った。各成分の分析はピアソンの相関係数やANOVAを求め,その有意差について検討する。

III. Results

1) Relationship of age with ERP measures

年齢とP300の頂点振幅,潜時は男女とも年齢と有意な関連性が認められなかった(Figure 1)。

2) Relationship of P300 to age (15years～)

若年層(15歳-59歳)を合わせてP300と年齢との関連性をみると,男女ともP300潜時において有意な相関が認められた。振幅は女性のみ負の相関が見られました(Figure 2)。

IV. Discussion

本研究の対象者においては各種のスケールよりスクリーニングされた健常高齢者であり,従来の研究報告の方法論上の疑問点をある程度カバーできたと思う。従来の研究結果と直接は比較できないが,若年者と比べるとP300の振幅は低下し,潜時は延長傾向であるが,加齢により直線的にP300の振幅低下,潜時延長を示すのではないことが示唆された。また,P300と年齢により変化するMMSとも明らか関連性がないことから,健常高齢者においてERP成分の規定要因は単なる年齢や性ではなく,頭部MRIによる脳の容積などの形態学的な要因との関連性も明らかにすることが課題として残っている。

V. Conclusions

若年と比較するとP300の振幅は低下し,潜時

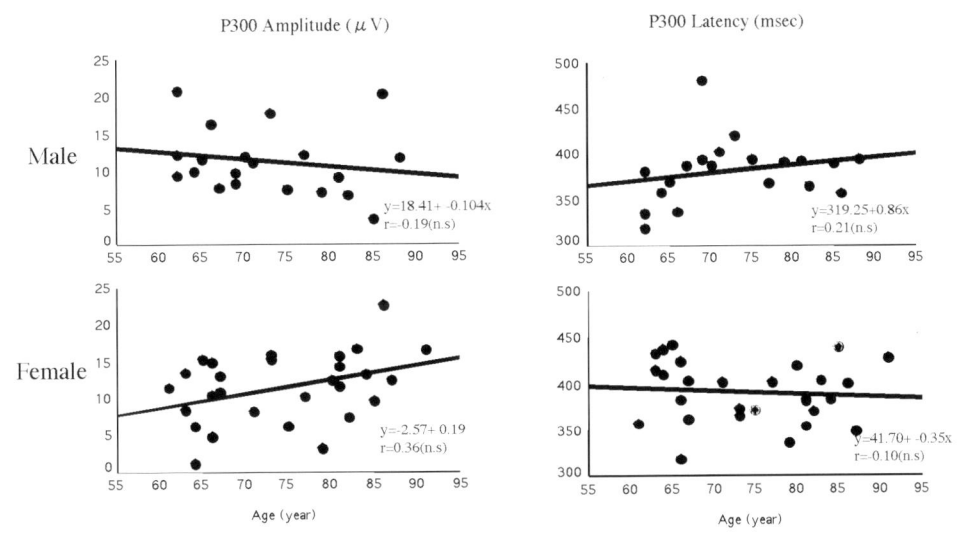

Figure 1 Regression analysis relating P300 Amp Lat(Pz) to age

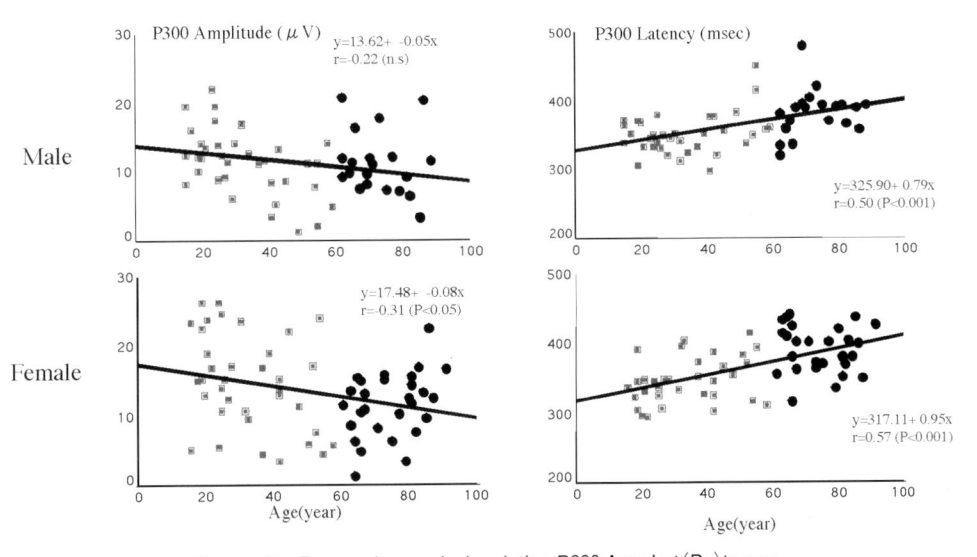

Figure 2 Regression analysis relating P300 Amp Lat(Pz) to age

は延長しているが，すべての高齢者が加齢により直線的にP300の振幅低下，潜時延長を示すのではないことが示唆された。健常高齢者P300変化を規定する要因を明らかにすることは痴呆の早期発見，予測に役立つと思われる。

*琉球大学医学部精神神経科学講座
Yu Jin, Ken-ichi Hiramatsu, Chikara Ogura, Hiroto Hokama, Shin Tanaka, Yoshinao Miyahara : Department of Neuro psychiatry, Faculty of Medicine, University of the Ryukyus.

**琉球大学付属病院地域医療部
Yuko Takeda : Division for General Medicine and Community Health Care, University hospital of the Ryukyus.

***琉球大学付属病院放射線部
Yoriyuki Shimazaki, Sadayuki Murayama, Nao Utsunomiya : Division for Radiology, University hospital of the Ryukyus.

うつ病の脆弱性指標としての事象関連電位N200異常
N200 abnormality in event-related potentials as a vulnerability marker for depression

川崎　俊彦[*1]　　小椋　　力[*1]　　小村　文明[*2]　　深尾　晃三[*3]
外間　宏人[*1]　　平野　　潔[*4]　　平松　謙一[*1]

I. 目　的

ヒトの認知異常を表す生物学的指標として事象関連電位(ERPs)がある。これまでうつ病に限らず様々な病態のERPsについて多くの報告がある。ところで，これまでERPsの異常については，それがその病態の状態に依存性(state dependent)なのか，素因に依存性(trait dependent)なのかを知ることが難しかった。だが素因依存性の，その病態に特異的な異常を発見する事が出来れば，その病態の発症前の診断，早期治療など予防に貢献することになろう。

うつ病の病前性格としては執着性格がよく知られている。そこでうつ病と執着性格および健常者のERPsを比較し，さらにうつ病の寛解時のERPsも比較することで，うつ病の素因依存性となる異常について調べてみた。

II. 対象と方法

うつ病者は36人で，DSM-III-Rの診断基準で大うつ病性障害の診断基準を満たすものであった。男性は21人で女性は15人，平均年齢は36.5±5.8歳であった。うつ病者と比較する健常対照者は36人のボランティアで，精神・神経疾患の既往や家族歴はないものであった。男性26人で女性10人，平均年齢は36.1±5.8歳であった。うつ病者のうち12人は寛解状態となった時点で再記録を行った。

執着性格者は，琉球大学在学中の学生378人を対象に行った下田式性格評価尺度で，執着性格の得点が14点以上であった21人(男性15人，女性6人で平均年齢は19.3±1.3歳)とした。執着性格者と比較する対照者は，性と年齢を一致させた44人

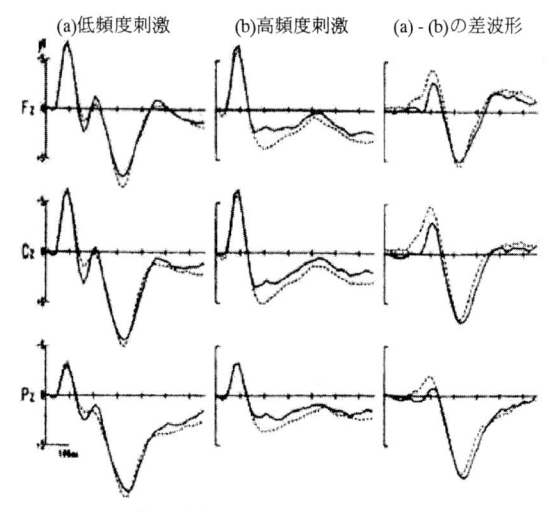

Figure 1　うつ病者(実線)および健常者(波線)のERPs

の健常者とした。男性は31人，女性は13人で平均年齢は20.5±1.4歳であった。

ERPsは，高頻度刺激を1kHz，80％，低頻度刺激を2kHz，20％とする聴覚oddball課題を用いた。両耳朶電極を基準とし国際10-20法に基づくFz，Cz，Pzの3箇所から記録した。

III. 結　果

うつ病と健常者，執着性格と健常者のそれぞれのERPsを測定し，比較してみた(Figure 1およびFigure 4)。うつ病患者の一部は寛解状態となってから再検し比較した(Figure 3)。N200成分は高頻度刺激でうつ病・執着性格で有意に誘発され(それぞれχ^2検定，Yate's補正で$p<0.05$，$p<0.05$)，平均波形でも健常者に比べて大きかった。Figure 2に示すように，うつ病ではN200の下位成分のうち低頻度刺激でのMMNは小さく，逆に高頻度刺激でのN2bは大きかった。寛

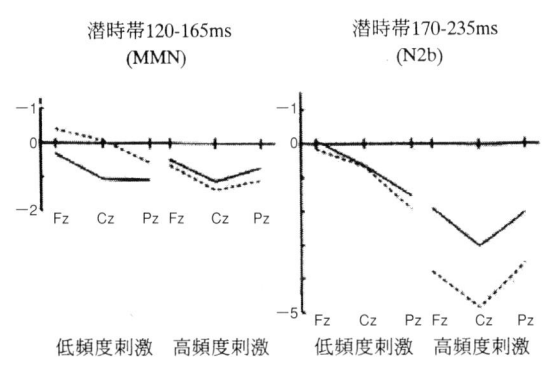

Figure 2 N200を前半・後半に分けたときの平均振幅実線がうつ病，波線が健常者。

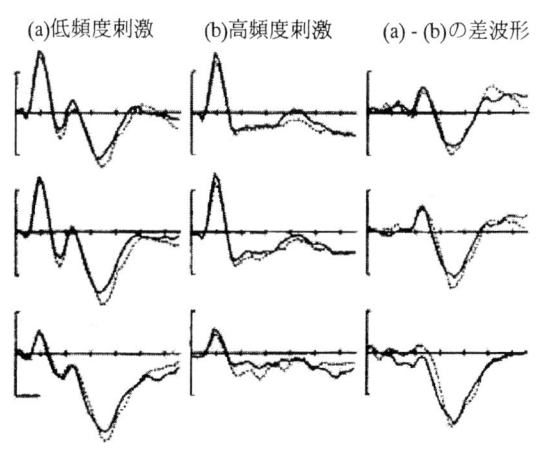

Figure 3 うつ病のうつ状態および寛解時の総加算平均波形実線がうつ状態，波線が寛解時。（n = 12）

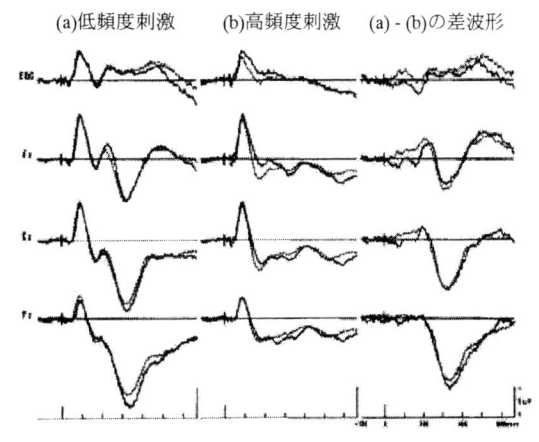

Figure 4 執着性格者および健常者の総加算平均波形実線が執着性格者（n = 21），波線が健常者。（n = 44）

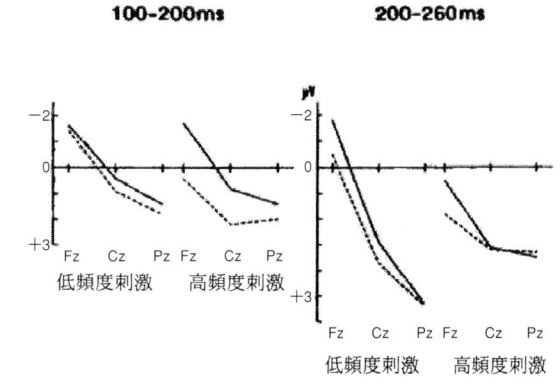

Figure 5 N200を前半・後半に分けたときの平均振幅実線が執着性格者，波線が健常者。

解状態のうつ病患者の病前病後のERPsを解析したところ，N200成分の前半後半とも有意な変化はなかった。Figure 5に示すように，執着性格でも同様に高頻度刺激でのN2bは大きかった。これらの所見は，うつ病の刺激を自動的に処理する過程の障害と，代償的なより意識的な刺激の処理過程の増強を示していると考えられる。N200のこれらの異常は，うつ病の発症前・寛解後を通じて見られることから，うつ病の生物学的マーカーとしての役割が期待できる。ただし，ERPは個人間のばらつきも大きく，多くの要因に左右されやすく，個人レベルでの発症マーカーとしてはまだ実用レベルではない。今後，個人レベルのうつ病発症の予測・発症の予防が可能となりうる程度の鋭敏度の向上などが今後の課題であろう。

---

*[1]琉球大学医学部精神神経科学講座
　Toshihiko Kawasaki, Chikara Ogura, Hiroto Hokama, Ken-ichi Hiramatsu : Department of Neuropsychiatry, University of Ryukyus.
*[2]島根県立湖陵病院
　Fumiaki Omura : Shimane Prefectual Koryo Hospital.
*[3]さわ病院
　Kozo Fukao : Sawa Hospital.
*[4]いずみ病院
　Kiyoshi Hirano : Izumi Hospital.

インドネシアのジャカルタ，ボゴール地区における精神分裂病患者の援助希求行動
－精神科治療への遅延と中断に焦点を当てて－

Help seeking behavior of patients with schizophrenia in Jakarta and Bogor, Indonesia, with special foci on delays and discontinuation of psychiatric treatments

Heriani*　　Sasanto Wibisono*　　Henny Wati*　　Grace Wangge*
Siti Munawaroh*　　Irmansyah*　　山本　和儀**　　新福　尚隆***

Introduction

Many schizophrenic patients do not come to psychiatric facilities at the onset of the illness. This is especially true in Indonesia and other Asian countries. Among previous studies, 50-60% of patients in mental hospitals were chronically ill and were admitted for the first time already in a chronic condition. They have sought various therapies before they were admitted to a mental hospital. Traditional and religious healers play an important role in the pathways to mental health care in Indonesia. To be able to develop a strategic plan in promoting early intervention in psychosis, we need to understand the patterns and major determinants of the health care seeking behavior of patients with mental illness and their families. The objectives of our survey were as follow : 1) To investigate the patterns of help seeking behavior of patients with schizophrenia and their families in Jakarta and Bogor ; 2) To clarify the characteristics of the patients and the decision makers of each pattern ; 3) To identify the decision makers and major determinant factors in selecting the type of management ; 4) To identify the factors related with delayed referral to psychiatric facilities ; 5) To identify the factors related with the discontinuation of psychiatric treatment.

Methodology

This was a survey of 141 consecutive new patients who met ICD-10 diagnostic criteria for schizophrenia who came to 3 mental hospitals as well as the department of psychiatry in a general hospital in Jakarta and surrounding areas. In addition, patients with schizophrenia who had discontinued medication for 1 year prior to the interview were also surveyed. Data was collected through : (1) a clinical interview with the patients, (2) interviewing the informants with a structured interview using an Interview Schedule.

Statistical Analysis : Simple frequencies were calculated for all variables and were analysed by Chi-square Test, Kosmogorov-Smirnov and Fischer exact test. P value of .05 was adopted for the statistical significance. All statistical analysis were conducted by SPSS ver 10.

Results and discussion

Only 43.3% of patients sought psychiatric treatment at first, while others sought various managements before they came to a psychiatric agent. The most common non-psychiatric management was traditional healers (31.2%). The interesting thing was that we still found 1.4% were either kept at home or *dipasung* (restrained at home), a practice usually found in remote areas. Most of these families utilized multiple agents (the median is 4 agents), only 6.3% used a single agent (Figure).

Reasons for delay were because they did not consider the patient's problem as serious, financial difficulty and did not know where to go. Patients

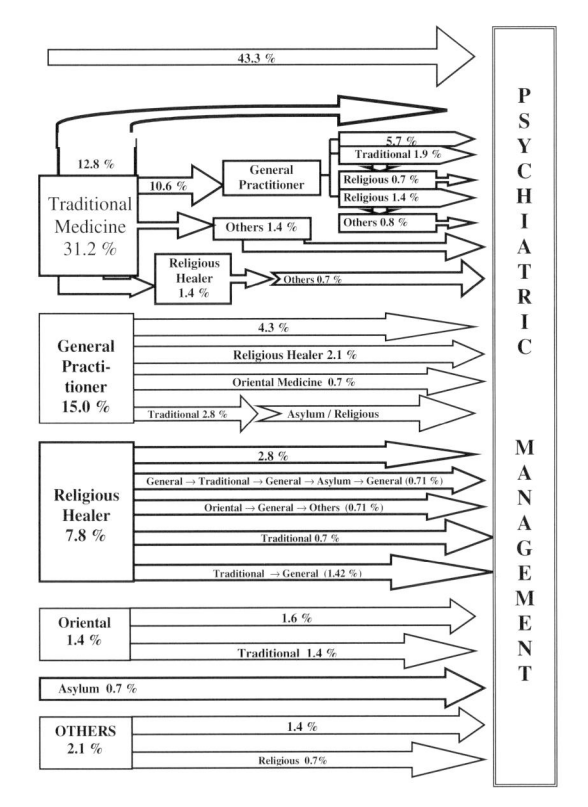

Figure Pathways before the first psychiatric management

living in rural areas tend to come later than patients living in urban or metropolitan areas did. Demographic factors related in delay in any type of management were patients' age and mode of onset. The older the patient and the more chronic the mode of onset, the more likely the delay. Delay to psychiatric agency was influenced by education, living area and distance to psychiatric facility.

The reason for not taking psychiatric management first was mostly (46.4%) because they did not know that it was a mental problem. The next common answer was that they thought the patient's problem could be managed better by agencies other than a psychiatric one, most commonly folk or religious healers (21.1%). This may be due to the family's interpretation of the patient's problem as caused by supernatural reasons. Another reason was financial burden.

The factors related to selecting an agent at first contact were education, living area, distance to psychiatric facility, and economy status. The higher educated and the higher the economy status, the more likely they selected psychiatric agents first. Patients from rural areas, low education, and older age tend to go to traditional or religious agents first.

After they have reached a psychiatric agent, only 59.4% continued the treatments. Reasons for discontinuation were mostly because the patient refused psychiatric treatment (29.4%); the patient was improved enough (28.2%), and unsatisfactory improvement (18.6%). Living in a rural area and far from psychiatric facilities, low education, informant's age, and previous experience with psychosis were found to be related to discontinuation to psychiatric managements.

We also did a follow-up study of the patients after the interview. We could only get data from 117 patients due to the incompleteness of address on the medical records. In the first month 85 (72.6%) still continue the treatment at the center. The number decreased to 69 (59%) in the second month, and to 59 (50.4%) in the third month.

Conclusion

The results suggest that we need to increase the awareness and enhance knowledge about psychoses and mental health in the community. We need to introduce lower budget psychiatric services that can meet the patient's demands nearer to the consumers. Traditional healers and other 'alternative' treatments still play an important role in managing psychoses and therefore should be considered in the mental health care system. Psychiatric services should be easily reached and can meet the patient's demand.

---

*Heriani, Sasanto Wibisono, Henny Wati, Grace Wangge, Siti Munawaroh, Irmansyah : University of Indonesia.
**琉球大学医学部精神神経学講座
　Kazuyoshi Yamamoto : Department of Neuropsychiatry, University of the Ryukyus.
***神戸大学
　Naotaka Shinfuku : Kobe University.

バリにおける精神医学の概念

Concepts of psychiatry in Bali*

Luth Ketut Suryani*

To understand a person requires three combined factors: mind, body and spirit. These are enmeshed and work together with the socio-cultural system and the environment. To be complete, they are all integrated with the Universal Spirit (fig. 1). The personal spirit is a mixture of energy of mother, father and God. The personal spirit manifests at conception (fig. 2). It is the source of knowledge, life and ability. This theory underlies all of Suryani's work.

Suryani's practice of psychiatry in Bali

Suryani's practice includes an in-patient hospital component used for acute care, especially for psychotic disorders. Treatment generally begins with pharmacological therapy, used only long enough to reduce symptoms, an average of one-month duration. Suryani's clinical practice and community activities are not typical of psychiatrists in Bali or Indonesia in terms of scope and techniques. The basis of all her works is mind-body-spirit-socio-cultural theory. The spirit aspect is incorporated in the total philosophy of all her activities[1]. Spirit is not a typical part of Western psychiatry. It is to be emphasized, she does not practice traditional healing and traditional healers do not practice psychiatry. In her private practice, she uses standard modern pharmacological therapy.

She also uses a unique technique of psychotherapy termed meditation psychotherapy. It involves inducing an altered state of consciousness, meditation and or trance, in both patient and herself as therapist. In this state, she works with repressed memories and may engage the patient and herself in communication with the patient's individual spirit and those of persons key to the patient's problems or mental disorder. In the hypnotic or trance state, the spirit works on the nuclear problem or basis of the problem. After the session the patient usually feels tired and requires a period of sleep to solidify reframed memories. After completion of therapy the patient's spirit continues to work, a process called "self-editing," for a period of three to four weeks to alleviate the problem(s).[2]

The use of this technique shortens the number of required sessions compared with standard psychotherapy. A therapy session takes up to one hour. The usual number of visits required is five, the maximum is seven. After completion of therapy, the patient is instructed to continue with regular medication at home and at community. Follow up of patients indicates the results are sustained. The technique is described in detail in another publication.[3]

She evolved the technique from clinical experience with hypnosis. Formal hypnotic induction is not required. It is particularly suitable to Balinese because trance is a part of daily living at home, in ceremonies and many other cultural activities.

Suryani's practice of psychiatry is not only for the individual but focuses heavily on group work for all age levels, from prenatal to old age, and is oriented primarily to prevention and education.

The author firmly believes that the basic strength and resiliency typical of Balinese culture will ultimately prevail in the face of the current crisis with its surge of social and mental health problems. To do so will require education and innova-

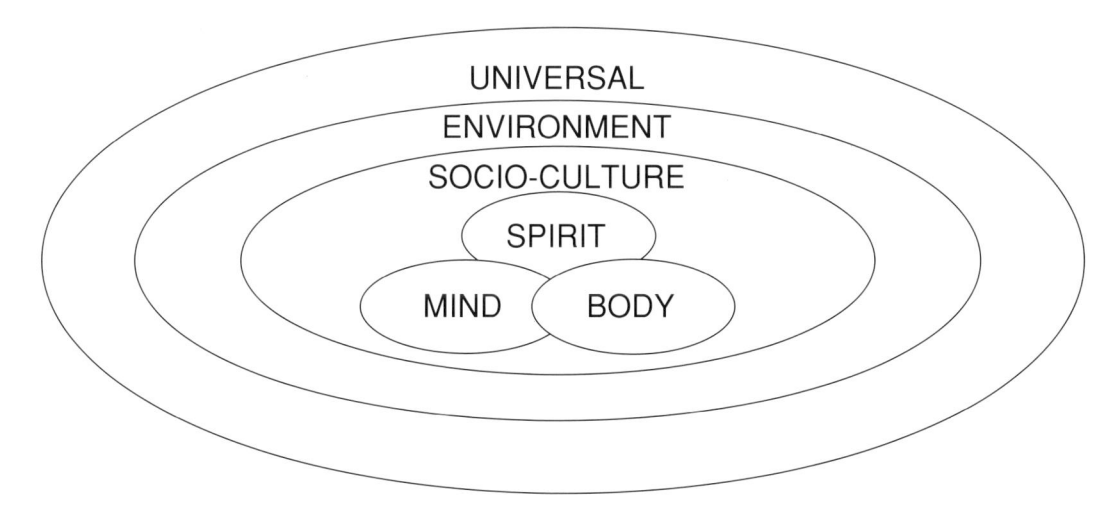

Figure 1 Suryani's concepts for a comprehensive theory

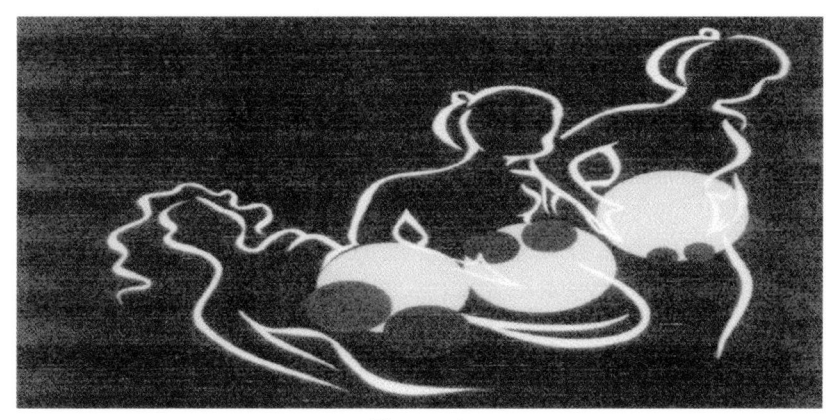

Figure 2

tive preventive and therapeutic methods applied at all levels of society.

References

1) Suryani, L. K. and Jensen, G. D. : Trance and Possession in Bali, Kuala Lumpur, Oxford University Press, 1994.
2) Suryani, L. K., Menemukan, Jati Diri dengan Meditasi. : Jakarta, PT Elex Media Komputindo, 2000.
3) Suryani, L. K. and Wrycza, P. Moksha. : A New Way of Life. Denpasar, PT Balipost, 1996.

---

*Presented at International Seminar on Integration of Traditional Healing and Modern Psychiatry in Asia, Denpasar - Bali, 23 November 2000.

*Luh Ketut Suryani, M. D., Ph. D. : Professor in Department of Psychiatry, Udayana University - Denpasar, Bali.

在日ラテンアメリカ精神障害者の治療と予防

Treatment and prevention of the Latin-American patients with mental disorders in Japan

阿部　裕*　　比賀　晴美**

The number of Latin-American immigrants has increased rapidly since 1990, and reached 280,000 persons in 2000. During the past 2 years, from April '99 to March 2001, 71 Latin-American patients came to Higa Clinic in Tokyo. There were 34 males, whose average age was 33.1 and 37 females, whose average age was 31.5. As regards each successive generation of Japanese Latin-Americans, the number of second generation Japanese Latin-Americans is 31, the number of those in the third generation is 26, the number of those in the forth generation is 3 and the number of pure Latin-Americans is 11. Their countries of origin ; 65 percent from Brazil, 20 percent from Peru, 6 percent from Argentina, 4 percent from Colombia, 3 percent from Honduras. Regarding their school education, 26 percent of patients graduated from universities, 36 percent finished the course of senior high school and 27 percent finished the course of junior high school. Almost all of them come from the Kanto area, especially Tokyo, Kanagawa, Chiba and Saitama. Many patients have already stayed in Japan for 6〜10 years and 62 percent of them live with their families and 34 percent of them live alone.

Next, pointing out the characteristics and care of the patients (Figure 1), first of all about 53 among 71 patients reported having suffered some specific provocation when they became sick, some of them had not only one provocation but two. One third of the 53 patients suffered from some kind of culture conflict. This point caused such problems as matrimonial conflict, family conflict and office conflict. In the cause of matrimonial conflict the difference of speed and degree of adapting themselves to the

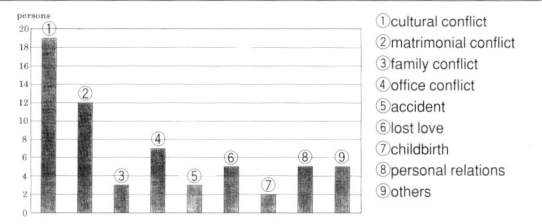

Figure 1　Provoking Factors of getting sick

①cultural conflict
②matrimonial conflict
③family conflict
④office conflict
⑤accident
⑥lost love
⑦childbirth
⑧personal relations
⑨others

Japanese culture and society brought about conflict between wives and husbands. Such matrimonial conflict had a close relation to the respective culture conflicts. In the case of family conflict the main problem was often related to the difference of life style and customs between the fathers and sons. Especially the problem of using different languages, where the parents speak their mother language and the child speaks Japanese makes for bad communication. In the case of office conflict the problems were often related to the bad understanding between them and their superiors. For example, they often interpreted a superior's advice as an injurious word.

Next, the diagnoses of the 21 out of 71 patients had previous mental illness. According to DSM-Ⅳ (Figure 2), 29 patients were diagnosed as having affective disorders, 12 patients diagnosed as schizophrenia, 15 patients diagnosed as anxiety disorders, 3 patients diagnosed as substance-related disorders, 5 patients diagnosed as adjustment disorders and seven diagnosed as others. Almost all of the case of affective disorder were females. It is supposed that the reason is because they have to work and to take care of children in a different environment and customs, and moreover they don't have so many places and occasions for releasing their stress in their daily lives with their families. In

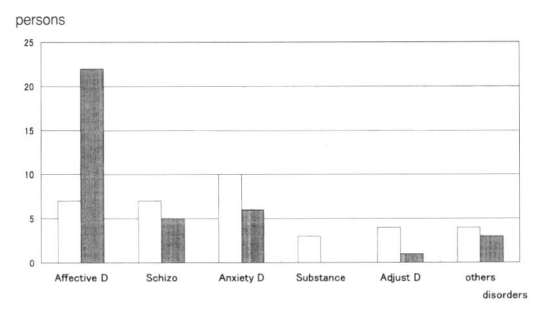

Figure 2 Diagnosis

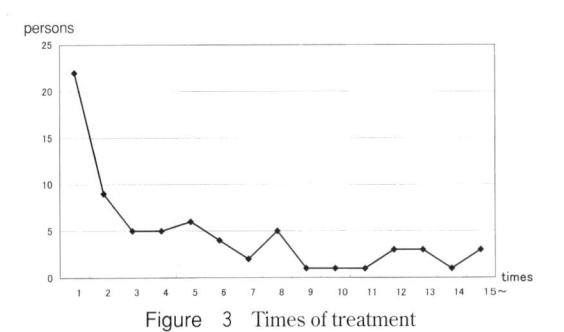

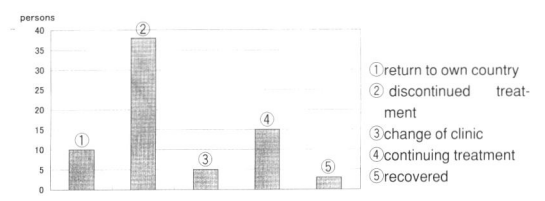

Figure 3 Times of treatment

Figure 4 Outcome of patients

① return to own country
② discontinued treatment
③ change of clinic
④ continuing treatment
⑤ recovered

the case of living alone the reason was that they were isolated from the Japanese society. The case of schizophrenia contained patients with acute psychosis and paranoid reaction. In the case of anxiety disorders, 6 showed panic disorders and 4 of these 6 were females. They had stayed in Japan for a long time, more than 5 years. In the adjustment disorders almost all of the patients were children. The others contained somatoform disorders, dissociative disorders and sexual disorders.

Next, as figure 3 shows, about half of outpatients stopped visiting the clinic within 4 times. There were 4 main reasons for this. One was because their house was situated far from the clinic. A second was because they couldn't be absent from their work. They felt that they couldn't be absent from work to continue treatment because their purpose for being in Japan was to earn money in order to go back to their own country. A third reason was because they had no support network to assist them in getting treatment. The fourth reason was that they didn't have national health insurance, so they stopped receiving the treatment when they got well a little. But recently, with the tendency to the settle down more people are continuing to visit the clinic because they want to work while receiving treatment. Looking at the outcomes of patients, figure 4 show that, 10 patients had returned to their country and received treatment there, 38 patients stopped the treatment, 5 patients changed to other clinics because of the long distance or the necessity of hospitalization, 15 patients are continuing to receive treatment, and 3 patients have been cured.

Among the affective disorders the number of discontinuation are remarkably high but there are also many cases of continuation. In the anxiety disorders there were also a lot of case of discontinuation. As for schizophrenia, most also continued their treatment in Japan or in their own countries, although some patients discontinued.

(CONCLUSION) (1) Almost all of the provoking factors of getting sick have relation to culture conflict, so for promoting the continuation of treatment and the prevention of relapse culture conflict needs to be seriously considered. (2) To promote the continuation of the treatment the construction of care service centers are need in each area. (3) In cases there are communication problems between a father and a son, there is need for collaboration with the schools or the persons concerned with the education in order to support the children. (4) A mental health service network for the Latin-American people is needed to help them to solve matrimonial and family conflicts.

*順天堂大学スポーツ健康科学部
　Yu Abe : School of Health and Sports Science, Juntendo University.
**比賀クリニック
　Haruyoshi Higa : Higa Clinic.

東海村臨界事故に関連した適応障害の一例

A case of adjustment disorder related to the critical accident at a unclear fuel conversion facility in Tokai village

中野　英樹* 　副田　秀二* 　中村　　純*

I. はじめに

東海村臨界事故は，1999年9月30日に茨城県東海村の核燃料物質加工施設で日本初の臨界事故である。作業員を含め数十人が被曝しそのうち2人が死亡する惨事となった人災であり，地域住民に対し，事故現場から半径350m圏内は避難勧告，半径10km圏内は屋内退避勧告という措置がとられた。本臨界事故に関連した適応障害の一例を報告する。

II. 症　例

初診時年齢32歳　女性　事務員（庶務）
主訴：不安，恐怖，食思不振
既往歴・家族歴：特記すべきことなし
生活歴・職歴：同胞2人の第2子。元来，臆病だが素直な性格。大学卒業後，入社9年目に同期入社の縁で知り合った夫（研究職）と幼少の娘との3人暮らし。本人及び夫ともに原子力施設での職員ではない。事故現場から職場・自宅ともに10キロ圏内にある。

現病歴：事故当日，東海村の臨界事故をテレビ報道で知り強い衝撃を受けた。さらに同日，原子力関連事故としてチェルノブイリ原発事故の映像を引き合いに出したテレビ報道を見た。その際，悪性疾患に罹患した児童の惨状を自ら及び家族の行く末のように感じ，出来るだけ遠くへ逃げたいという気持ちになった。しかし翌日，娘を他県にある実家に預け，本人は仕事への責任感から恐怖を圧して自宅へ戻り，なんとか出勤はした。徐々に不安，食思不振，不眠，放射線被曝についての恐怖，心臓がザワザワする感じなどの症状が増悪していったため夫の勧めで職場の健康管理センターへ相談した。

初診時現症（10月8日）：不安・食思不振・不眠がみられ，臨界事故の話題になると泣き出すなど感情が不安定だった。エチゾラム1.5mg/日を処方した。

2回目診察（10月20日）：「ここから離れたい。テレビで安全だと言っても，本当かどうか判らない」と心配そうな表情であった。しかし，夫や実家の姉からは「心配のしすぎ」と言われ仕方なく実家から娘を引き取った。

3回目診察（11月3日）：不安・恐怖感は若干軽快したが，「食材が放射能に汚染されているのでは」と，一人でいる時はチョコレートを食事代わりとする日もあった。食思不振とあわせて体重が1カ月間で4kg減少した。また「事故関連の記事を見ると，感情のコントロールがつかない」と話した。

4回目診察（11月17日）：通勤以外は極力屋内で過ごしていた。自分の心情を周囲の者に理解してもらえず孤立感を抱き，入眠困難が続いた。

5回目診察（12月1日）：不安・恐怖感，入眠困難は軽快傾向となり，エチゾラム0.5mg/dayにてコントロール可能となった。外出への抵抗感も弱まったが，茨城県産の食材は汚染への恐怖から購入出来なかった。職場でも事故のことばかりを考え，上司に叱責されることもあった。

6回目診察（1月14日）：「事故の話は家族ともしない。報道での安全宣言も疑っている。工場内の被曝者が亡くなったという報道に涙が止まらなかった」と，事故の話題にふれると涙を流した。

7回目診察（2月1日）：「やっとテレビでの事故関連の報道にも馴れてきた。でもその話題は拒否反応が出てしまう」と話し，東海村へ近づくこ

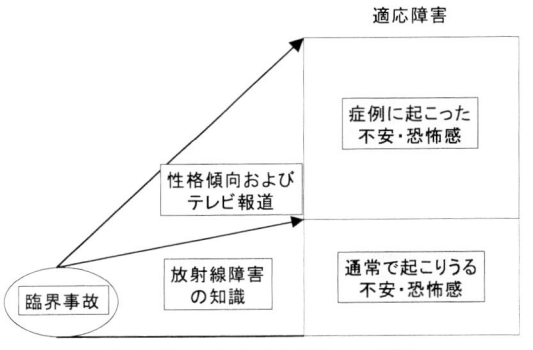

図　誘因による適応障害への影響

とは極力避けていたが，日常生活への支障はさほど目立たなくなった。

その後の経過：4月に再診の予約を入れていたが，本人から「調子が良いため受診をキャンセルしたい」と電話があった。再び不調となれば連絡をもらう形としたが，1年以上たった時点でも連絡はない。

III．考　察

1．診断について

外傷性のストレス要因が光景として視覚的に認識されえないけれどもその存在についての情報がストレスを生み出す場合(不可視トラウマ)，これは厳密にいえばDSM-IVのPTSDのA基準には該当しない[1]。そのため診断を不安と抑うつ気分の混合を伴う適応障害(DSM-IV)とした。しかし不可視トラウマによってPTSDを生ずる可能性があるとする考え方もある[2]。

2．誘因について

1）放射線障害の知識

放射線障害の特徴から「当初は症状がなくても，後から重篤な身体的悪影響が進展するかもしれない」という心配を抱くことは通常でもありうるが更に後述する条件が加わった。

2）報道内容

テレビ報道でチェルノブイリ原発事故の映像が恐怖心を助長した。送り手としては参考としての映像であっただろうと思われるが，当時者にとっては不必要な恐怖心をあおられ，あたかも自らの行く末を示しているかのように感じられた。

3）性格傾向

臆病という性格傾向のため他事故の惨状の映像という報道内容を目にしたことで放射線被曝への恐怖が相乗的に強まった(図)。

IV．まとめ

放射線被曝のような不可視トラウマの場合には，当事者に提供される情報によっては不安や恐怖心に強い影響を与え適応障害を引き起こす可能性がある。

参考文献

1）佐藤親次，岡田幸之：東海村臨界事故での心理ケア経験．心と社会，No. 100；183-188, 2000.
2）Scringar, C. B. : PTSD. Diagnosis, Treatment and Legal Issues. 2nd ed., Bruno Press, New Orleans, L. A., p.63-79, 1988.

---

*産業医科大学医学部精神医学教室
Hideki Nakano, Shuji Soeda, Jun Nakamura : Department of Psychiatry, School of Medicine, University of Occupational and Environmental Health.

パニック障害患者の coping と QOL
Coping and quality of life in patients with panic disorder

竹内　龍雄*　　日野　俊明*

I. はじめに

coping はパニック障害（以下 PD）の転帰の予測因子の一つとされ[1]，第2次・3次予防に関係する。PD 患者に特徴的な coping として，情動中心対処，逃避型，社会支援模索型が多いことが指摘されており[5,8,9]，われわれも確認している[2]。一方，PD 患者の quality of life（以下 QOL）の低下が指摘されており，われわれの調査では「自立のレベル」領域の QOL の低下を認めている[6]。

本報告では，われわれの行った2つの調査結果から，両者の関係を検討し，特に社会支援模索型 coping のもつ意味について考える。

II. 調査1，PD 患者の coping[2]

表1は，1997.11～98.10に帝京大学医学部附属市原病院精神神経科外来を訪れた PD 患者を対象に，SCI[4]を用いて行った coping の調査結果である（PD 患者67例（男25，女42），平均年齢40.7±13.7歳，健常被験者315名（男140，女175），平均年齢38.3±11.9歳）。表1に示すとおり，対処ストラテジーでは「情動中心型」が，対処型では「社会的支援模索型」と「逃避型」が，それぞれ PD 群が対照群に比べて平均得点が有意に高くなっている。なおこの表にはないが，広場恐怖を伴うものと，伴わないものとで比べると，伴うものの方が逃避型が有意に高かった。

III. 調査2，PD 患者の QOL[6]

表2は，1996.6～11に同じく当科外来を訪れた PD 患者を対象に，WHOQOL-100[7]を用いて行った QOL の調査結果である（PD 患者31例（男13，女18），平均年齢37.9±12.2歳，健常被験者68名（男28，女40），平均年齢38.1±11.1歳）。表2に示すとおり，「全般的な生活の質」と「自立のレベル」で，PD 群が対照群に比べ有意に得点が低かった。

IV. 考　察

PD 患者の coping については，問題解決型が少ない，情動中心型が多い，逃避型が多い，などの点で多くの報告が一致している[5,8,9]。社会的支援模索型も特徴の一つにあげられているが，多いという報告[9]と，少ないという報告[3]がある。われわれの調査1では，情動中心型，逃避型が有意に高得点で，この点は多くの文献報告と一致し，社会的支援模索型も有意な高得点を示した[2]。

QOL については，PD 患者で低下しているとの報告が多く，われわれの調査でも QOL 全般の低下が見られた[6]。ただし「自立のレベル」の低下を指摘した報告はなく，われわれ独自の結果であった。

情動中心型，逃避型 coping の高値は，ストレスによる不安などの情動に伴う苦痛の処理に追われ，問題（原因）解決に向かうことが少なく，不安や恐怖に立ち向かわず，認知的・行動的に回避しようとする傾向を示すと考えられる。特に広場恐怖を伴うものにこの傾向が強いことは，広場恐怖が回避行動そのものであるところから，当然の結果とも言えよう。

社会的支援模索型の高値については，文献では低いとする報告もあり，検討を要する。原因の一つに調査対象の重症度の違いが考えられる。入院例など比較的重い症例を対象を主とした報告では低く，一般住民など軽い例を対象とした報告では高い傾向が見られ，われわれの対象も後者に属する。社会的支援模索型は主として問題解決型対処に属するので，症状が重い場合，前述と同様に問

表1　PD患者のcoping(SCIによる)[2]

	PD患者 (n=67)		健常被験者 (n=315)	
	mean	SD	mean	SD
問題解決型	29.3	9.5	26.6	10.6
情動中心型	29.4*	9.5	25.1	8.2
計画型	7.7	3.6	7.5	3.9
対決型	6.1	3.1	5.8	2.9
社会的支援模索型	7.2**	3.6	4.9	3.5
責任受容型	7.6	3.2	7.5	4.1
自己コントロール型	7.7	2.9	7.2	3.1
逃避型	7.0**	3.2	4.8	2.5
離隔型	6.3	2.9	6.3	2.9
肯定評価型	7.9	3.7	7.7	3.5

*$p<0.05$　**$p<0.01$

表2　PD患者のQOL(WHOQOL-100による)[6]

	PD患者 (n=31)		健常被験者 (n=68)	
	mean	SD	mean	SD
身体的領域	2.98	0.58	2.95	0.50
心理的領域	2.90	0.48	3.11	0.56
自立のレベル	2.91*	0.57	3.51	0.52
社会的関係	3.10	0.61	3.14	0.52
生活環境	3.15	0.52	3.18	0.53
精神性・宗教・信条	2.95	0.98	3.21	0.73
全般的な生活の質	2.63*	0.88	3.20	0.47

*$p<0.05$

題解決に向かうことが少なくなり，低下すると考えられる。

次に社会的支援模索型copingのもつ意味を考える際に，QOLとの関係に注意すべき点について指摘したい。われわれの調査2から，パニック障害患者では「自立のレベル」領域のQOLが低いのが特徴であった。社会的支援模索型は，ソーシャル・サポートを利用することにより，ストレスに対処し適応をはかる方法であるが，そのことは同時に，周囲に依存する問題解決方法でもあることを意味する。すなわち社会的支援模索型copingは，適応や不安の克服に有利な一面と，自立性を損ない，QOLを低下させる一面との二面性をもつと考えられる。従って，個々の症例ではこの点での見極めが必要であろう。具体的には，自立的対処法の修得，自助グループの利用等の重要性が示唆される。

V. 結　論

PD患者の治療では，問題解決をめざし，回避せず，積極的対処を促すことが，ストレス対処の点から望ましい。

ソーシャル・サポートの利用は，適応に有利な一面と，自立のレベルを下げ，QOLを低下させる可能性があることに注意する必要がある。

文　献

1) Cowley, D. S., Flick, S. N., Roy-Byrne, P. P. : Long-term course and outcome in panic disorder : a naturalistic follow-up study. Anxiety, 2 ; 13-21, 1996.
2) 日野俊明, 竹内龍雄, 池田政俊ほか：パニック障害の対処様式について(続報)—「ラザルス式ストレスコーピングインベントリー」を用いた検討—. 精神科治療学, 14 ; 1403-1407, 1999.
3) Hoffart, A., Martinsen, E. W. : Coping strategies in major depressed, agoraphobic and comorbid in-patients : a longitudinal study. Br. J. Med. Psychol., 66 ; 143-55, 1993.
4) 日本健康心理学研究所：ラザルス式ストレス・コーピング・インベントリー(SCI). 実務教育出版, 東京, 1996.
5) Roy-Byrne, P. P., Vitaliano, P. P., Cowley, D. S. et al. : Coping in panic and major depressive disorder : Relative effects of symptom severity and diagnostic comorbidity. J. Nerv. Ment. Dis., 180 ; 179-83, 1992.
6) 竹内龍雄, 林　竜介, 池田政俊ほか：パニック障害患者のQuality of Life—WHOQOL-100を用いた調査から—. 日社精医誌, 6 ; 149-158, 1998.
7) 田崎美弥子, 野地有子, 中根允文：WHOのQOL. 診断と治療, 83 ; 2183-2198, 1995.
8) Vitaliano, P. P., Katon, W., Russo, J. et al. : Coping as an index of illness behavior in panic disorder. J. Nerv. Ment. Dis., 175 ; 78-84, 1987.
9) Vollrath, M., Angst, J. : Coping and illness behavior among young adults with panic. J. Nerv. Ment. Dis., 181 ; 303-308, 1993.

---

*帝京大学医学部附属市原病院精神神経科
Tatsuo Takeuchi, Toshiaki Hino : Department of Psychiatry, Ichihara Hospital, Teikyo University School of Medicine.

知的障害者の不適応予防のための施設の心理的機能についての若干の考案

Some considerations on psychological function of institution for preventing maladaptation of intellectually disabled people

平野　潔*

I．はじめに

　知的障害の原因，成人した彼らの障害の程度や質も様々であり，知的障害者更生施設で生活している者も多い。精神科薬物が必要とされる激しい行動傷害からささいな問題まで，様々な不適応や精神症状を示す入所者も多い。そのため，身体的症状や精神症状の治療のために，医療機関との連携（受診・入院）とともに，施設内での心理学的援助の方法に対するニードはかなり高い。

　今回，演者は，2つの施設において，3年間臨床心理学的視点から月1回のコンサルテーションを行う機会があった。

　方法は，入所者と施設のスタッフ（時に家族）を交えての同席面接を行い，知的障害者との初回面接で，面接者に起きた連想を素材として，その「意味」をスタッフとともに連想を広げ討議していく方法を行った。面接と討議は精神分析的視点―面接者の逆転移を素材とした主観的視点―から行った。

　その結果，再適応過程に及ぼす施設の精神機能（mental function）をもった器としての心理的機能，不適応に至った背景など幾つか理解が得られた。

II．施設の心理的機能

　症例検討会の中で，スタッフとともに発見できた施設がもつ7つの心理的機能について報告したい。

　1）対象としての施設

　無反応，意味不明な発語など，スタッフは関わりを持ちにくいことが多いが，その空しさから逆に，自分を統合する外部の対象の必要性を実感でき，彼らの基本的な存在感を保証している対象としての役割に気づくことが重要になる。移行対象，対象a，鏡像，部分対象などの原初的対象の意味を施設は担っている。

　2）解読する機能を担った環境としての施設

　行動傷害，欲動の表出に対して，意味というフィルターで解読していくことが，症状の緩和に役に立つ。

　3）主体の倫理的存在の危機とその回復

　現実的欠如（障害）のために，環境は与えていく存在として見られがちであるが，「現実的欠如（障害）を持った人は周囲を豊かにする」という彼らの倫理的存在を再認識する役割を施設は持っている。

　4）言語的環境の中に位置づけるということ

　彼らは言語機能が低下していることもあって，自分を言語で表現できないことが多いので，施設のスタッフ自体も，次第に行動レベルでの指導という働きかけが多くなりやすい。どうしても語る主体としての彼らの存在が忘れがちになるので，彼らをめぐって，語ることが必要になる。

　5）施設における存在領域と説明モデル

　施設は福祉的措置によって，社会的居場所というただ1つの器ではなく，表に示したような4つの存在領域と説明モデルの中で生きている主体的存在として文脈を広げて見ていく機能を持っている。

　6）精神機能をもった施設

　彼らの身体的存在を受け入れた施設は，社会的存在保護環境は，物理的存在保護環境，精神的存在保護環境である。特に，スタッフが言葉によって自らの機能を内省することで，施設自体が精神

表　施設における入所者の存在領域と説明モデル

		説明モデル(言語体系)とアプローチ			
		Biological Approach based on Medical Model	Psychological Approach based on Psychological Model	Sociological Approach based on Social Model	Philosophycal Approach based on Philosophycal Model
存在領域	Ⅳ. 倫理的存在	身体的存在の可能/不可能 生命 life/live ●後どれくらい生きられるか	精神的存在の可能/不可能 Psychic Reality/desire ●本人の望みの実現可能性	社会的存在の可能/不可能 自律性 ●社会の中で生きていけるか	Philosophy 存在根拠 存在の必要性・意味
	Ⅲ. 環境的存在(母胎)	環境/医学 生物学的環境 物理の化学的環境 身体の存在保護的環境 ●生きてきた,生きている環境の状況で語られる存在	環境/心理 心理学的環境 対人状況言語的環境 精神の存在保護的環境 ●周囲の人々の理解や反応(の歴史)で語られる存在	Sociology 社会的環境 福祉,衣食住,戸籍,社会制度 社会的存在保護的環境 Social Work ●周囲の社会的状況で語られる存在	環境Ⅹの倫理
	Ⅱ. 精神的存在	精神/医学 精神医学(Psychiatry) 精神症状 精神医学的状態像 精神医学的診断 ●精神症状で語られる存在	Psychology Psychological Assesment/Test Psychotherapy ●自我によってFrustrationを表現する存在	精神/社会 社会的精神 精神の社会性 Social therapy ●社会的不適応で語られる存在	欲望の倫理
	Ⅰ. 身体的存在	Biology 生物学的身体 Somatic therapy ●身体の病気や症状で語られる存在	身体/心理 心理学的身体 (身体像) ●心を抱いた身体の動きで語られる存在	身体/社会 社会的身体 身体の社会性 ●HandicapとAutonomyで語られる存在	身体の倫理

機能(mental function)をもった器となっている。環境側の言葉と精神機能が,彼らの「心mind」を生成していく。

7) 6つの器の機能をもった施設
①現実的存在を可能にする現実的環境
②鏡像的二者関係の中で人と繋がった存在を保証する機能
③許容範囲の設定(法,禁じ手,手順,役割)によって身体的,精神的,社会的秩序を守る機能
④表現方法,作業課題によって,何かする,できる自尊心を高める機能
⑤語る存在を保証する言語的環境(象徴的世界)
⑥一人できること/できないことの判断を通して自律性を体験する機能

この6つのうち,どの機能が優勢になるか,逸脱しているか,どの対象が必要で過剰(固着し停滞していること)なのかを理解でき,介入方法の視点が整理できた。

Ⅲ. 不適応予防と援助

1. 不適応の発生

1) 知的障害者(主体)は,環境との間の「意味あるつながり」を容易に喪失しやすく,「無いこと」の強度が高くなり,精神機能の容量を越えてしまう時,象徴と出会えず,発語(言葉)の低下,1語文(S1)への固着(holophrase),欲動の高まり,欲求の制止状況,心身症,習癖といった問題行動に繋がりやすい。

2) 長期間の適応行動の歴史のある入所者の場合,障害をめぐる倫理(彼らの存在根拠)が危機に陥ったこれまでの状況(環境の失敗)がある。

乳幼児以来,環境と個体からのニードとの不整合や出会い損ないというアクシデントの積重によって自分としてうまくやれること(自律性:autonomy)をめぐる悪戦苦闘の歴史などがみられた。

2. 援　助

1) 4つの存在領域と説明モデルの多様な存在の中で,身体療法(薬物療法)に加え,施設の精神機能を再賦活化するために必要な施設の心理的機能を明確化することが,彼らに必要な援助方法であった。

2) 施設側のスタッフの同一性—変わりない姿勢を維持すること—という施設の心理的機能が彼らの同一性を守り,不適応予防に繋がると思われた。環境が「意味」をもった目で絶えず抱え,言葉で入所者について語り合っていくことが絶えず必要とされるのではないかと思われる。

3) 施設は障害者に現実的居場所,社会的居場所を提供しながら,同時に心理学的にみると施設自体が精神機能を持っていることがわかった。精神分析的発達論と,日常の生活指導の「意味」と繋がる時,彼らの不適応予防や回復に重要な貢献をしてくることがわかった。

---

*医療法人和泉会いずみ病院
　Kiyoshi Hirano : Izumi-Hospital, Okinawa.

日本における周産期精神医学（1）
―産後早期の気分障害とその危険因子についての多施設研究―

Perinatal psychiatry in Japan (1) —Multi-centre prospective study of early postpartum mood states—

山下　洋* 　吉田　敬子* 　上田　基子* 　田代　信維*

Aim of the study

1) To investigate whether the very early mood disturbance link to the early onset of postnatal depression.

2) To investigate risk factors of early mood disturbance, especially focused on obstetric factors which have been very little studied in systematic ways.

3) To show guideline to detect early onset of postnatal depression by obstetric staff rather than psychiatrists

Sampling

14 hospitals which are tertiary and teaching hospitals took part in this project. In an obstetric ward in each hospital, recruitment continued until 20 women had agreed to participate. Fourteen Hospitals sent back to our centre 252 completed questionnaires during the first postnatal days. 226 out of 252 patients (89.7%) filled out the questionnaires at one-month postnatal outpatient clinic.

Methods

The questionnaire we developed for this project consists of three parts as follows ;

1) On admission and around delivery ; a Consent Form, Basic demographic information, Obstetric and Neonatal factors.

2) Maternity blues scale (Blues scale ; Stein, 1980) During the first 5 days ; Self report questionnaire, total score of eight or more on any one of the first five postnatal days, indicates maternity blues.

3) Edinburgh Postnatal Depression Scale (EPDS ; Cox et al., 1987) given on the fifth postnatal day and again at one month postnatally. An EPDS score of 9≧ at 1 month indicates a probable case of postnatal depression.

Results

Incidence of Maternity blues and Postnatal depression ;

79 of the 226 patients (35.0%) had Maternity blues. 46 of the 226 patients (20%) had postnatal depression (EPDS≧9) at one month postnatally.

Relationship between Postnatal depression and possible risk factors ; The relationship between postnatal depression and other factors is demonstrated in Table 1.

Relative factors of postnatal depression (EPDS≧9 on 1 month) were as follows ; Maternity blues (79 ; 37%) (OR=4.4　95% CI ; 2.2-8.7), EPDS≧9 on the 5th postnatal day (59 ; 26%)) (OR=13.0　95% CI ; 4.8-38.6), Maternal complication (OR=3.2　95% CI ; 1.6-6.2)

Summary and clinical implication

1) The incidence of postnatal depression using the EPDS in our multi-centre study (20%) is similar to the ones reported in the United Kingdom and European countries.

2) The high score of EPDS on the fifth postnatal day could usefully predict later postnatal depression at one month.

3) Obstetric complications are significantly related to later postnatal depression at one month.

Table 1 Relationship between Postnatal depression and possible risk factors (Proportion (%))

	Day 5			1 month		
	EPDS≧9	EPDS<9	Comparison	EPDS≧9	EPDS<9	Comparison
Sex of Baby	32/59(54)	97/167(58)	NS	25/46(54)	104/180(58)	NS
Primiparous	32/59(54)	80/167(48)	NS	27/46(59)	85/180(47)	NS
History of Pregnancy loss	25/59(42)	41/167(25)	p=0.010	16/46(35)	50/180(28)	NS
Caesearian section	8/59(14)	9/167(5.4)	p=0.041	4/46(8.7)	13/180(7.2)	NS
Low birth weight (<2.5kg)	9/59(15)	13/167(7.8)	NS	6/46(13)	16/180(8.8)	NS
Bottle feeding only	6/59(10)	17/167(10)	NS	2/46(4.3)	21/180(12)	NS
Maternal Complication	36/59(61)	61/167(37)	p=0.001	30/46(65)	67/180(37)	p=0.001
Neonatal Complication	16/59(27)	17/167(10)	p=0.002	10/46(22)	23/180(13)	NS
Stein scale≧8	48/59(81)	31/167(19)	p<0.0001	29/46(63)	50/180(28)	p<0.0001
EPDS≧9 at 5th day				32/46(69)	27/180(16)	p<0.0001

4) Postnatal depression could be prospectively monitored from very early postnatal days while mothers are still in obstetric ward.

References

1) Cox, J. L. et al. : Detection of postnatal depression : Development of the 10 item Edinburgh postnatal depression scale. Br. J. Psychiatry, 150 ; 782-786, 1987.
2) Stein, G. : The pattern of mental change and body weight change in the first postpartum week. J. Psychosomatic Research, 24 ; 165-171, 1980.

---

*九州大学医学部神経精神科
Hiroshi Yamashita, Keiko Yoshida, Motoko Ueda, Nobutada Tashiro : Department of Neuropsychiatry, Graduate School of Medical Science, Faculty of medicine, Kyushu University.

日本における周産期精神医学(2)
―産後うつ病の女性の地域におけるスクリーニングと介入に関する研究―

Perinatal psychiatry in Japan(2)―Screening and intervention of postnatal depression in community―

上田　基子* 　吉田　敬子* 　山下　洋* 　田代　信維*

Background and objectives

It was found a much higher percentage of women in need of assessment for postnatal depression(PND) (Yoshida et al., 1997 ; Yamashita et al., 2000) than previously recognized in Japan(Okano et al., 1998). The incidence of PND is around 15%, which is uncommon but often overlooked. In Japan neonatal home visit system from community health centres is well organized, however it is not used to detect mothers with possible psychiatric problems. Then we planned a project to implement community PND screening with the Edinburgh Postnatal Depression Scale(EPDS ; Cox et al., 1987) at a neonatal home visit program of our local community health centre. The aim of the study is(1) to screen and care mothers with PND using EPDS in association with the home visit system in community, (2) to investigate the efficacy of the screening and care system and give some guideline for mother-infant mental health.

Method

Our subjects were the mothers received a neonatal home visit from our health centre which was in cooperation with our study. The center is one of seven health centres in our city, Fukuoka, which has more than 1,300,000 residents. There are approximately 1,800 births each year in our catchment area, and about 450 of 1,800 births are received the neonatal home visit. The existing home visit service is applied to mother-baby dyads where (1) with low-birth weight of less than 2,500 grams, (2) first born babies with birth weight of less than 2,800 grams, (3) babies with perinatal or pediatric problems, (4) mothers with socio-economical problems, (5) mothers who request home visit.

One hundred mothers were asked to participate in our study. All of them were Japanese who gave birth between August 27, 1998 and April 6, 1999. EPDS were carried out on the first visit(12～109 days), 6 months and 12 months postnatally. The risk factors of onset of depression, such as lack of support and past psychiatric history were also investigated. The women whose EPDS scores were 9 (cut-off point in Japan ; Okano et al., 1996 ; Yamashita et al., 2000) or above were followed up by community health visitors. At 12 postnatal month, the Japanese translated non-patient version of the Structured Clinical Interview for DSM-IV (SCID ; American Psychiatric Association, 1994) was applied to the 70 mothers, who were fully followed up, by psychiatrists.

Result

The mean age of the 100 women was 29.7 years (range 19~42 years), and 77% of them were primiparous. The average number of children was 1.30 (range 1~3), all but one was married. The average month of delivery was 38.5 months. Between 70 women interviewed with the SCID and 30 women who didn't, no significant differences were found in age, gestational age at delivery, mood of delivery either forceps or Caesarean section, baby's birth weight, and past psychiatric history. The women who were not interviewed were more likely to be multiparous (p=0.033) and not to have had babies' pediatric problems which need to be hospitalized or operated during the 12 months after delivery.

Sixteen out of 100 women (16%) scored the EPDS being 9 or above were detected at the first home visit. During the 12 month postnatal follow-up period, 19 out of 70 women (27%) were categorized as SCID depressive cases, 12 with a major depressive disorder and 7 with a depressive disorder not otherwise specified. Twelve out of 19 depressive cases had an onset within one week postnatally (10 major depressive disorder and 2 depressive disorder not otherwise specified). Between 19 depressive cases and 51 non-depressive cases, there were no statistically differences in demographic characteristics, mood of delivery, baby's birth weight. Babies' pediatric disease which required either outpatient treatment or admission during one year after birth were significantly associated with depressive disorders found in the mothers (p=0.001). Especially proportion of baby's admission were much higher in depressed mothers (42%) compared to non-depressed mothers (6%).

Discussion

Screening depressed mothers using already well organized neonatal home visit is available for care of mother-baby dyads in terms of mental health. Majority of depression had their onset within one week postpartum, therefore if we wish to use the existing neonatal home visit system not only for monitoring babies but also for detecting depressive mothers, we would like to suggest the first home visit by health visitors better to be carried out within the first couple of postnatal weeks. And whenever babies have some pediatric problems and checked, it is prudent to simply ask mother's feeling in combination with using the EPDS for welfare of mothers and infants. This study became a clue of early intervention of PND by health visitors of the local community health centre.

References

1) American Psychiatric Association : Diagnostic and Statistical Manual of Mental Disorders. American Psychiatric Press, Washington, D.C., 1994.
2) Cox, J. L., Holden, J. M., Sagovsky, R. : Detection of postnatal depression. Development of the 10-item Edinburgh Postnatal Depression Scale. Br. J. Psychiatry, 150 ; 782-786, 1987.
3) Okano, T., Murata, M., Masuji, F. et al. : Validation and reliability of Japanese version of EPDS (Edinburgh Postnatal Depression Scale). (in Japanese with English summary) Arch. Psychiat. Diagn. Clin. Eval., 7 ; 525-533, 1996.
4) Okano, T., Nomura, J., Kumar, R. et al. : An epidemiological and clinical investigation of postpartum psychiatric illness in Japanese mothers. J. Affect. Disord., 48 ; 233-240, 1998.
5) Yamashita, H., Yoshida, K., Nakano, H. et al. : Postnatal depression in Japanese women. Detecting the early onset of postnatal depression by closely monitoring the postpartum mood. J. Affect. Disord., 58 ; 145-154, 2000.
6) Yoshida, K., Marks, M. N., Kibe, N. et al. : Postnatal depression in Japanese women who have given birth in England. J. Affect. Disord., 43 ; 69-77, 1997.

---

*九州大学医学部神経精神科
Motoko Ueda, Keiko Yoshida, Hiroshi Yamashita, Nobutada Tashiro : Department of Neuropsychiatry, Graduate school of Medical Science, Faculty of Medicine, Kyushu University, Fukuoka.

日本における周産期精神医学（3）
―理解と認識：国際比較文化研究から―

Perinatal psychiatry in Japan(3)—Perception and cognition : From a international cross-cultural study—

吉田　敬子*　　上田　基子*　　山下　洋*　　田代　信維*

Background and objectives

Mental health problems in perinatal period are still misunderstood or under-recognized by pregnant and postnatal women, their families and maternal health care professionals due to a lack of education for perinatal psychiatry and of sharing their knowledge.

The aim of the study is to highlight the common and different perception between the women, families and professionals and to improve efficacy of mental health care based on mutual understanding about perinatal psychology and psychiatry.

Method

This study is part of EU and international cross-cultural research on postnatal depression. Data of the postnatal women in four focus groups of total 17 women(age ranged from 25~37 years old, 5~8 postnatal months, all married and housewives, none of them were working)and three key informants in each categories(3 fathers, 3 grandmothers, 6 health professionals ; 1 psychiatrist, 1 pediatrician, 1 obstetric clinician, and 3 health planners) were collected through one local health center of Fukuoka city.

Qualitative method is to describe from the point of view of subjects being studied, to find the meaning rather than measuring, and to emphasis on a comprehensive or holistic understanding.

Results

Data highlighting different perceptions related to Japanese specific cultural perception were as follows. 1)Happiness during pregnancy ; Having a baby boy, Socially accepted, attending a traditional ceremony for pregnancy, Being proud of having a pregnant daughter(grandmother)2)Unhappiness during pregnancy ; Husband's affair during wife's absence. 3)Happiness after birth ; being accepted by mother-in-law(Focus group). All the summaries obtained from the key informants are in Table 1. 4)understanding postnatal depression ; Many focus group mothers confused as maternity blues(Table 2). Fathers and grandmothers did not know much so they did not give any particular answer. The Clinicians did not really recognize postnatal depression precisely, explaining that they were not educated about perinatal psychiatry. The planners were much less knowledgeable and were not aware of importance of these issues, lacking a concrete policy.

Discussion

The perinatal women in Japan are in an unique situation from the cross-cultural point of view. Living standards and medical technology are highly Westernized, whilst they are still following the traditional ideas and customs of childbirth. It is meaningful to look into the gaps in the themes extracted between the postnatal mothers of focus groups and other key informants including their family members and medical／health professionals.

References

1) Sato, T., Sugawara, M., Toda, M., Shima, S. and

Table 1 Qualitative data from focus group mothers／Relatives

1. What brings happiness to women?		2. What brings unhappiness to women?	
During pregnancy	After birth	During pregnancy	After birth
Feeling foetus Pregnancy itself Became pregnant, conceived Healthy condition Physical (body) change Increasing family menber Building up family Husband's happy reaction Having child Having boy Socially accepted (Father) Being fertile (Grandmother)	Baby's growth and development Baby's smile Being together with baby Baby's facial expression Listening to baby's voice, Baby care Elder child is caring baby Husband is caring baby Communication with baby and husband Breast-feeding Accepted by mother-in-law Socially accepted Going to shrine with baby (Father)	Morning sickness Tiredness (physically) Fear of delivery Feeling irritable Have to leave work Limited daily activity Not supportive work atmosphere for pregnant women Limited social life Too exhausted baby care Under control ; should not eat particular food, drink alcohol etc. Husband's love affair during wife's absence during Satogaeri bunben (Grandmother)	Baby unwanted Having baby for family as wife's duty Burden of baby care, tiring Loss of honeymoon period Having difficulty in baby care Bothered by baby Less social life No time for oneself Physical, hormonal unbalanced Changed marital relationship, Father rather than husband Interference by mother-in-law Little support from husband Pain after having C／S Insufficient breast-milk

Table 2 Qualitative data from focus group mothers／Relatives

3. Understanding PND	4. What can be done to help?
Blues Being apathy Tearfulness Moody Committing child abuse Neurosis Being stuck at home Abandon baby Not clear in mind Being irritable Can not sleep Having distress with husband	Listening to mother Emotional support from husband and family Being together with husband, husband's existence Midwifery support Pediatrician's advice Talk other mothers rather than psychiatrist, Chatting with young mothers Counseling (Telephone counseling) Midwifery home visit Visiting friend Escaping baby care for a little while

Kitamura, T. : Rearing related stress and depressive severity. The Japanese J. Psychology, 64 (6) ; 409-416, 1994.

2) Yamashita, H., Yoshida, K., Nakano, H., Tashiro, N. : Postnatal depression in Japanese women—Detecting the early onset of postnatal depression by closely monitoring the postpartum mood- J. Affect. Disord., 58 ; 145-154, 2000.

3) Yoshida, K., Marks, M. N., Kibe, N., Kumar, R., Nakano, H., Tashiro, N. : Postnatal depression in Japanese women who have given birth in England. J. Affect. Disord, 43 ; 69-77, 1997.

---

*九州大学医学部神経精神科
Keiko Yoshida, Motoko Ueda, Hiroshi Yamashita, Nobutada Tashiro : Department of Neuropsychiatry, Graduate School of Medical Science, Kyushu University.

婚姻後に精神障害を発症または再発した離婚調停事件の当事者について

Divorce settlement cases involving the onset and/or recurrence of psychiatric disorder after marriage

神川千賀子*

I. はじめに

家庭裁判所の調停は，調停委員が主体となって裁判官との評議をもとに，当事者間の調停を進める。調査官や，医務室技官は，必要に応じて裁判官の命令を受けて，調査や調停で当事者に直接に関わる。家庭裁判所で，医務室技官が調査や調停に立ち会うことを「立会（りっかい）」と表現する。当事者の診断と援助という裁判官の命令によって立会するが，精神障害が推測される当事者が調停というストレスフルな状況下におかれる時，精神障害の再発や症状の悪化を予防するためにも，調停の進行について，医務室技官の意見を調停委員会へ述べている。また，精神障害を発症している当事者や，心理的な傷として精神障害をわずらっている当事者に，医務室技官は適切に対応していく必要がある。最も医務室技官が当事者に直接関与することが多い夫婦関係調整事件には，離婚と円満解決となる調停がある。これらの事件の当事者について，5年間の概観と私の考察したことを述べたい。

II. 夫婦関係調整事件とは

まず始めに，家庭裁判所の夫婦関係調整事件の流れを簡単に説明する。申立人が，申立ての時点で離婚の意思がはっきりしているとき，「夫婦関係調整事件（離婚）」，となるが，調停が開始されても，調停の進行中に，申立人がもう一度やり直そうという気持ちに変わるときもあり，「円満解決」，つまり，夫婦としてやっていく合意ができるときもある。また，その反対の場合，「夫婦関係調整事件（円満解決）」を申し立てても，相手方にその意思が無い場合，申立人の気持ちが離婚へと変化し，「離婚」となる場合もある。いずれの場合も「成立」となると，調停条項を取り決めて終結する。「不成立」になる時は，地方裁判所に訴訟を起こすことができる。申立てが「取り下げ」で終わる場合は，調停条項はなく，ある程度当事者同士が納得し，このまま同居し，あるいは別居のままで良いというときである。当事者の精神状態が悪く，調停継続不可能なときは，まれに「成さず」という結果になる（図1を参照）。

III. 5年間に立会した夫婦関係調整事件調停の当事者の概観

平成8年4月から平成13年3月の5年間に夫婦関係調整事件で直接関わった当事者は48人，26事件であった。私が関与したこれらの事件に限っていうと，離婚か円満解決の調停は離婚調停85％，離婚の申立人で精神障害のある妻36％，離婚の相手方で精神障害のある夫27％，離婚，円満解決ともに精神障害があると思われる当事者が申立人か相手方になる割合はそれぞれ約50％，調停の時点で精神障害があると思われる当事者は67％であった（グラフ1を参照）。年齢は30代，婚姻後10年以内に申し立てる当事者が多く，申立て時の婚姻形態は，別居88％，夫婦間の子の数は2人が多かった。当事者の精神障害は，分裂病圏や躁鬱病が約半数，境界性人格障害や性格的問題，家庭内暴力，アルコール依存など人格的な問題に関わる障害もあった（グラフ2を参照）。家族間対立は半数以下，精神福祉医療に関与していない当事者は45％で，外傷性ストレス障害，妄想性障害，性格の偏りによる家庭内暴力などの当事者であった。精神障害や性格の偏りやアルコール依存や薬物使用などによる暴力は29％だった。調停の結果は，

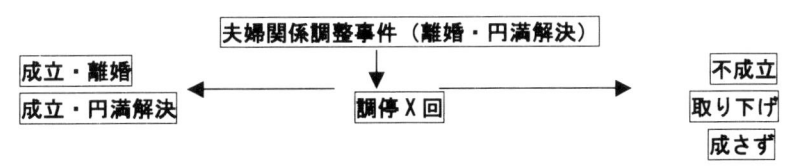

図1　夫婦関係調整事件の流れ

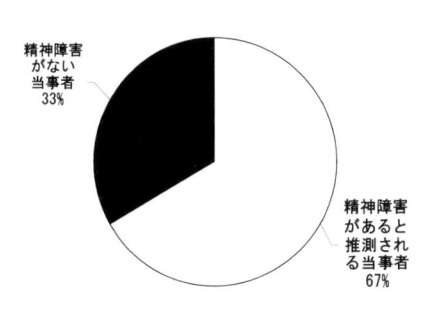

グラフ1　精神障害があると推測される当事者

- 精神障害がない当事者 33%
- 精神障害があると推測される当事者 67%

グラフ2　当事者の推測される精神障害等(割合)

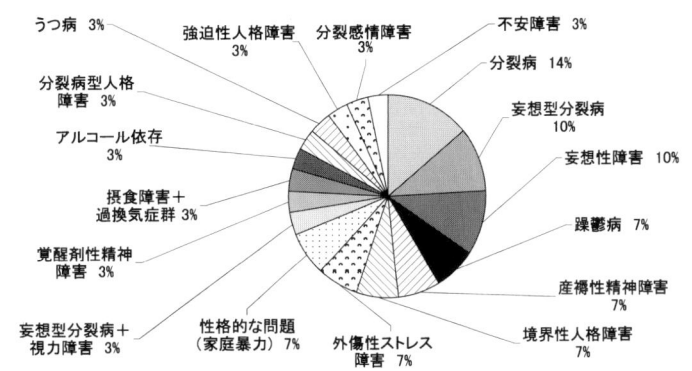

- うつ病 3%
- 強迫性人格障害 3%
- 分裂感情障害 3%
- 不安障害 3%
- 分裂病型人格障害 3%
- 分裂病 14%
- アルコール依存 3%
- 妄想型分裂病 10%
- 摂食障害＋過換気症群 3%
- 妄想性障害 10%
- 覚醒剤性精神障害 3%
- 躁鬱病 7%
- 妄想型分裂病＋視力障害 3%
- 産褥性精神障害 7%
- 性格的な問題(家庭暴力) 7%
- 境界性人格障害 7%
- 外傷性ストレス障害 7%

取り下げ37%，不成立31%，成立28%(離婚3件，別居・婚費2件，円満解決2件)であった。精神障害があっても単独で離婚の成立や養育費などを決められる当事者もある。約2割の当事者に代理人か家族がついたが，離婚成立はその3分の1であった。大部分の夫婦が子を有し，精神障害のある当事者が子を抱え込むこともあった。

IV. 考　察

家庭裁判所は，精神障害の予防という観点からは，その機能を担うところではないが，当事者や家族から調停の継続を期待される場所になることが多く，医務室技官が，当事者や家族に医療機関へ出向くように助言することも多い。調停の進行のために当事者の精神状態を把握し援助や助言をする医務室技官の立会の意味を5年間の結果などから考察した。①精神障害がある当事者が，入院や症状の悪化で調停を中断することなく調停を最後までやり通せるように配慮された取り扱いを受け，社会的生活者として健康な当事者と公平に取り扱われる。②精神障害のある当事者が，何らかの医療や福祉の関与のもとで精神的あるいは具体的な生活上の援助をうけながら子の養育や仕事が継続できるよう，調停の期間中に医療機関や保健所とのつながりを当事者や家族が持つように助言し，当事者の精神障害の予防的働きが，家庭裁判所から，医療機関へ移行して，精神障害のある当事者が，何とか落ち着いて生活できる時期に調停を終結させる。

以上のように裁判官や調停委員に対し当事者について意見を述べる場合，精神障害のある当事者の精神障害の予防という観点も含めた意見も述べる必要があると考えた。

＊大阪家庭裁判所医務室技官
Chikako Kamikawa：Medical Office of Osaka Family Court.

月経前不快気分障害の診断基準(DSM-IV)を用いた検討
―看護婦861人を対象としたアンケート調査より―

Premenstrual dysphoric disorder (PMDD) among Japanese nurses

尾鷲登志美*　大坪　天平*　田中　克俊**　松丸憲太郎*　岡島　由佳*　上島　国利*

I. はじめに

月経前不快気分障害(premenstrual dysphoric disorder : PMDD)は，DSM-IV の研究用基準案に取り上げられた病態で，既に1930年代に提唱され[2]，1950年代より一般的に知られている月経前症候群(premenstrual syndrome : PMS)や月経前緊張症とは区別して用いられる。PMSは，月経前黄体期に身体または精神症状が1つ以上存在するものを指しているのに対し，PMDDは著しい抑うつ気分，著しい不安，著しい情緒不安定，活動に対する興味の減退を基本とする11項目の症状のうち5項目以上をほぼ同時に満たし，さらに社会的生活に支障を来し，連続2回以上前方視的に症状が確認されて初めて診断される。

上記のように，PMDDは重症度や，その結果生じる障害などからPMSとは明らかに区別できる。PMSに関する報告は散見するものの，PMDDに関する本邦の報告は少ない。今回我々は，PMDDの実態を把握するとともに，PMDDと性格傾向の関連等について検討したので報告する。

II. 対象と方法

昭和大学病院および昭和大学病院附属東病院に勤務する看護婦861名；平均年齢27.0±5.9(20～50歳)を対象に，DSM-IVにおけるPMDD診断基準(研究用基準案)に準じた質問票，Hospital anxiety depression scale (HADS)[6]，NEO five-factor inventory (NEO-FFI)[5]による自己記入式評価を実施した。調査前に研究の目的と方法を説明し，全員から文書にて同意を得た。

III. 結　果

1. PMDDの診断

PMDD 診断基準における各症状11項目中，5項目以上を満たす者154人(17.9%)，5項目以上を満たし，かつ，社会生活において支障をきたす者51人(5.9%)，過去2回の月経前に症状を認めPMDD 診断基準を満たす者36人(4.2%)であった。

2. 年齢別PMDDの診断

20～24歳の4.3%，20～29歳の3.6%，30～34歳の4.4%，35～39歳の6.5%，40～44歳の5.3%，45～50歳の0%がPMDDの診断基準を満たした。

3. PMDD群と非PMDD群の比較

PMDDの診断基準を満たす36人(PMDD群)と満たさない825人(非PMDD群)の間で比較を行ったところ，年齢，NEO-FFIの開拓性，愛想のよさ，誠実さの得点において有意差は認めず，HADSの抑うつ得点，不安得点，NEO-FFIの神経質得点においてPMDD群が非PMDD群に比較して有意に高く，また，NEO-FFIの外向性得点がPMDD群において有意に低いという結果を得た(表)。

IV. 考　察

今回の我々の調査では，4.2%の女性がDSM-IVのPMDDの診断基準(研究用基準案)を満たした。これは，諸外国で報告されているPMDDの有病率(3～8%)とほぼ同等である。

今回の調査では，PMDD群と非PMDD群の間

表 PMDD 群と非 PMDD 群の比較

	PMDD	非 PMDD 群	P (t 検定)
年齢（歳）	26.9±5.1	27.5±7.1	0.64
HADS　　抑うつ	7.4±4.2	5.2±3.4	0.003
HADS　　不安	9.6±4.3	6.7±3.6	0.000
NEO-FFI　神経質	30.1±6.9	25.6±6.7	0.000
NEO-FFI　外向性	22.2±5.2	24.7±6.1	0.009
NEO-FFI　開拓性	28.1±4.5	27.7±4.5	0.42
NEO-FFI　愛想のよさ	27.3±4.7	28.7±4.6	0.082
NEO-FFI　誠実さ	24.9±5.8	26.5±5.6	0.11

で，HADS の抑うつ得点，不安得点，NEO-FFI の神経質得点，外向性得点において有意な差が認められた。海外の文献では，PMDD では他の精神疾患（特に大うつ病）の併存率が高いという報告が多く[1]，特に分娩後のうつ病や反復性の大うつ病との関連が示唆されている。今回の調査結果からも，PMDD 群で将来大うつ病が併存する可能性が非 PMDD 群に比べて高い事が予想される。気分障害の好発年齢が中高年であることを考慮すると，今後の縦断的な検討が必要であると考えられた。

PMDD の各症状（抑うつ気分，不安，情緒不安定，易刺激性など）に選択的セロトニン再取り込み阻害薬（SSRI）が有効との知見が集積されつつあり[3,4]，米国では fluoxetine が 2000 年 11 月に，PMDD もしくは重症の PMS の治療薬として認可された。PMDD は社会的な障害を伴う重篤な疾患であるが症状緩和が可能な疾患である。PMDD を早期から発見，診断し治療が必要であると思われる。

V. まとめ

861 名の看護婦（平均年齢 27.0±5.9 歳）を対象にアンケート調査を実施したところ，PMDD の診断基準（DSM-IV 研究用基準案）を 4.2％が満たした。

文　献

1) Endicott, J. : History, evolution, and diagnosis of premenstrual dysphoric disorder. J. Clin. Psychiatry, 61(supple 12) ; 5-8, 2000.
2) Frank, R. T. : The hormonal basis of premenstrual tension. Arch. Neurol. Psychiatry, 26 ; 1053-1057, 1931.
3) Steiner, M. : Premenstrual syndrome and premenstrual dysphoric disorder : guidelines for management. J. Psychiatry Neurosci, 25 ; 459-468, 2000.
4) Yonkers, K. A., Halbreich, U., Freeman, E., et al. : Symptomatic improvement of premenstrual dysphoric disorder with sertraline treatment : a randomized controlled trial. JAMA, 278 ; 983-988, 1997.
5) 吉村公雄，中村健二，大野裕ほか：5 因子モデルによるパーソナリティの測定-NEO Five-Factor Inventory (NEO-FFI) の信頼性と妥当性．ストレス科学，13(1) ; 45-53, 1998.
6) Zigmond, A. S., Snaith, R. P. : Hospital Anxiety and Depression Scale. 精神科診断学，4 ; 371-372, 1993.

---

*昭和大学医学部精神医学教室
Owashi, T., Otsubo, T., Matsumaru, K., Okajima, Y., Kamijima, K. : Department of Psychiatry, Showa University School of Medicine.
**(株)東芝安全保健センター
Tanaka, K. : Principal Office Medical Center, Toshiba Corporation.

摂食障害の予防活動
―女子大キャンパスをベースにして―

Preventive activities against eating disorders—From the experiences in a woman's university

生野　照子[*]　北村　圭三[*]　頼藤　和寛[*]　丸島　令子[*]

　我が国では摂食障害の本格的な予防活動はまだ試みられていない。今回我々は，女子大学のキャンパスをベースにした予防活動を開始したので報告する。活動としては，1回および継続的な講義を実施して"体重や体型に関する意識が変化するか""やせ願望を抑制できるか"を調査し，続いて，学生参加による実際的な予防活動を開始した。

I. 1回の特別講義による啓発活動

　大学1回生の女子174名を対象とし，2000年4月～6月に実施。調査方法は，講義開始前にEAT26と「体重や体型に関するアンケート」を行い，その後の約60分間で"体重の重要性""やせの害""摂食障害とは""摂食障害の重篤性"について講義した。講義終了後に再度アンケートに回答を求め，2カ月後にも再調査をして啓発効果の持続について調べた。2カ月後の回答者は156名である。

　結果：①EAT26は，30点以上が6名。因子別得点では，ダイエット因子が平均5点で最も高かった。②講義の内容は全体的によく理解された。とくに"痩せが及ぼす心身への弊害"に反応が大きかった。2カ月後にも84%の学生が講義内容を覚えており，やはり"心身の弊害"が印象に残っているとする学生が多かった。③講義直後は体重や体型に関する意識が変化し，"重い体重だ・太っている""体重・体型に不満"とする学生が減少した。しかし，2カ月後にはこれらの結果は元に戻っていた。④外見へのこだわりは2カ月後に逆に増加し，こだわる理由は"外観をよくしたいから"が最も多かった。⑤ダイエット行動は2カ月後に減っていたが，有意ではなかった。

　考察：1回の講義によっては，①「摂食障害やダイエットに関する知識の増加」が期待される。②心身に及ぼす弊害について教えることが効果的である。③体重や体型に関する意識は予防教育の影響を受けやすいが，少なくとも2カ月後にはもとに戻る可能性がある，などが判明した。つまり，1回の講義だけでは"体重や体型へのこだわり"を減らすことが難しく，2カ月以内のブースターセッションが必要と考えられた。

II. 継続的講義による啓発活動

　2000年10～12月にかけて計11回の継続的講義を実施。対象者は女子大生87名。調査方法は，Fat Phobia Scale（FPS），EAT40，EDIを用いて受講前後のやせ願望や摂食行動に関する変化を調べた。検定はWilcoxnの符号付検定。講義内容は集中講義と同じであるが，グループディスカッションやビデオ学習を付加し，グループ毎の自主的調査や実験も行った。講義終了時の感想では「摂食障害はダイエットだけではなく心の病だということが分かった」というのが52.6%，「摂食障害者がいたら助けてあげたい」というのが40.4%であり，この結果からは学生たちは講義によって知識を得るだけでなく，摂食障害の本質的な部分まで理解したかのように思われた。

　結果：①FPSは，受講前の平均は158点とやや高値であり，学生たちの肥満恐怖はやや強いことが分かった。受講後は159.4点であり，肥満への認識に変化は見られなかった。因子分析によって抽出された，悪印象・非親和的・攻撃的・依存的・非創造的の5因子に関しても，平均点に若干の推移は見られたものの有意差は無く，受講前後に変化がないことが分かった。②EAT40では，受講

前では総得点が30点以上の者が10％であり，ダイエット因子は9点以上が18.2％，過食及び食物に没頭する因子は2.8点以上が17％，食事のコントロール因子は2.5点以上の者が19.2％であった。これも，受講前後に有意差はみられなかった。③EDIの総得点は，受講前は50点以上の者が32.3％，受講後は37.1％であり，有意差はみられなかった。

考察：講義による受講生の変化は有意でなく，感情的あるいは知識的な改善はあったが，実際のダイエット行動の予防に結びつけるには難しいことが分かった。これらの一因としては，季節が秋になって食欲が増し，ダイエットや外見を意識する時期になったことも考えられる。

以上，特別・継続講義ともに，知識面での改善はみられても，実際のダイエット行動ややせ願望を変容させることは難しいことが実証された。講義でダイエット行動を変えることの難しさは欧米での予防活動で既に指摘されてきたが，知識教育だけでなく，より実際的な活動が必要であることが今回の試行でも確認された結果であった。したがって，他の予防活動との併用が不可欠であると考え，学生参加を含めた実際的な予防活動を開始した。

Ⅲ．学生参加による予防活動

まず教員による予防活動グループを結成し，予算を申請した。同時に，大学の医務室及び学生相談室との連携体制を作り，地域とも連携して講演活動を行った。次いで学生の自主的運営による「ED会」という会合を結成した。スタッフは教員や学生15名であり，学生が中心となって世話役となり，摂食障害について学習したり，友達同士で話し合ったり，教員と共に個人的な相談にも応じる会合である。摂食障害に興味がある人，摂食障害の知人を援助したい人，摂食障害に悩んでいる人など誰でも気軽に参加できる会合であり，週1回で月に3回開催，うち1回は摂食障害本人だけによるセルフヘルプグループとして行っている。1回は約45分間であり，5～10名の参加者がある。スタッフはポスターを掲示して参加を呼びかけたり，啓発用のパンフレットを作成して入学式で配布し，1回生のうちから摂食障害に対する意識を促そうと試みている。参加者のアンケートからは，ダイエットや摂食障害の考え方が変化したという結果を得ており，学生による自主的活動は有意義な成果をあげていると考えられる。現在は講演会の開催など多面的な活動を展開しつつあり，今後は地域や，中学，高校とも連携してプログラムを進めていく予定である。

---

*神戸女学院大学人間科学部
Teruko Ikuno, Keizou Kitamura, Kazuhiro Yorifuji, Reiko Marusima : Kobe College School of Human Sciences.

女子大学生における摂食障害傾向と環境要因との関連

Relationship between tendency to develop on eating disorder and environmental factors among female university students

石田　彩子[*1]　　伊達真理子[*2]　　渡邉　陽子[*3]　　吾妻　ゆみ[*4]
稲富　宏之[*4]　　田中　悟郎[*4]　　太田　保之[*4]

Introduction

After World War II, Japan has become one of the leading economic powers in the world, and today it is enjoying an age of repletion. With the mass media perpetually concentrating on diets, and "being slender" portrayed as one of the criteria for social estimation, cases are often reported of an extreme desire for being slim or of abnormal eating habits leading to eating disorders, especially among the younger generation who are easily influenced by these trends. However, society has not yet reached a consensus concerning the decisive factors which aggravate the tendency toward eating disorders. We have conducted an investigation of female college students concerning the factors, which link individual feelings towards environments at home, school and society to a tendency to develop eating disorders.

Subjects and methods

We distributed self-reporting questionnaires to 225 female college students who agreed to the aim and method of our research. Of these, 175 replies were valid (78%). As criteria, we used : 1) the Eating Disorder Inventory-2 (EDI-2)[1] to evaluate comprehensively the eating behavior and psychological features of patients with eating disorders ; 2) FACES-III[4] to measure the level of "cohesive force of emotional ties among family members" and "ability to change the power structure and roles among family members" ; 3) the Scale of Characteristic Behavior of Good Girls[3] to measure the degree of desire to be favored by others in controlling their own feelings and thoughts ; and 4) the Scale of Social Environment Factors[2] to measure the tendencies towards "anxieties concerning academic performance and the future," "respect for appearance," and "the independence and social participation of women".

Results and discussion

Conducting a factor analysis (varimax rotation) of the EDI-2, we obtained nine factors : "the desire to be slim", "abnormal eating habits", "loss of self-confidence", "human distrust", "self-hatred", "self-uncertainty", "perfectionism", "rejection of maturity", and "self-destruction". Of these, two factors "the desire to be slim" and "abnormal eating habits" were considered to have a link to abnormal eating behavior, and the total score of the two factors became signs of an eating disorder tendency. The results of multiple regression analysis with setting the score of eating disorder tendency as a dependent variable and Body Mass Index (BMI), FACES-III, characteristic behavior of good girls, anxieties for academic performance and future, respects for appearance and independence and social participation of women as independent variables ($R = 0.652$, $R^2 = 0.425$, $F(9.166) = 13.628$, $p = 0.001$). It was also found that BMI ($\beta = -0.571$, $p = 0.05$), characteristic behaviors of good girls ($\beta = -0.150$, $p = 0.05$), anxieties for academic performance and future ($\beta = 0.126$, $p = 0.05$) and respects for appearance ($\beta = 0.186$, $p = 0.01$), had a significant independent effect on eating disorder tendency.

Considering the significant influence of "respect for appearance" and the "characteristic behavior of good girls", a strong tendency to seek the approval of others and an inability to find self-esteem were presumed. In today's competitive society, people are often compared with others according to numbers, and those who have grown up in such circumstances tend to evaluate themselves by something accurate and obvious. Since body size can be measured by numbers and can be controlled by diet and exercise, it could be easily chosen as a criterion to receive respect from others.

It is natural and necessary to confirm one's self-ability and self-value, but it has meaning when one can find these through self-respect. When a girl is always concerned with what other people think and views self-esteem through comparing numbers, this could overstrain her and stress could lead to risky behavior such as eating disorders. For those who have a strong sense of respect for appearance, since one's face and body size are superficial, even people who are just passing by could also be competitors. Although the concept of "good appearance" differs according to the person, "being slim" tends to be highly regarded due to the influence of mass media. Since the subjects of this study are of the age when they are sensitive to fashion and are very careful about their own appearance, they could be very easily influenced by such social current of the times.

Perfection and obsessive dispositions were viewed in relationship to the "characteristic behavior of good girls". A person with a strong inclination to possess such a disposition seems unwilling to compromise her goal, even when continuing the diet could lead to eating disorders. In addition to this, a current trend in which dieting is accepted as part of one's normal daily behavior also seems to be affecting the situation.

In the "characteristic behavior of good girls" and "the anxiety concerning academic performance and the future", perfectionist and obsessive tendencies were suggested and it seems that such strong tendencies could produce great anxiety and that eating disorders could be a psychological mechanism to ease such anxiety.

We also found that higher one's BMI, the higher the tendency to have an eating disorder. In a way, it seems natural that a person with a high BMI has a strong desire to be slim and tries a strict diet in a society in which being slim is admired. Since the subjects of this study were female college students, there were not many clinical cases of extremely skinny people with abnormal desires to lose weight.

References

1) Garner, D. M., Olmstead, M. P., Polivy, J. : Development and validation of a multidimensional eating disorder inventory for anorexia nervosa and bulimia. Int. J. Eat Disord, 2 ; 15-34, 1983.
2) Kobayashi, Y., Matsuoka, K., Kurita, H. : Relationship between Tendency toward Eating Disorders and Environmental Factors in Female High School Students. Seishin Igaku, 41 ; 821-829, 1999 (in Japanese).
3) Munakata, T. : Burnout and relevant measures. In : (eds.), Monou, H., Hayano, J., Hosaka, T. et al. : Type A behavior. Seiwa Shoten Publishers, Tokyo, p218-235, 1993 (in Japanese).
4) Olsan D. H., Portner J., Lavee Y. : Family Adaptability & Cohesion Evaluation Scales Ⅲ. Family Social Science, Minnesota, 1985.

[*1] 西脇病院
Ayako Ishida : Nishiwaki Hospital.
[*2] 野副病院
Mariko Date : Nozoe Hospital.
[*3] 和白病院
Yoko Watanabe : Waziro Hospital.
[*4] 長崎大学医療技術短期大学部
Yumi Agatsuma, Hiroyuki Inadomi, Goro Tanaka, Yasuyuki Ota : School of Allied Medical Sciences, Nagasaki University.

青年期女性における摂食障害の早期徴候と Self-esteem の関係
The relationship between early signs of eating disorders and self-esteem in adolescent women

塚本　美奈*

Ⅰ．緒　　言

　摂食障害は青年期に始まり潜在的に生命の脅威となる疾患である。先行研究では，摂食障害は潜行し治療が難しいことが示されている。だから，早期発見と予防はより安全な介入方法であると考えられる。摂食障害の予防において，一つの介入ポイントは Self-esteem を高めることである。そこで，この研究は札幌市とその近郊に住む青年期女性の摂食障害の早期徴候と Self-esteem のレベルを知りその関係を明らかにすることを目的とした。

Ⅱ．方　　法

　データ収集は札幌とその近郊に住む13歳から22歳までの青年期女性に質問紙を用いて行った。2000年7月の12日間に札幌の中心部に位置する大通り公園にて，便利標本抽出により対象を集めた。質問紙はフェイスシート，摂食態度調査表-26（EAT-26），そして Rosenberg Self-esteem Scale（RSS）で構成した。分析は347名の回答についてSPSSを使用して統計処理を行った。青年期を3つの群に分けて，13歳から15歳を青年期前期，16歳から18歳を青年期中期，そして19歳から22歳を青年期後期とした。EAT-26の得点から，20点以上を得点した女性を摂食障害の早期徴候を示す者とした。RSS の得点により Self-esteem のレベルを‘低い’，‘中等度’，そして‘高い’の3つのレベルに分けた。

Ⅲ．結　　果

　対象全体の12.1％が摂食障害の早期徴候を示していた。さらに，青年期前期では12.5％，青年期中期では16.1％，そして青年期後期では5.2％の女性が摂食障害の早期徴候を示していた。（Figure 1参照）。RSSの得点の平均値は各青年期とも中等度の Self-esteem レベルの範囲内であった。しかし，年齢を経るほど低い Self-esteem レベルの女性の割合が大きい傾向がみられた。（Figure 2参照）。対象全体では低い Self-esteem レベルの女性の中に摂食障害の早期徴候を示している者が多い傾向はみられたが有意水準5％で統計的な差はなかった。（Figure 3参照）。青年期中期では低い Self-esteem レベルの女性の中に摂食障害の早期徴候を示している者が多いことに有意差がみられた。（Figure 4参照）。

Ⅳ．考　　察

　青年期は外観を気にし，身体サイズや形に目を向けやすい時期である。また，心理的にも身体の変化を受け入れていくこと，両親からの心理的な独立，進路の選択，そして個人としての価値基準の確立を含む発達課題を達成しながら成長している。そして，それらは不安や葛藤の原因になる場合がある。このような心理的変化が摂食態度に影響すると考えられる。摂食障害の予防や早期発見のためには青年期の早い時期から介入していくことが大切である。Self-esteem は自己の価値や愛好への主観的な評価である。低い Self-esteem レベルの女性の中に摂食障害の早期徴候を示している者が多かったことから，自己に向けられた否定的な感情は摂食態度と結びつくと考えられる。摂食障害の予防に関する因子として Self-esteem は大切である。今後，Self-esteem に影響する因子を理解するための研究がさらに必要である。

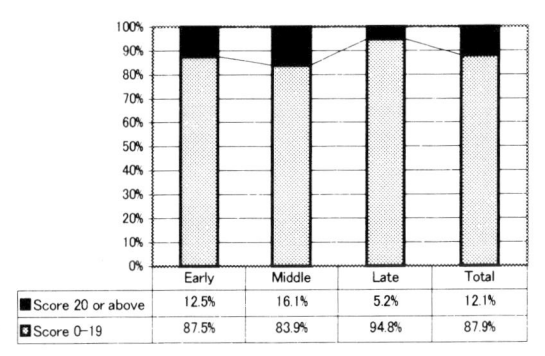

Figure 1 Early signs of eating disorders in adolescent women

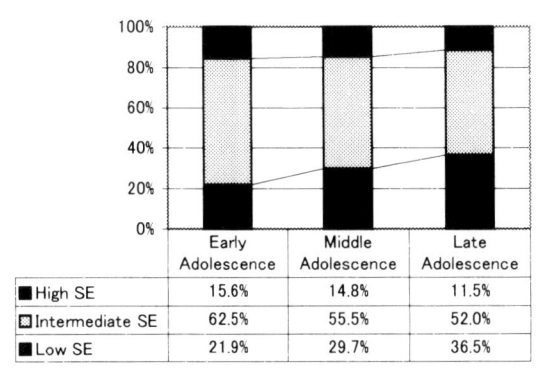

	Early	Middle	Late	Total
■ Score 20 or above	12.5%	16.1%	5.2%	12.1%
□ Score 0-19	87.5%	83.9%	94.8%	87.9%

Figure 2 The level of self-esteem among three adolescent groups

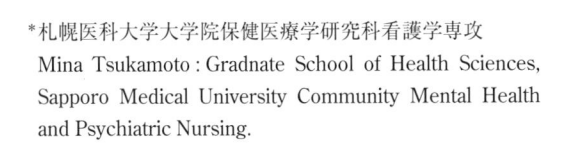

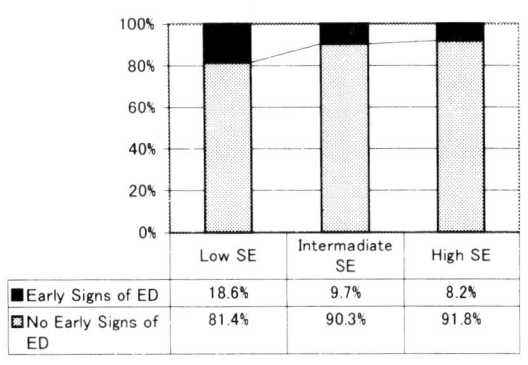

	Early Adolescence	Middle Adolescence	Late Adolescence
■ High SE	15.6%	14.8%	11.5%
□ Intermediate SE	62.5%	55.5%	52.0%
■ Low SE	21.9%	29.7%	36.5%

Figure 3 Early signs of eating disorders & level of self-esteem in total adolescents

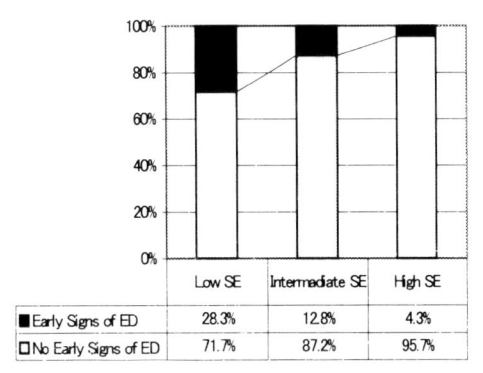

	Low SE	Intermadiate SE	High SE
■ Early Signs of ED	18.6%	9.7%	8.2%
□ No Early Signs of ED	81.4%	90.3%	91.8%

Figure 4 Early signs of eating disorders & level of self-esteem in middle adolescents

	Low SE	Intermediate SE	High SE
■ Early Signs of ED	28.3%	12.8%	4.3%
□ No Early Signs of ED	71.7%	87.2%	95.7%

*札幌医科大学大学院保健医療学研究科看護学専攻
Mina Tsukamoto : Gradnate School of Health Sciences, Sapporo Medical University Community Mental Health and Psychiatric Nursing.

医学生の喫煙開始防止には入学後早期の介入が必要
Earlier intervention prevents medical students from smoking

武田　裕子*　　佐藤　浩昭**　　高橋　秀人**　　小椋　力*　　大塚　盛男**　　関沢　清久**

I. 背　景

　先進国の中でも，わが国の喫煙率は高い（男性55.2％，女性13.3％）。男性医師の喫煙率も欧米に比べると非常に高く，25～37％と報告されている。喫煙の健康被害は喫煙者自身のみならず周囲の非喫煙者にも及ぶことから，医師には患者教育を行うことが求められている。しかし，喫煙する医師は禁煙指導に消極的であるという報告がある。

II. 目　的

　医学生の喫煙の実態，喫煙予防・禁煙教育に対する意識や態度を調査し，医学生自身の喫煙開始防止や禁煙の方策・課題を明らかにする。

III. 方　法

　筑波大学の医学生1年生から6年生の約600名を対象に，無記名自記式アンケート調査を1999年12月に実施した。調査票は，国際肺疾患予防連合（IUATLD）が，1985年に国際調査を実施した際に開発したものを用いた[2]。調査項目は，医学生の喫煙習慣，非喫煙の動機，喫煙関連疾患に関する知識，喫煙に関する患者教育に対する意識や態度，喫煙対策への関心や意見で，これらに若干の質問項目を付加した。付加した項目は，両親の喫煙歴の有無，大学構内で教員や医師の喫煙を見かけたことがあるか，構内における喫煙やタバコの販売制限に関する意見である。

IV. 結　果

　医学生611名（男子417名，女子194名）のうち574名（男子385名，女子189名）から回答を得た（回収率94％）。回答者の年齢は，18～24歳が536名で25歳以上は37名，調査時点での喫煙率は，男子22.6％，女子8.5％であった。一度でも喫煙したことがあると答えた学生は，男子39.5％，女子17.5％に上った。喫煙経験者のうち，77％が20歳前に喫煙を開始またはタバコを試したことがあると回答した。また，医学部入学後に喫煙を開始あるいは試した学生が100名いたが，そのうち87％は1，2年次であったと答えている。禁煙した学生は80名であったが，その89％が21歳以下で喫煙を中止している。

　われわれの調査では，医学生の両親の喫煙率は父親が57.5％，母親8.8％であった。両親の喫煙の影響を，学生を3群に分けて比較した。全く喫煙したことのない非喫煙者（n＝389），過去に6カ月以上喫煙していたが現在は禁煙している禁煙成功者（n＝17），6カ月以上喫煙している喫煙者（n＝67）の3群である。その結果，母親の喫煙率は3群で差がなかったが，父親の喫煙には表1に示すような差が見られた。さらに大学構内で教員や医師の喫煙を見かけたことがあるかという質問には，見かけたと答えた学生は喫煙者に有意に多かった（表1）。

　タバコを吸わないあるいは吸うべきではないと考える理由を尋ね，全くその通りまたは理由として挙げてよいと答えた学生の割合を上記の3群で比較したところ，「自分自身の健康を守るため」「自らを厳しく律するため」「出費を抑えるため」という項目で有意差が認められた（表2）。禁煙成功者と喫煙者の2群で有意差があった回答は，「タバコの煙で具合が悪くなったことがある」で，喫煙者に多かった（表3）。また，禁煙成功者の8割以上が医学部構内の喫煙制限を望んでいた。

表1 両親や教師の喫煙と医学生の喫煙習慣

	非喫煙者 (n=389)	禁煙成功者* (n=17)	喫煙者** (n=67)	(χ^2検定)
父親が喫煙者	54.3%	82.4%	64.2%	$p=0.03$
医師・医学部教員の 喫煙を見かけたことあり	81.9%	82.4%	95.5%	$p=0.02$

*禁煙成功者:以前は毎日喫煙していたが禁煙して6カ月以上経過
**喫煙者:6カ月以上毎日喫煙

表2 タバコを吸わない・吸うべきではない理由

	非喫煙者 (n=389)	禁煙成功者 (n=17)	喫煙者 (n=67)	(χ^2検定)
自分の健康を守る	95.9%	100%	86.4%	$p=0.004$
自分を厳しく律する	14.7%	17.7%	31.8%	$p=0.003$
出費を抑える	43.8%	58.8%	68.7%	$p=0.001$

表3 禁煙成功者と喫煙者の回答で有意差を認めた項目

	禁煙成功者 (n=17)	喫煙者 (n=67)	(χ^2検定)
たばこで具合が悪くなったことがある	35.3%	65.2%	$p=0.026$
医学部構内での喫煙は制限されるべきでる	88.2%	41.5%	$p=0.026$

V. 考 察

1985年のIUATLDによる調査と比較すると,男子医学生の喫煙率は不変もしくは減少しているものの女子医学生の喫煙率の著しい増加が見られる[1]。医学部入学後に喫煙を試した,あるいは経験した学生は100名おり,喫煙歴はあるが現在は喫煙していない学生の約9割が21歳までに中止している。従って医学生の喫煙開始防止,禁煙には入学後早期の介入が必要であることが明らかとなった。喫煙者は,タバコによる体調不良や自制心のなさを感じており,経済的負担も自覚していることから,単にタバコの害を説くだけの介入では不充分と考えられる。構内の喫煙制限など環境の整備も求められる。

文 献

1) 森 亨:医学生における喫煙と健康に関する意識調査. 昭和61年度健康づくり研究委託費喫煙と健康調査研究班(班長 尾島忠男)報告書, 1987.
2) Tessier, J. F. et al.: Smoking habits and attitudes of medical students towards smoking and anti-smoking campaigns in fourteen European countries. Eur. J. Epidemiol., 5 ; 311-21, 1989.

---

*琉球大学医学部附属病院地域医療部
 Takeda Y, Ogura C : Ryukyu University Hospital, University of the Ryukyus.
**筑波大学
 Satoh H, Takahashi H, Ohtsuka M, Sekizawa K : University of Tsukuba.

医学生は構内の禁煙環境と禁煙教育カリキュラムを求めている

Medical students requested a smoke-free environment and curriculam to promote effective smoking cessation and prevention

武田　裕子* 　佐藤　浩昭** 　高橋　秀人** 　小椋　　力* 　大塚　盛男** 　関沢　清久**

I. 背　景

タバコ依存症としての喫煙に対する治療法の研究が進んでいる。包括的な喫煙対策には，喫煙予防のための健康教育，禁煙しやすい環境づくり，喫煙者に対するニコチン依存症の治療と禁煙支援が必要とされる。この中で医師の果たす役割は大きく，患者教育やタバコ依存症の治療に関する知識やスキルを備えた医師の養成が求められている。

II. 目　的

患者教育に役立つ行動変容の技術やカウンセリングスキル，ニコチン置換療法等に関する教育の推進に効果的な医学部カリキュラムについて検討すべく，筑波大学の医学生約600名を対象に喫煙習慣，知識，禁煙教育に対する意識や態度を調査する。

III. 方　法

方法は一般演題2D-19に記載した通りである。無記名自記式アンケート調査を1999年12月に実施した。調査票は，国際肺疾患予防連合（IUATLD）が，1985年に国際調査を実施した際に開発したものを用いた[3]。喫煙に関する患者教育に対する意識や態度，喫煙対策への関心や意見を訪ねた。

IV. 結　果

医学生611名（男子417名，女子194名）のうち574名（男子385名，女子189名）から回答を得た（回収率94%）。全く喫煙したことのない非喫煙者は389名，過去に6カ月以上喫煙していたが現在は禁煙している禁煙成功者が17名，6カ月以上喫煙している喫煙者が67名であった。この3群で，患者教育に対する態度，意識に差があるかを調べたのが表1である。状況の異なる3人の患者に対して，医師として禁煙について話したり勧めたりするかという設問である。まず，喫煙によって生じる疾患に罹患している，あるいは喫煙によって何らかの症状を呈している患者，次に，症状はないが喫煙と健康の関係に興味があり，自分から質問してきた患者，最後に，喫煙しているが何の症状もなく特に自分から話題にすることもない患者の3人である。1番目と2番目の患者に対しては，どの医学生もほぼ100%禁煙教育を行なうと回答したが，3番目の無症状・無関心の患者に対しては，しばしば，あるいは時々教育すると答えた割合は，喫煙者の学生に低い傾向が見られた。

喫煙対策に対する関心・意見・態度について，非喫煙者と毎日喫煙者を比較したのが表2である。「医師が禁煙の重要性を解らせるべき」「医師は喫煙の害を知らせるべき」など，医師の積極的な関与に対して肯定的な意見は非喫煙者に多く，統計学的に有意な差が認められた。医学部構内でのタバコの販売禁止については，非喫煙者の7割が賛成したのに対し，喫煙者では2割以下であった。しかし，「禁煙教育を行なうのに十分な基礎知識を持っている」と感じているのは喫煙者に多かった。

約9割の学生が，もし有効な禁煙法があれば積極的に患者教育を行なう」と答えており，「患者を教育できる特別なトレーニングが必要」と感じている学生は約7割で，この2つの項目については非喫煙者と喫煙者で差がなかった。

表1　患者教育に対する態度の違い

	非喫煙者 (n=389)	禁煙成功者 (n=17)	喫煙者 (n=67)	(χ^2検定)
喫煙関連疾患(＋)/症状(＋)	98.4%	100%	100%	p=0.51
喫煙関連疾患(－)/関心(＋)	97.6%	97.0%	100%	p=0.77
喫煙による症状(－)/関心(－)	53.8%	43.8%	29.4%	p=0.05

表2　喫煙対策に対する関心・意見・態度

	非喫煙者 (n=389)	喫煙者 (n=67)	(χ^2検定)
医師が禁煙の重要性を解らせるべき	88.5%	75.4%	p=0.004
医師は喫煙の害を知らせるべき	89.3%	78.1%	p=0.012
医学部構内でのタバコの販売禁止	69.1%	16.7%	p=0.001
禁煙教育の基礎知識を持っている	15.7%	26.6%	p=0.03
有効な禁煙法があれば積極的に指導	87.4%	92.3%	p=0.26
患者指導のための教育が必要	73.7%	67.7%	p=0.31

V. 考　察

　患者教育に関する態度調査では，喫煙による症状がなく，特に禁煙に関心のない患者に対して禁煙教育を行なうとした医学生は約半数に留まり，また喫煙する学生では特に少ない傾向が見られた。喫煙者の方が患者教育に消極的であるという傾向は，86年の森らの調査[2]，アジア9カ国，ヨーロッパ14カ国，オーストラリア，旧ソビエト連邦の調査でも示されている[1]。日本医師会と国立公衆衛生院による全国調査でも，喫煙しない医師ほど患者の禁煙指導を進めやすいという結果が示され，医師の喫煙予防が患者に対する禁煙教育の推進につながることが示唆されている。

　我々の調査から，喫煙の予防や禁煙に医師が関わるべきであると多くの医学生が考えているものの，それに必要な基礎知識に乏しいと感じており，患者指導のための教育が必要と感じていることが明らかとなった。有効な禁煙法があれば積極的に患者教育を行なうと回答した学生が約9割に上ることから，卒前医学教育の充実が強く求められる。さまざまな段階で，例えば薬理学や医療経済学，行動科学など多様な側面からタバコ依存の問題点と医師の果たす役割について取り上げ，知識のみならず患者指導などの臨床的スキルを修得できるカリキュラムの作成が望まれる。

文　献

1) Crofton, J. W. et al. : Medical education on tobacco : implication of a worldwide survey. Medical Education, 28 ; 187-196, 1994.
2) 森　亨：医学生における喫煙と健康に関する意識調査. 昭和61年度健康づくり研究委託費喫煙と健康調査研究班（班長　尾島忠男）報告書, 1987.
3) Tessier, J. F. et al. : Smoking habits and attitudes of medical students towards smoking and anti-smoking campaigns in fourteen European countries. Eur. J. Epidemiol., 5 ; 311-321, 1989.

＊琉球大学医学部附属病院地域医療部
　Takeda Y, Ogura C : Ryukyu University Hospital, University of the Ryukyus.
＊＊筑波大学
　Satoh H, Takahashi H, Ohtsuka M, Sekizawa, K : University of Tsukuba.

多飲水と水中毒に関する予防医学的考察
―当院入院患者調査を通して―

Prevention considerations in polydipsia and water intoxication—Through research on inpatients—

徳田　毅[*]　　浦崎千恵子[*]　　前田　並恵[*]　　兼城　賢作[*]　　新垣　淑巳[*]
名城　真治[*]　　久場　兼功[*]　　豊里　明[**]　　森園修一郎[**]

I. はじめに

1938年に低ナトリウム血症を伴う精神分裂病の報告以来,精神科領域の疾患において,多飲水及び水中毒の存在が広く認められるようになった。しかし今なお原因不明で有効な治療手段がなく,予防医学的なアプローチが主体となっている。

今回我々は,当院入院患者を対象に疫学的調査を行い,患者背景及びその臨床特性について検討を試みた。

II. 対象と方法

平成13年5月時点の当院入院患者を全て対象とした。

調査方法はカルテ調査及び面接に加え,国立療養所犀潟病院の多飲水患者スクリーニング表(図1)を用いて,看護スタッフから情報収集を行った。また本研究では,医師の診察に基づいて,多飲水・水中毒の病態と診断された者を多飲水患者とした。

III. 全体的な背景

当院はベッド数239名の精神科単科の病院で,今回の対象数は213名。内訳は精神分裂病患者が最も多く全体の85%を占めていた。男性が多い傾向にあった。

IV. 多飲水患者の割合

この中で,実際に多飲水の診断を受けていたものは,213名中53名で,全体の25%を占めていた。これまでの研究で報告されている割合の範疇にあった。

V. 多飲水患者と対照群との比較

まず,多飲水の診断はない患者群(以下,対照群とする)と多飲水の患者群との間で,平均年齢・血清ナトリウム値・罹病期間・在院日数の比較を行った。

平均年齢において,対照群の平均年齢は55.2歳であるのに対し,多飲水患者群は49.5歳と若年の傾向にあった。

血清ナトリウム値については,対照群の平均が140mEq/l,多飲水群が135mEq/lと,多飲水群で低値であった。

罹病期間の比較検討では,両群とも28年で,ほぼ同様であった(図2)。

在院日数であるが,対照群も2665日に対し,多飲水患者は3164日と長期化の傾向があった(図3)。

VI. 病的多飲水患者スクリーニング基準について

次に我々は,多飲水患者の行動そのものに着目した。一様に多飲水患者と言っても,その行動形式についてはさまざまな様式があるからである。

今回の研究では,1995年の犀潟病院の研究報告で提唱されている「病的多飲水患者スクリーニング表」を用いて,多飲水患者の行動パターンを分析した。それによると「コップ保持」「蛇口飲水」等が多いが,全体的に様々なパターンを示すことがわかった。

着目すべき点は,このスクリーニング表を全症例に当てはめた所,入院患者の半分以上が多飲水関連行動にあった。

①コップ保持	いつもコップを持っている。
②ボトル保持	ボトルを用意して飲水する。
③コーヒーや清涼飲料水の多量摂取	コーヒーや清涼飲料水を飲む回数，摂取量が多い。またタバコを立て続けに吸うことがあり，その時にコーヒーや清涼飲料水などの摂取が多い傾向がある。
④衣服の濡れ	衣服が絶えず濡れており，水を飲んでばかりいると考えられる。
⑤ポットややかんの独り占め	病棟で出すポットややかんを独り占めする。いつもポットややかんの近くにいて，一日中「お茶飲み」をしている。
⑥持続飲水	コップまたはボトルを使用して，やかんやボトルに汲んだ水をいつまでもやめる様子もなく，あおるように飲んでいる。または水道の前に立ち止まり飲水している。
⑦蛇口飲水	水道の蛇口に口をつけて飲水する。
⑧強行引水	制止しても無視して飲み続けたり，怒って反抗したりする。
⑨隠れ飲水	多飲を注意すると，トイレや洗濯場などの通常の飲水場でない所で隠れて飲水する。
⑩汚水飲水	保護室に隔離すると，トイレの水を流して便器から手で汲んで飲んだり，ポータブルトイレに溜まった自分の尿を飲んだり，尿をトイレットペーパーにかけて，それを食べたりする。散歩に出ると道端の溜まり水を飲んだりする。
⑪自発的な訴え	尋ねれば多飲水の事実を認める。自分からよく飲むと言う。
⑫その他	＜いつも氷をなめている＞＜トイレに行く回数が多い＞＜投薬の時に，薬を飲むための水分の量が多い傾向がある＞など水を多く飲んでいる何らかの証拠がある。

（国立療養所・犀潟病院の基準を参照）
図1　病的多飲水スクリーニング表

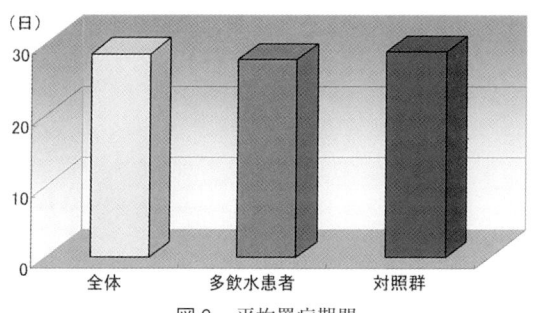

図2　平均罹病期間

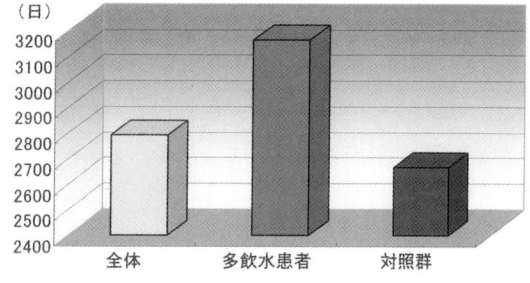

図3　平均在院日数

Ⅶ．考　察

本研究の結果を中心に2点の考察を行う。

まず1つめは，罹病期間と在院日数の比較検討である。多飲水群と対象群で，罹病期間にはほとんど差がなかったが，在院日数において相違がみられた。これは入院の長期化が多飲水行動になんらかの影響があることが示唆された。

2つめは，多飲水関連行動表での検討について行う。今回この行動表を用いたところ，実際に診断されている多飲水患者数と，行動表にて多飲水関連行動を疑われた数に相違が見られた。これは多飲水患者を過剰に診断している可能性，つまり偽陽性の可能性を否定できない。しかし現時点では多飲水に対する有効な手段はないため，基準を緩くして早期に発見したほうが，臨床上有効であると考えたので，今回の結果を採用した。

またこの多飲水行動関連表において，潜在的な多飲水患者の存在も示唆された。

本研究において，多飲水患者の疫学調査及び行動表を用いての評価をすること，つまり予防医学的な対応が，現時点では有効な手段だと考える。

Ⅷ．おわりに

1) 当院における多飲水患者の疫学的調査を行った。

2) 多飲水患者は全体の25％であった。

3) 対照群との比較で，平均年齢・在院日数・ナトリウム値に相違があった。

4) 特に在院日数の長期化が，多飲水患者に影響があるものと考えられた。

5) 多飲水関連行動表を用いて，患者の行動様式を評価することが，予防医学的に有効と考えられた。

---

*沖縄中央病院
　Tsuyoshi Tokuda, Chieko Urasaki, Namie Maeda, Kensaku Kaneshiro, Yoshimi Arakaki, Shinji Nashiro, Kenko Kuba : Okinawa Chuoh Hospital.
**琉球大学医学部精神神経科学講座
　Akira Toyosato, Shuichiro Morizono : Department of Neuropsychiatry, University of the Ryukyus.

一般人群と精神障害者群の生活習慣病有病率の比較より障害者群の予防，治療について

Comparison of general group and mental disorder group—Prevention about life style-related diseases

角谷　嘉紀*　中村　伸*　田頭政三郎*　中村　聰**

Ⅰ．はじめに

精神障害者は身体疾患への認識の低さから生活習慣病を有していても治療困難例を認める。また精神障害者の生活習慣病の実態調査，及び一般人との対比の報告は極めて少ない。しかも過去の報告は一般群が国民栄養調査によるものであったり地域，検査時期の一致はしていないものが多かった。そこで沖縄県内に於いて，およその時期を一致させて精神科入院者群(以下入院群)95名と一般人群107名の40歳以上男性の糖尿病，高血圧，高脂血症，肥満の有病率を比較した。

Ⅱ．対象と方法

40歳以上の男性
O病院精神科入院中の95名(開放病棟54名，閉鎖病棟42名)以下入院群。　平均年齢61.1歳±9.9歳
検査時期：平成12年12月1日から平成13年1月31日
沖縄県T地区医師会人間ドック受診者107名以下一般群。　平均年齢50.2歳±7.2歳
検査時期：平成13年1月1日から1月31日(図1)

1) 糖尿病　空腹時血糖値110mg/dl以上かつ／または食後2時間血糖値140mg/dl以上
2) 高血圧　収縮期圧140mmHgかつ／または拡張期圧90mmHg以上
3) 高脂血症　総コレステロール値220mg/dl以上
4) 肥満　BMI 25以上

上記の基準をみたすもの，及び既に治療を受けているものを有病群とする，従って糖尿病，高血圧は境界域も有病群とする。

Ⅲ．結　果

1) 糖尿病については入院群が有病率24%，一般群が17%で有意差はなかった。
2) 高血圧については入院群が29%，一般群が21%で有意差はなかった。
3) 高脂血症については入院群が20%，一般群が29%で有意差はなかった。
4) 肥満については入院群が有病率22%，一般群が47%で有意差を認めた。入院群で開放病棟群と閉鎖病棟群を比較すると有病率はそれぞれ33%，7%で有意差を認めた。(図2，図3，図4)

Ⅳ．考　察

糖尿病，高血圧，高脂血症では入院群と一般群で有意差はなかった。糖尿病，高血圧については境界域を含めたため境界域を含めない群間で比較してみたが有意差はなかった。入院群で開放病棟群と閉鎖病棟群を比較したがこれら三疾患に有意差はなかった。

肥満だけが入院群と一般群で有意差を認めた。さらに入院群においても開放病棟群と閉鎖病棟群で肥満に関し有意位差を認めた。図には示していないが一般群と開放病棟群の比較では有意差はなかった。

開放病棟群ではかなり自由にお菓子，ジュース等の高カロリーの食品が買い食いできその結果が肥満につながっていると考えた。これまでは入院群の肥満及び体重が増加傾向にある患者にはその旨を伝え，低カロリー食にしたり，体をなるべく

図1 対象

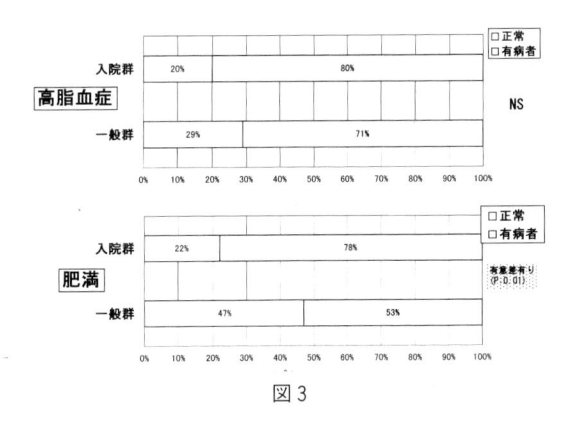

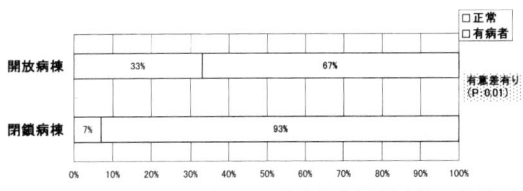

図2

図3

図4 肥満：入院群での開放病棟と閉鎖病棟の比較

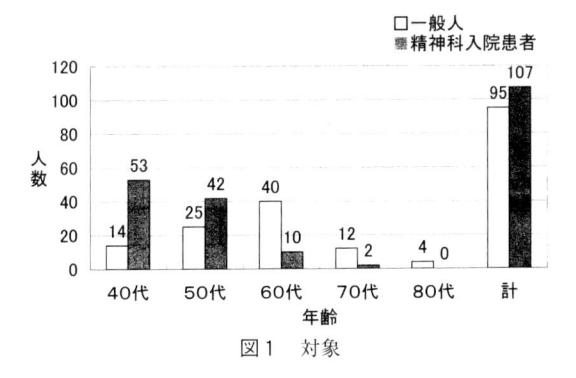

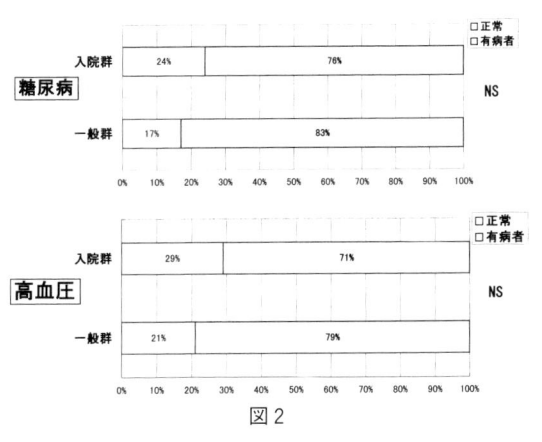

動かすことを勧めてきたが，開放病棟群での肥満の有病率の高さから，これだけでは不十分であると考えられた。

糖尿病，高血圧，高脂血症，肥満が揃うと死の四重奏といわれ，これら四疾患が一つ加わるごとに将来の脳卒中や虚血性心疾患に罹患する率が増すことが知られている。また，肥満が他の三疾患の発症因子とされている。このことから開放病棟群の肥満の予防が他の三疾患の防止，ひいては将来の脳卒中，虚血性心疾患の予防にもつながると推察される。

今後は肥満とそれがもとになり起こりやすくなる疾患，将来の脳卒中，虚血性心疾患の危険について平易で具体的な説明を行い，食生活が食事療法のみの問題でないことを説くなどの生活指導を行うことを予定している。

---

*オリブ山病院
　Yoshiki Kadoya, Shin Nakamura, Seizaburou Tagami :
　Oribuyama Hospital.
**中部地区医師会立成人病検診センター
　Satoshi Nakamura : Medical Examination Center.

精神分裂病患者の緩和ケア病棟における日常生活動作の低下の予測について

Predicting ADL deterioration in schizophrenic patients in palliative care unit

上間　一* 又吉　嘉伸* 田頭　政三郎* 与那原宣彦**

I. 目　的

　癌の末期で緩和ケア病棟に入院した精神分裂病患者は，病状が進行しても比較的日常生活動作が低下せず，死亡直前になって，急速に日常生活動作が低下する傾向があることに気づいた。このことは，癌の末期の精神分裂病患者のケアにおいて，あわてることなく対処するために，また患者の家族への病状説明においても，重要なことであると思われた。

　そこで，当院緩和ケア病棟に入院した癌末期の精神分裂病患者と一般の患者の間で，歩行・食事・応答の日常生活動作の低下から死亡までの期間において違いがみられるかを検討した。

II. 対　象

1) 精神分裂病群

1995年5月より2001年5月までに当院緩和ケア病棟で癌によって亡くなった精神分裂病患者9人。
・年令：34歳〜85歳（平均62.5歳）
・性別：男性4人，女性5人

2) 対照群

2000年12月より2001年5月までの6カ月間に当院緩和ケア病棟で癌によって亡くなった精神分裂病でない患者34人。
・年令：29歳〜96歳（平均70.5歳）
・性別：男性18人，女性16人

III. 方　法

カルテより，下記の3項目について調査した。
1) 歩行不能から死亡までの期間（日）
2) 食事摂取不能から死亡までの期間（日）
3) 応答不能から死亡までの期間（日）

ただし，当院緩和ケア病棟入院時より歩行不能および食事摂取不能，応答不能の患者は，原則として除外した。

IV. 結　果

1) 歩行不能から死亡までの期間について
　精神分裂病群は13.3日で，対照群の20.8日に較べて短かったが，有意差はみられなかった。

2) 食事摂取不能から死亡までの期間について
　精神分裂病群は6.56日で，対照群の8.88日に較べて短かったが，有意差はみられなかった。

3) 応答不能から死亡までの期間について
　精神分裂病群は1.20日で，対照群の1.82日に較べて短かったが，有意差はみられなかった。

V. 考　察

　歩行不能，食事摂取不能及び応答不能から死亡までの期間のいずれにおいても，精神分裂病群は対照群に較べて短かったにもかかわらず，有意差がでなかったのは，精神分裂病群の症例数が少なかったこと，および対照群の中に，アルコール性精神病や老年性の精神障害，器質性の精神障害等の精神分裂病と似た経過を示す症例が含まれていたためと思われる。

　また，精神分裂病群が対照群に較べて，日常生活動作の低下から死亡までの期間が短い傾向がみられた原因としては，抗精神病薬が何らかの意味で苦痛緩和に作用したことや，精神分裂病による自己認識の障害が，癌による肉体的苦痛を，自己の苦痛と捉えられなくして，ぎりぎりまで日常生活動作が低下しなかったことなどが考えられる。

　今後，症例数を増やしての検討が必要である。

*オリブ山病院
Hajime Uema, Yoshinobu Matayoshi, Seizaburou Tagimi : Oribuyama Hospital, Okinawa.
**沖縄リハビリテーションセンター病院
Nobuhiko Yonahara : Okinawa Rehabilitation Center Hospital.

精神障害者の身体合併症の外科的治療に際しての危険因子に関する検討
―術後せん妄の予防―

Risk factors in surgery for neuropsychiatric patients
―Prevention of postoperative delirium―

宮里　洋[*]　王　継軍[*]　宮平　良尚[*]　福田　吉顕[*]
村上　忠[*]　平松　謙一[*]　小椋　力[*]

　精神障害者が身体疾患で手術を受ける場合，外科医と精神科医の連携による心身両面からのアプローチが必須である。今回我々は，琉球大学医学部附属病院における精神障害者の身体合併症手術の現状および課題について報告する。また，術後せん妄についてretrospectiveに解析し，予防的見地から若干の考察を加え報告する。

対象と方法

　琉球大学医学部附属病院において1999年4月1日から2001年1月31日までの22か月間に，身体疾患を合併し，手術を施行された精神障害者21例（26手術例）を対象とした。患者の身体疾患に対する理解の程度や治療に対する態度を的確に把握するため，以下に示す中村ら（1994）の評価尺度（一部改変）を用い，5段階に分類した。
1．身体疾患をよく理解し，検査，治療に協力的。
2．精神症状ゆえに身体疾患への理解に問題があるが，身体管理上問題はない。
3．精神症状のため検査，治療にやや支障があり，時に応じて隔離，拘束，薬物等を要する。
4．精神症状が活発で身体疾患を全く理解せず非協力的。ほとんど常時，隔離，拘束することで検査，治療が可能である。
5．治療を完全に拒否し，いかなる手段でも治療の継続が困難である。

　術後せん妄に関しては，その要因を検討する目的で年齢，抗精神病薬用量，手術時間および麻酔時間について調べた。

　統計はStudent's t 検定，χ^2 検定を用いて解析した。

結　果

　症例の内訳は男性12例（44.3±18.3歳），女性9例（47.2±14.9歳）の合計21例（45.6±16.6歳）であった。手術症例はのべ26例（男性17例，女性9例，45.6±16.6歳）であった。1例以外すべて全身麻酔下の手術であった。精神疾患の内訳は精神分裂病が13例（61.9%）と最も多く，以下，精神遅滞2例（9.5%），痴呆2例（9.5%）等であった。手術を要した身体疾患26例の内訳は，骨折が最多で7例（26.9%），次いで眼科疾患5例（19.2%），以下，腎不全，乳癌および褥創各2例（7.7%）等であった。身体疾患理解度・治療態度による評価尺度では，術前は，grade 1：4例（15.4%）；grade 2：12例（46.2%）；grade 3：7例（26.9%）；grade 4：2例（7.7%）；grade 5：1例（3.8%）であった。一方，術後では，grade 1：6例（23.1%）；grade 2：12例（46.2%）；grade 3：5例（19.2%）；grade 4：3例（11.5%）；grade 5：0例（0%）であった。Grade 1，2に属する身体管理上問題のない症例は術前61.6%から術後69.3%へ増加し，また，grade 3以上に属する身体治療上かなりの困難のあった症例は術前38.4%から術後30.7%へと減少したが，これらの差は有意ではなかった。

　手術後の身体疾患の転帰は，治癒16例（61.5%），軽快89例（30.8%），不変2例（7.7%）

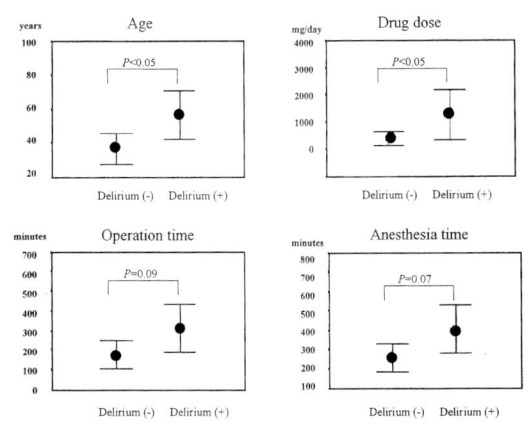

Figure 1　Predicting Factors in Post-op. Delirium

で，死亡例はなかった。

　術後せん妄は26手術例中4例(15.4%)に認められた。せん妄を生じた4例は全例精神分裂病であった。せん妄を生じた群では，患者の年齢(p<0.05)およびchlorpromazine等価換算した抗精神病薬用量(p<0.05)が有意に高かった。また，手術時間(p=0.09)および麻酔時間(p=0.07)が長いほどせん妄が生じやすい傾向を認めた(Figure 1)。

考　察

　概して，身体疾患に対する理解度の不良なgrade 3以上は精神科病棟での管理が中心となることが多かったが，その場合でも，呼吸器，循環器系の身体的問題が生じやすい術後急性期を身体科管理とすることは必要かつ実際的と思われた。手術後の身体疾患の転帰は，治癒および軽快の両者で約92%を占め，死亡例はなかった。これらの結果は一般患者の手術成績に比較しても遜色はないものと考えられる。

　術後急性期の合併症の中で最も頻度が高いものの1つがせん妄であり，本研究においても15.4%に認められた。精神障害者の術後せん妄の発症の危険因子として年齢および抗精神病薬の服用量があげられた。また，手術時間および麻酔時間が長いほどせん妄が生じやすい傾向を認めた。従来，一般患者の術後せん妄発症の危険因子として，1) 60歳以上，2) 血液学的所見の異常，3) 4時間以上の手術時間，4) 術後合併症の出現，5) 体液バランスの変化などがあげられており(浅川と平沢，1998；佐藤ら，2000)，我々の結果はこれらの報告の一部と同様であった。

　術後回復期には，手術侵襲や麻酔による影響がほぼ消失し，患者も環境の変化に適応し，代わって本来の精神疾患による精神症状が前景に立つか，時に一過性増悪を認める(柏瀬ら，1984)。今回，脳外科手術後28日に皮下シャントチューブを自己切断した器質性精神障害の1例，および整形外科手術後17日にwrist cutした神経症(適応障害)の1例を経験した。手術というイベントが一段落した時点においても精神科的治療を継続することが重要と思われた。

文　献

1) 浅川理，平沢秀人：術後せん妄の臨床．一瀬邦弘編：精神医学レビュー26 せん妄，ライフサイエンス，東京，1998.
2) 柏瀬宏隆，石井弘一，片山義郎．精神障害者の手術．臨床精神医学13；417-422, 1984.
3) 佐藤晋爾，鈴木利人，川西洋一ほか：術後せん妄の病態に関する臨床的研究—prospective study—．臨床精神医学29；1341-1349, 2000.
4) 中村誠，野村総一郎，郷原道彦ほか：精神障害者の術前術後管理MPUでの経験．精神医学，36；1251-1257, 1994.

---

*琉球大学医学部精神神経科学講座
Hiroshi Miyazato, Wang Jijun, Yoshinao Miyahira, Yoshiaki Fukuda, Tadashi Murakami, Ken-ichi Hiramatsu, Chikara Ogura : Department of Neuropsychiatry University of the Ryukyus.

一般在宅高齢者における認知障害と MRI 所見

MRI findings and cognitive impairment among community-dwelling elderly subjects

古賀　寛[*,**]　杠　岳文[**]　尾籠　晃司[*]　一宮　厚[*]
遠藤　光一[**]　比江島誠人[**]　八尾　博史[**]

I. はじめに

　近年わが国は超高齢社会をむかえ, 医療面の進歩・改善と共に社会保障制度上も介護保険制度の制定など, 国をあげてその対策が進められている。特に痴呆に関してはその予防方法や早期発見・早期治療, 援助方法などが重要であり, それらに焦点を当てた対策が今後さらに必要とされると考えられる。

　痴呆の予防については, わが国では久山町研究以外に一般住民を対象とした長期のコホート的研究がいまだなされていない。我々は国立肥前療養所において, 平成7年に地域住民を対象とした頭部 CT による健診を始め, 平成9年からは脳 MRI 健診を行い, ライフスタイルや身体状況が認知機能低下や脳血管障害にいかに関わっているかを解析し, それらの予防につながる危険因子の解明に努めている。今回はその第一報として認知障害と定量的 MRI 所見について報告する。

II. 対象と方法

　対象は明らかな痴呆を有しない地域在住の高齢者254名で, 全員が60歳以上であり, 平均年齢は 73.9 ± 6.8 歳であった。全例に頭部 MRI 検査を行い, 既往歴の聴取, 血液一般・生化学検査を施行し高血圧, 糖尿病などの脳血管障害の危険因子の評価を行った。また知的機能検査として Mini-Mental State Examination (MMSE) を施行した。対象者の MMSE の平均は 26.0 ± 3.3 点であり, 得点の低い者も数名みられたが, それらの者も自立した生活が自宅で出来ており, DSM-IV の痴呆の診断基準をみたすような明らかな痴呆といえる者はいなかった。対象者の中で MMSE23点以下の者を認知障害有りと判定し, 認知障害の無い群と比較した。

　MRI 画像の測定は, 白質病変については T2 強調画像で高信号域, T1 強調画像で等信号域を示したものについて FLAIR 法画像を用い, 画像の density を分けてそのピクセル数をカウントする semi-automatic 法を用いて, 面積を定量的に測定した。そしてその白質病変の面積を頭蓋骨内縁の面積で除したものを%WML とした。また白質病変測定と同じスライスレベルでの脳実質の大きさを T2 強調画像を用いて定量的に測定し, これを頭蓋骨内縁の面積で除したものを%Brain とし, 脳萎縮の指標とした。また脳梗塞はその有無と個数について全脳レベルで定性的に評価した。脳梗塞は T2 強調画像で高信号域, T1 強調画像で低信号域を示し, 直径が5mm 以上の大きさの病変を有意な脳梗塞と判定した。

　さらに従属変数を認知障害の有無, 独立変数を MRI 画像上の異常所見を含む臨床検査所見としてロジスティック回帰分析を行った。

III. 結　果

　画像所見の定量的測定の結果は, %WML は $0.37 \sim 29.7\%$ であり, 平均は $5.61 \pm 4.44\%$ であった。また%Brain の測定結果は $66.1 \sim 94.6\%$ で, 平均は $82.3 \pm 6.4\%$ であった。また有意な脳梗塞は54名 (21.3%) に認められた。

　これら MRI 画像の測定結果と臨床所見をもとに在宅高齢者の認知障害に影響を与える因子について調べた。MMSE が23点以下の認知機能低下群は46名 (18.1%) いた。認知障害を有する群は有しない群に比べて, 有意に高齢 (78.0y vs 72.9y, $p<0.0001$) で教育歴が短く (7.4y vs 8.7y, $p<$

0.0001)，高血圧の既往が多かった(46.2% vs 32.8%，p=0.013)。また血液ヘマトクリット値の平均は低かった(36.4% vs 38.6%，p=0.0012)。さらに認知障害を有する群では，MRI画像上の定量的白質病変の程度が大きく(8.25% vs 5.03%，p<0.0001)，脳の容積は有意に小さく(79.0% vs 83.1%，p<0.0001)，脳梗塞の割合は高かった(30.8% vs 18.0%，p=0.014)。ロジスティック回帰分析の結果，認知障害に影響を及ぼす有意な因子は白質病変(Odds ratio：OR 1.575, 95% confidence interval：CI 1.123〜2.208)，脳萎縮(OR：0.761, CI：0.587〜0.987)，教育歴(OR 0.682, CI 0.544〜0.855)であった。

IV. 考　察

今回我々は在宅で問題なく生活をしている高齢者の認知障害に影響を与える因子について，MRI画像の定量的所見等を用いた研究を行い，認知機能障害に対しては白質病変，脳萎縮，教育歴が関連があると結論した。以前我々がCTを用いて在宅高齢者を対象とした同様の研究を行った際には，認知機能障害には加齢と脳梗塞，それに白質病変の関与が示唆されたが，今回は認知障害に影響を与える因子としては白質病変と脳萎縮が重要であった。一般住民を対象とした臨床研究はこれまでにもいくつかあり，特に痴呆の有病率や発症因子に注目した報告は多いが，それらは白質病変や無症候性脳梗塞などといったある特定の病変の出現頻度や危険因子，あるいはその病変と認知障害との関連をみたものが多い。今回のように一般的な認知障害に影響する要因について広く調べることは，まだ報告例は少ないが痴呆の原因の解明や予防という点から重要と思われる。

今後我々の研究プロトコールでは，MRIを用いて5〜10年毎のコホート研究を30年以上にわたり行う予定であり，更に症例数を増しながら痴呆発症の危険因子を詳しく調べ，予防や早期発見に役立てたい。

＊九州大学大学院医学研究院精神病態医学教室
　Hiroshi Koga, Koji Ogomori, Atsushi Ichimiya：Department of Neuropsychiatry, Fuculty of Medicine, Kyushu University Hospital.

＊＊国立肥前療養所・情動行動障害センター・臨床研究部
　Hiroshi Koga, Takefumi Yuzuriha, Koichi Endo, Shigeto Hiejima, Hiroshi Yao：Hizen National Hospital.

編者略歴

小椋 力（おぐら　ちから）

昭和12年	鳥取県に生まれる
昭和37年	鳥取大学医学部卒業
昭和42年	鳥取大学大学院医学研究科修了
	鳥取県岩見町立浦富病院精神科（精神科医長）
昭和44年	鳥取大学医学部助手
	同年8月，鳥取大学医学部付属病院講師
昭和50年	鳥取大学医学部講師
昭和51年	米国ロチェスター大学医学部留学（2年間）
昭和56年	鳥取大学医学部助教授
昭和59年	琉球大学医学部教授，現在に至る
平成10年	琉球大学医学部附属病院長（2年間）

第11回国際事象関連電位学会会長（平成7年）
日本社会精神医学会会長（平成8〜9年）
日本精神障害予防研究会代表世話人（平成8年〜）
日本臨床精神神経薬理学会会長（平成8〜9年）
日本精神神経学会会長（平成9〜10年）
日本臨床薬理学会理事長（平成11年〜）
「国際精神保健シンポジウム in 沖縄」会長（平成12年）
第1回日本国際精神障害予防会議会長（平成13年）

精神障害の予防をめぐる最近の進歩

2002年3月29日　初版第1刷発行

編　者　小　椋　　力
発行者　石　澤　雄　司
発行所　㈱星　和　書　店
　　　　東京都杉並区上高井戸1-2-5　〒168-0074
　　　　電話　03(3329)0031（営業部）／　03(3329)0033（編集部）
　　　　FAX　03(5374)7186

Ⓒ2002　星和書店　　　　Printed in Japan　　　　ISBN 4-7911-0477-3

| 誰にでもできる精神科リハビリテーション | 野田文隆、蜂矢英彦 責任編集 | A5判 272p 3,650円 |

東京武蔵野病院精神科リハビリテーション・マニュアル

| 精神科リハビリテーション実践ガイド | M.Y.エクダヴィ、A.M.コニング 著 東雄司、岩橋正人、岩橋多加寿 訳 | A5判 192p 2,600円 |

病院から地域へ―社会復帰を援助するために

| 新しいコミュニティづくりと精神障害者施設 | 大島巌 編著 | B5判 344P 2,816円 |

「施設摩擦」への挑戦

| これからの精神医療と福祉 | 西山詮 編著 | A5判 216P 2,600円 |

世田谷区の復帰施設の実態調査を紹介し、現状と問題点を探る

| 痴呆の基礎知識 | 宮里好一 著 | 四六判 264p 2,200円 |

医学的知識・ケア・予防法をわかりやすく

発行：星和書店　　価格は本体(税別)です

心の地図 上 〈児童期―青年期〉 こころの障害を理解する	市橋秀夫 著	四六判 296p 1,900円

心の地図 下 〈青年期―熟年期〉 こころの障害を理解する	市橋秀夫 著	四六判 256p 1,900円

家族のための精神分裂病入門 精神分裂病を患っている人を 理解するために	エィメンソン 著 松島義博、荒井良直 訳	四六判 240p 1,500円

みんなで学ぶ精神分裂病 正しい理解とオリエンテーション	D.ヘル 他著 植木啓文、曽根啓一 監訳	四六判 256p 2,330円

精神分裂病はどんな病気ですか？ 原因、治療、援助、予後等をやさしく解説	D.ショア 編 森則夫、丹羽真一 訳	四六判 120p 1,340円

発行：星和書店　　　　　　　　　価格は本体(税別)です

〈2001年 改訂新版〉
こころの治療薬ハンドブック
1薬剤を見開きでわかりやすく解説

青葉安里、
諸川由実代 編

四六判
224p
2,600円

心病む人への理解
家族のための分裂病講座

遠藤雅之、田辺等 著

A5判
148p
1,845円

SSTコミュニケーショントレーニング
患者への理解と敬意、信頼関係を基礎に

山本タカタ著
福間病院山本SST研究会 訳

A5判
172p
1,900円

わかりやすいSSTステップガイド　上巻
基礎・技法編

ベラック他 著
熊谷直樹、
天笠崇 監訳

A5判
264p
2,800円

わかりやすいSSTステップガイド　下巻
実用付録編

ベラック他 著
熊谷直樹、
天笠崇 監訳

A5判
96p
1,800円

発行：星和書店　　　　　価格は本体(税別)です

初期分裂病
分裂病臨床の客観的診断基準の確立

中安信夫 著

A5判
152p
2,670円

初期分裂病／補稿
分裂病の早期発見、早期治療

中安信夫 著

A5判
288p
4,800円

対談　初期分裂病を語る
その概念と臨床像、ケースカンファランス

中安信夫 編著

四六判
112p
1,650円

増補改訂　分裂病症候学
記述現象学的記載から
神経心理学的理解へ

中安信夫 著

A5判
上製函入
244p
13,000円

宮﨑勤精神鑑定書別冊
中安信夫鑑定人の意見

中安信夫 著

A5判
上製函入
640p
15,000円

発行：星和書店　　　　　　価格は本体（税別）です

治療のテルモピュライ 中井久夫の仕事を考え直す	星野、滝川、五味渕 他著	四六判 264p 2,800円
中井久夫選集 **分裂病の回復と養生** 「最終講議」補論他珠玉の論文満載	中井久夫 著	四六判 280p 2,800円
中井久夫共著論集 **分裂病／強迫症／精神病院** 最重要論文を一挙収録	高、住野、高谷、 内藤、中井、永安 他著	A5判 216p 3,300円
精神病治療の開発思想史 ネオヒポクラティズムの系譜	八木剛平、 田辺英 著	四六判 296p 2,800円
精神療法の旅路 分裂病治療の半世紀	阪本健二 著 岩井圭司 編	A5判 396p 12,000円

発行：星和書店　　　　　価格は本体(税別)です